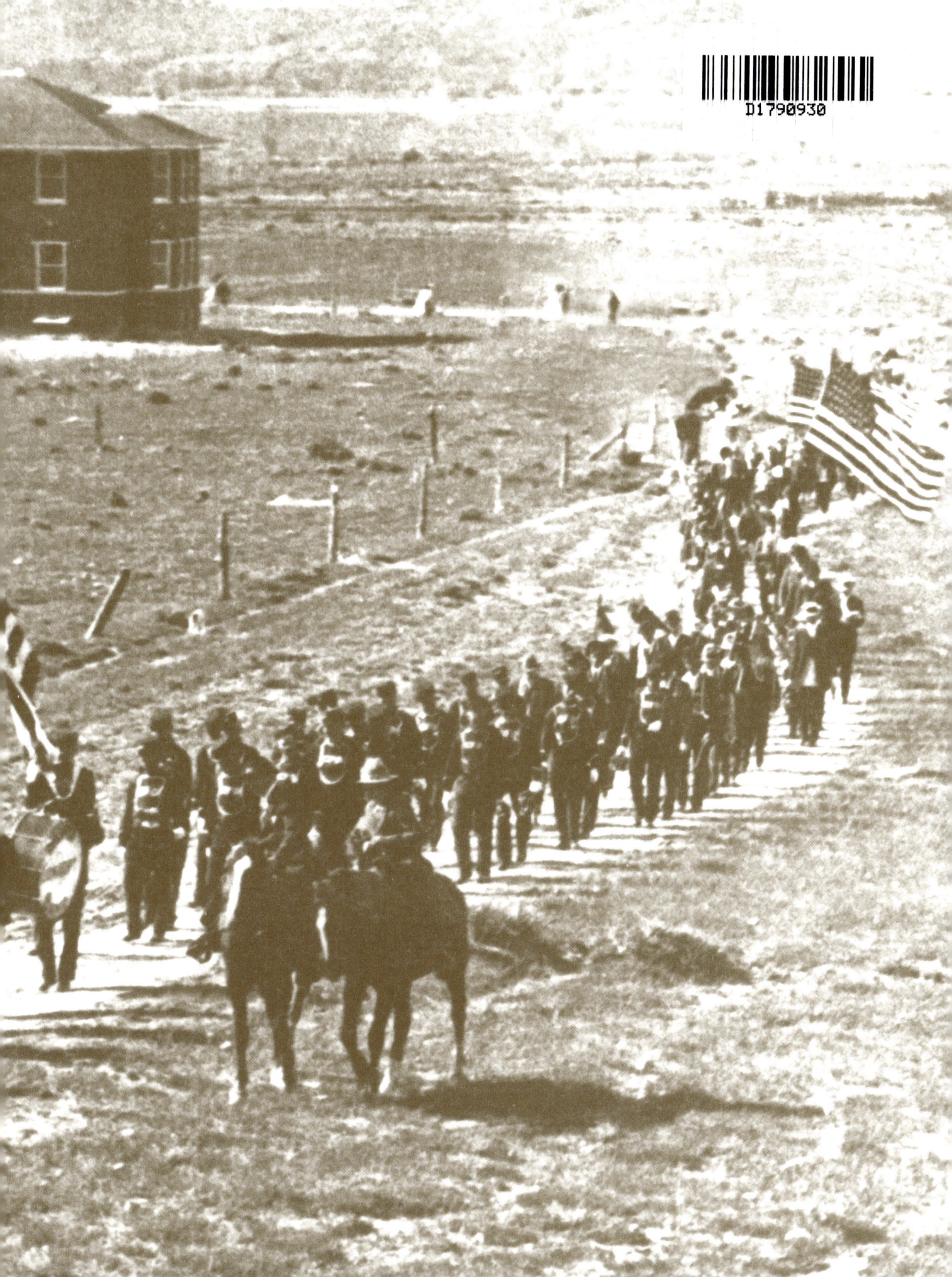

Wyoming Medical Center
A CENTENNIAL HISTORY

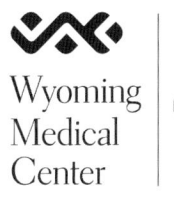
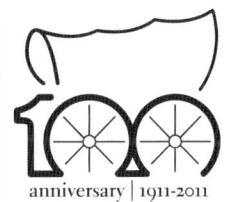

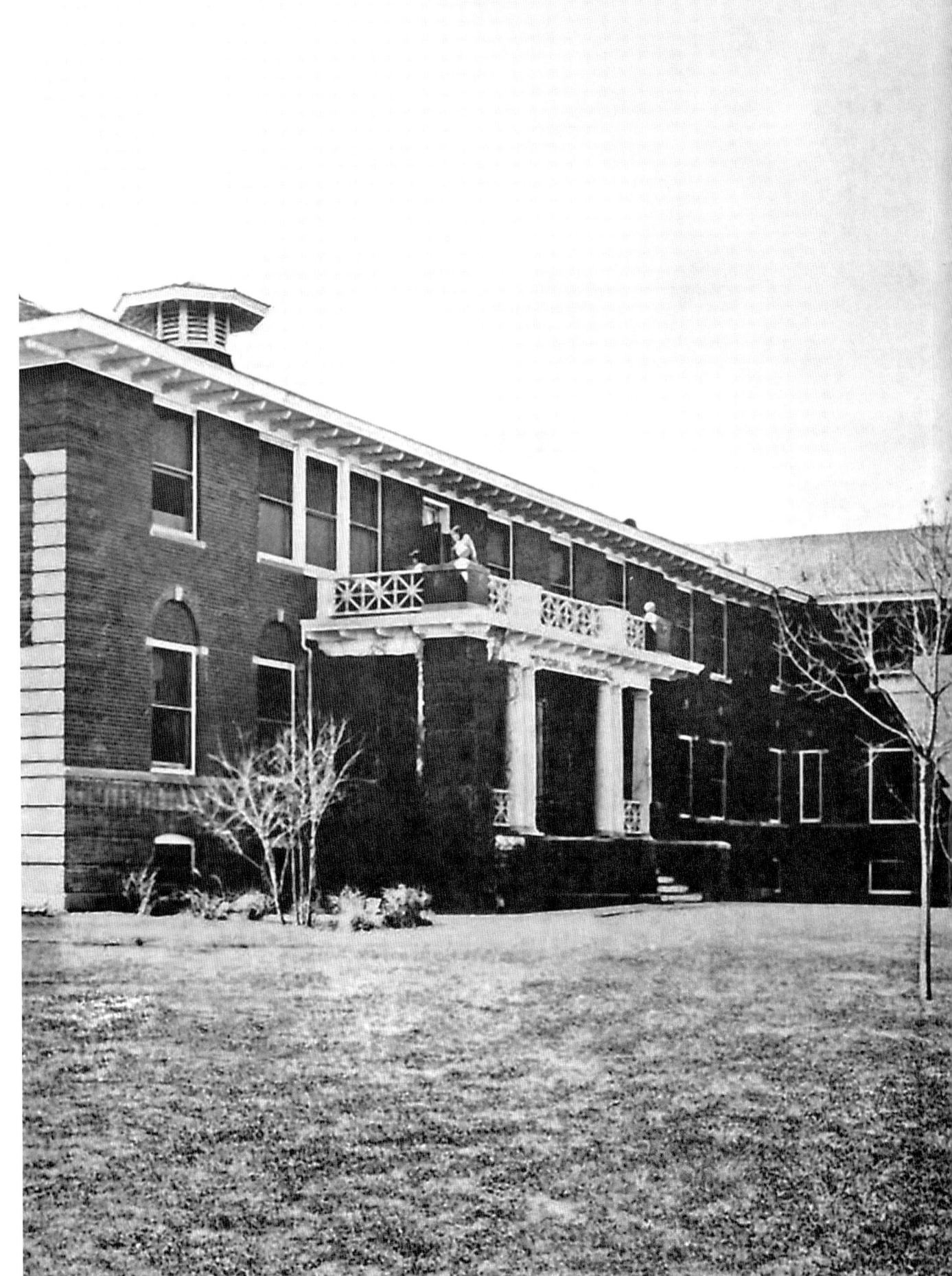

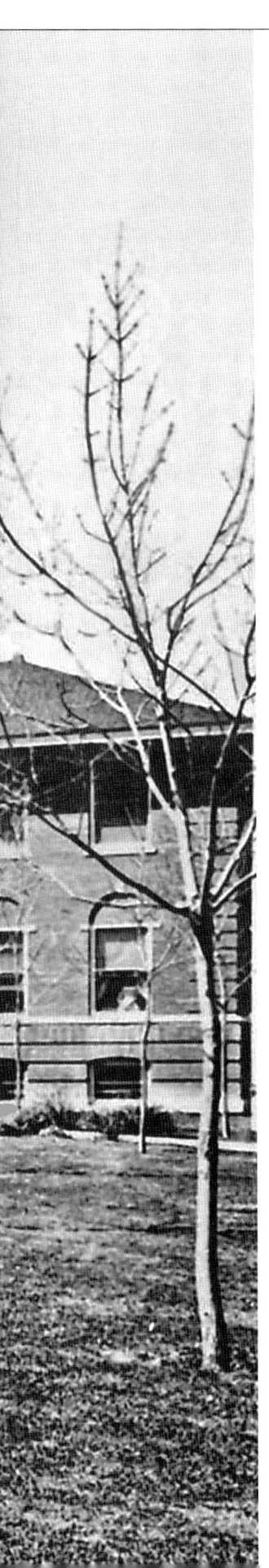

Wyoming Medical Center
A CENTENNIAL HISTORY

by Rebecca A. Hunt, Ph.D.

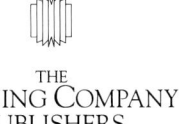

THE
DONNING COMPANY
PUBLISHERS

DEDICATION

This book is dedicated to my parents Warren and Sara Weaver, to my children Kate Miller, Aaron Hunt, and Cam Luecke, and of course to Geoffrey.

Copyright © 2010 by Wyoming Medical Center

All rights reserved, including the right to reproduce this work in any form whatsoever without permission in writing from the publisher, except for brief passages in connection with a review. For information, please write:

The Donning Company Publishers
184 Business Park Drive, Suite 206
Virginia Beach, VA 23462

Steve Mull, *General Manager*
Barbara Buchanan, *Office Manager*
Heather L. Floyd, *Editor*
Stephanie Danko, *Graphic Designer*
Priscilla Odango, *Imaging Artist*
Katie Gardner, *Project Research Coordinator*
Tonya Hannink, *Marketing Specialist*
Pamela Engelhard, *Marketing Advisor*

Ed Williams, *Project Director*

Library of Congress Cataloging-in-Publication Data

Hunt, Rebecca A., 1952-
　Wyoming Medical Center : a centennial history / by Rebecca A. Hunt.
　　p. cm.
　Includes bibliographical references and index.
　ISBN 978-1-57864-655-5 (hardcover : alk. paper)
　1. Wyoming Medical Center—History. 2. Wyoming Medical Center—History—Pictorial works. 3. Hospitals—Wyoming—Casper—History. 4. Hospital care—Wyoming—Casper—History. 5. Medical personnel—Wyoming—Casper—History. 6. Casper (Wyo.)—History. 7. Casper (Wyo.)—Social conditions. I. Title.
　RA982.C223W84 2011
　362.1109787'93—dc22

2010041444

Printed in the United States of America at Walsworth Publishing Company

Table of Contents

6	Acknowledgments	
7	Introduction	
8	**CHAPTER ONE**	Before the Hospital: Up to 1909
18	**CHAPTER TWO**	Casper Gets Her Hospital: 1909 to 1920
30	**CHAPTER THREE**	The Hospital Grows: 1921 to 1940
44	**CHAPTER FOUR**	The War Years and Beyond: 1941 to 1959
64	**CHAPTER FIVE**	From Memorial Hospital of Natrona County to Wyoming Medical Center: 1960 to 1986
100	**CHAPTER SIX**	Wyoming Medical Center: 1986 to 2010
134	Selected Bibliography	
138	Index	
144	About the Author: Rebecca A. Hunt, Ph.D.	

Acknowledgments

A pictorial history is a special type of book. It relies heavily on archival sources and private collections. This project would not have been possible if Elaine Hough had not had the foresight to save thousands of photographs and documents from Wyoming Medical Center. Then she was wise enough to donate them to the Western History Center at Casper College. Thank you, Elaine.

I would like to thank retired Western History Center Archivist Kevin Anderson for making the still-unprocessed collection available. Michelle Bahe and Rick Young at the Fort Caspar Museum supplied me with some early photographs that added to the pictorial content. Alice Weaver collected and then donated a number of early photos to me for the project.

I was fortunate to have colleagues and family who tackled reading various stages of the manuscript. Geoff Hunt and James Whiteside looked it over with historians' eyes and gave me valuable input. Tim and Debi Weaver, longtime employees at Wyoming Medical Center, provided names and dates for photographs and checked the facts on the manuscript. My sister-in-law Suzanne Short came for a visit and ended up reading the whole thing. She provided a completely outside view and told me when it did not make sense. Finally, the Centennial Committee, Mike Phillips, Shauna VanderLinden, and the administrators at Wyoming Medical Center took the time to read as well.

I would also like to thank my editor Heather Floyd for being a gentle noodge who gave me the extra time I needed when my father unexpectedly died in the middle of the project. I appreciate how anxious this made you and how graceful you were.

Finally, my family gave me the space and time to write, a luxury when I was juggling teaching, grandchildren, and life in general. You all made it possible to write the words that commemorate this remarkable institution.

All photographs are from the Wyoming Medical Center collection at the Western History Center at Casper College unless otherwise labeled.

Introduction

"We can chart our future clearly and wisely only when we know the path which has led us to the present." Adlai Stevenson

A nurse holds a small child recovering from a bout of influenza. Her diligent care and expert training give her the edge over the disease, bringing the child back from the brink. This is the caring side of medicine in the early twentieth century.

A young doctor sits in a booth carefully directing robotic hands over a sleeping patient. The microsurgery the DaVinci Robotic Surgical System is about to perform will make the patient's surgery quick and safe and recovery faster. This is twenty-first-century medicine at its most creative.

These images come from the beginning and end of a century of health care. While robots did not help with surgery in 1911, nurses were and still are a mainstay of care in 2010. What both images have in common is that they occurred in a hospital. A hospital is a vital necessity to a community. It provides medical care for residents, oversees health issues, and serves the needs of the surrounding area. In Wyoming, a full service, comprehensive hospital is even more important because towns are few and far between and highly specialized medical facilities and personnel are not always locally available to rural residents. In the twenty-first century, Wyoming Medical Center in Casper fulfills all the classic roles of a community hospital and many more besides.

But this was not always true. In the nineteenth century, people saw hospitals as "pest houses," a place to go to die. When Natrona County came into existence, Casper did not have a hospital. Many people used home remedies and "nurse" was part of a wife and mother's job description. Doctors, when called upon, often delivered babies and most other medical care in peoples' homes. Occasionally, a doctor or nurse acquired a building and turned it into a private hospital. Public hospitals came later.

Many towns had serious problems with water quality and sewage issues, and they suffered periodic epidemics of such things as diphtheria, whooping cough, or cholera. This is the story of a hospital, a town, and a corps of trained caring professionals. This is the story of the facility we now call Wyoming Medical Center.

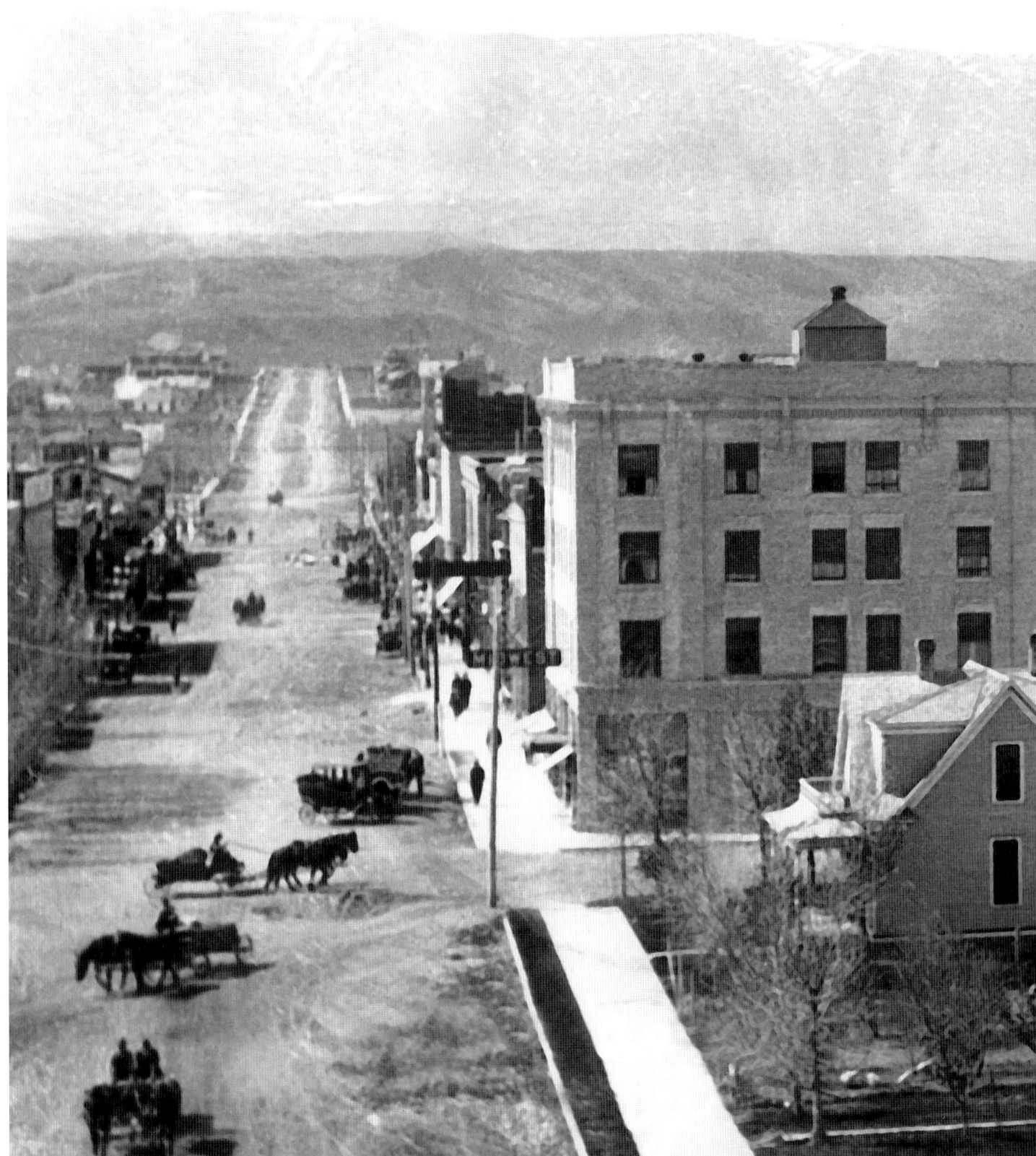

CHAPTER ONE

Before the Hospital
UP TO 1909

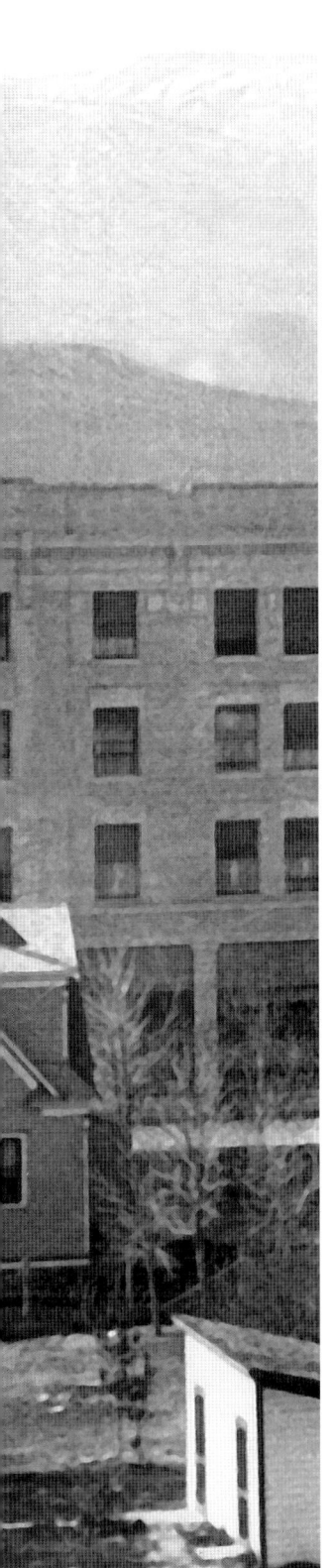

The first residents of Central Wyoming were nomadic American Indians, members of Plains tribes such as the Lakotas, Cheyennes, Arapahos, and Shoshones. Tribal healers used natural remedies to take care of illnesses and wounds. The women worked together to deliver babies and see children through the trials of childhood. After they resettled onto reservations, government agents and church missionaries introduced them to Western medicine.

From the 1830s into the 1860s, migrants passed through the Platte River country but few, other than former fur trappers and their families, lived in the area. The Platte Bridge Station military post, established in the 1860s, was the first large-scale settlement. Post surgeons provided care, often in a very desultory and non-professional manner. This was an era when more soldiers died of diseases and accidents than of wounds received in battle. Medical records at military posts showed that everything from influenza to malnutrition could be debilitating and sometimes fatal.

Travelers coming west on the Oregon, Overland, and Mormon trails succumbed to typhoid, cholera, dysentery, and other communicable diseases as well as accidents and misadventure. The West was not necessarily a healthy place; on the other hand, as many children followed their families across the plains, fresh air, plain food, and lots of exercise brought a rosy bloom to their cheeks. Mothers often suffered from overwork, and many gave birth in a tent or the back of a wagon, attended by the other women of their community on wheels. Overland diaries recorded the births and sometimes deaths of these mothers and babies. The wonder is not that people died on the trail. The wonder is that so many survived.[1]

Wyoming became a territory on July 25, 1868, and it achieved statehood on July 10, 1890.[2] Natrona was carved out of Carbon County and Casper was incorporated on April 9, 1889.[3]

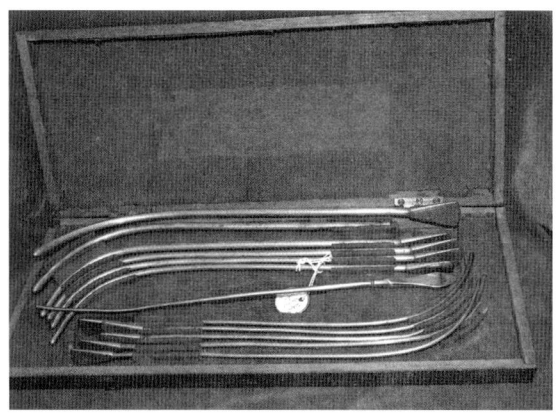

Military physicians used kits like this to treat battle wounds. Most soldiers died of illness. *Author's collection.*

The town of Casper predated the county. The Fremont, Elkhorn and Missouri Valley Railway Company platted the town in June of 1888, and the first buildings went up that summer.[4] By the fall, owners had moved from their original sites. The first building to move from A and First streets and McKinley and Jefferson streets to the new location in the vicinity of Center and Second streets was Robert White's saloon.[5] Alfred Mokler described these early buildings in his 1922 *History of Natrona County, Wyoming, 1888–1922.* He said, "By 1889 Casper had four saloons, four restaurants, one with a candy store and a harness shop, four livery stables, one grocery, one weekly paper, a bank, [and] a combined jeweler, doctor, barber."[6]

Early Casper had a highly mobile population of fewer than one hundred people.[7] Some of the town leaders included Peter Nicolaysen, A. J. Cunningham, Peter Demorest, Philip Watson, Wilson Kimball, George Mitchell, Mathew Campfield, and Alexander McKinney.[8] Campfield, Casper's earliest African-American resident, was a barber. His shop was on the west side of Center Street next to Kimball's drugstore.[9] More people lived on the neighboring cattle ranches owned by county leaders Joseph Carey and Bryant Brooks. Sheep ranches dotted the countryside in the areas not already taken by the cattle ranchers. In fact sheep, around 2 million strong, outnumbered people for much of the county's early period.[10]

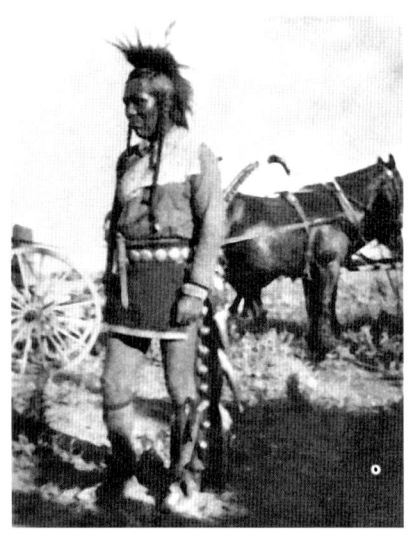

This young Shoshone man visited Casper in 1903. *Author's collection.*

As early as 1891, the Natrona County Commission appointed the first county physician to oversee medical issues throughout the county. Dr. W. W. Miller made $125 a year for taking on the task of monitoring countywide public health issues such as water safety, garbage cleanup, and epidemics.[11] This supplemented the money he made in his private practice.

As citizens created a town government, one early appointed position was that of town physician. J. L. Garner, M.D. was the company doctor on the Fremont, Elkhorn and Missouri Valley Railway. In 1895, he became the first town medical officer, serving until he was replaced by Dr. John Leeper in 1896. Town officials then appointed Garner again the next year.[12]

EARLY HEALTH CHALLENGES

Residents in the 1890s did not have a steady supply of good water. Most got it from the town well, on the west side of Center Street. They brought barrels and dipped the water with a bucket from the well. In June 1891, the town added a wooden pump for easier access. Others got their water from the Platte, from Garden Creek, or from Elkhorn Creek. Some people dug wells, but outhouses set up near water sources were a constant danger as they polluted the water supply. Piles of garbage, dead animals, and sewage overflows also created hazardous health conditions. Water-borne diseases soon began to kill Casper residents, especially children.[13]

In April 1892, the city approved a $3,000 bond to build a unified water system. By October 1893, they realized they had underestimated the cost and needed to hold a special election to get voters to approve an additional $30,000 bond for the project.[14] The city was still without a central water supply in 1895, when Fred Seeley began hauling it in barrels from Garden Creek and selling them at thirty-five cents a barrel.[15]

On August 24 of that year, the project to bring water from Elkhorn Creek finally began. A settling pond south of town held the creek water and then steel pipes brought it to people's residences. Although the system became fully functional on May 26, 1896, alkali soon began to decay the pipes. The city then began replacing all of the pipes with cast iron.[16] Even with these improvements it would be years before Casper had consistently good water throughout the city. Alfred Mokler noted that Casper got a sewer system in June of 1903.[17]

During the nineteenth century, the only disease that doctors had developed a vaccine for was smallpox. This meant that people, especially children, were subject to epidemics of diseases now controlled by vaccines.

In the summer of 1893, scarlet fever swept through the county. The *Natrona Tribune* recorded the August death of two-and-a-half-year-old Lilly Trollop at Bates Hole and noted that two other Trollop children were ill with the disease.[18] Another newspaper reported the death of one-year-old William Jones in Casper.[19] That same month Maren Nicolaysen and Johnnie Homan died of what the newspaper called *cholera infantum*, which could have been salmonella poisoning.[20]

December 1895 brought an outbreak of diphtheria that closed the Natrona County schools until January 30, 1896. Town physician Dr. John Leeper instituted a general quarantine of all those with the disease that lasted until early March. At one point, the illness forced the closure of all churches. Many families left town, but by early summer, most had returned.[21]

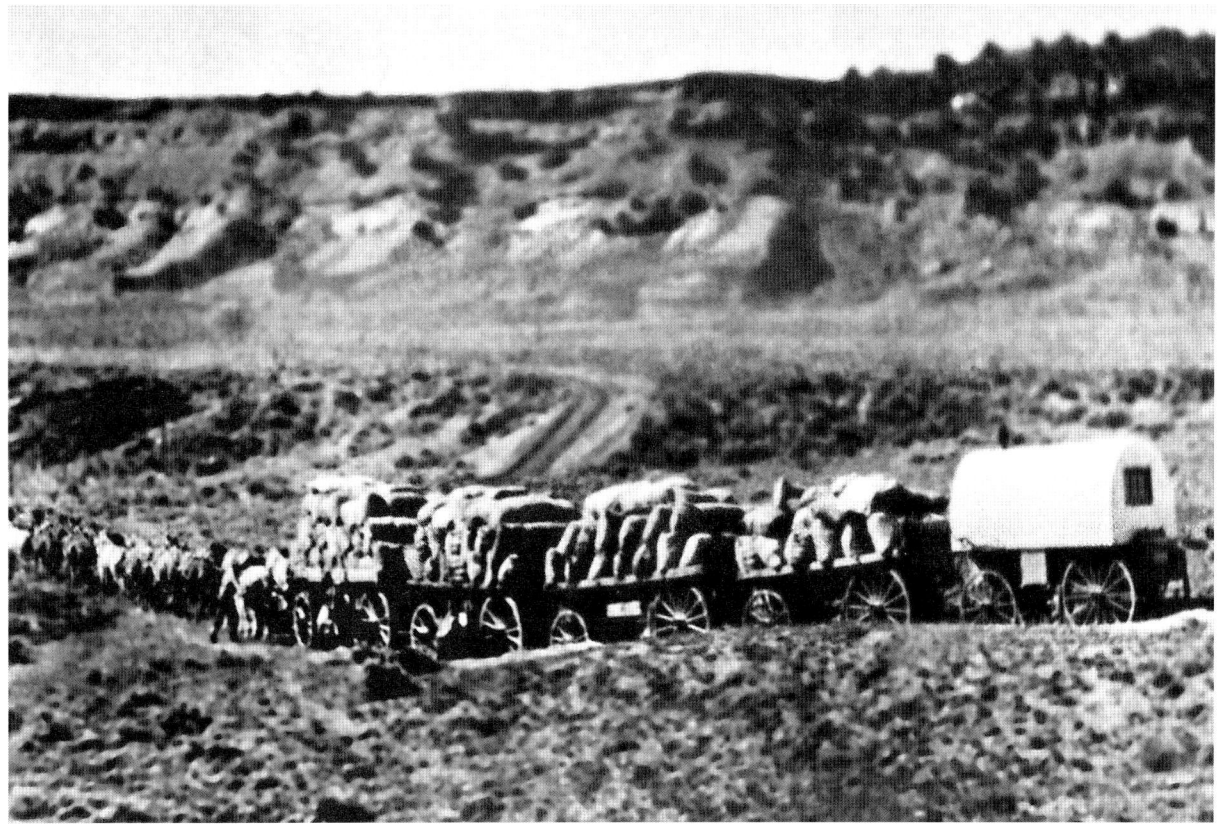

Wool was one of the county's chief exports. These wool wagons transported wool to the train station. *Author's collection*.

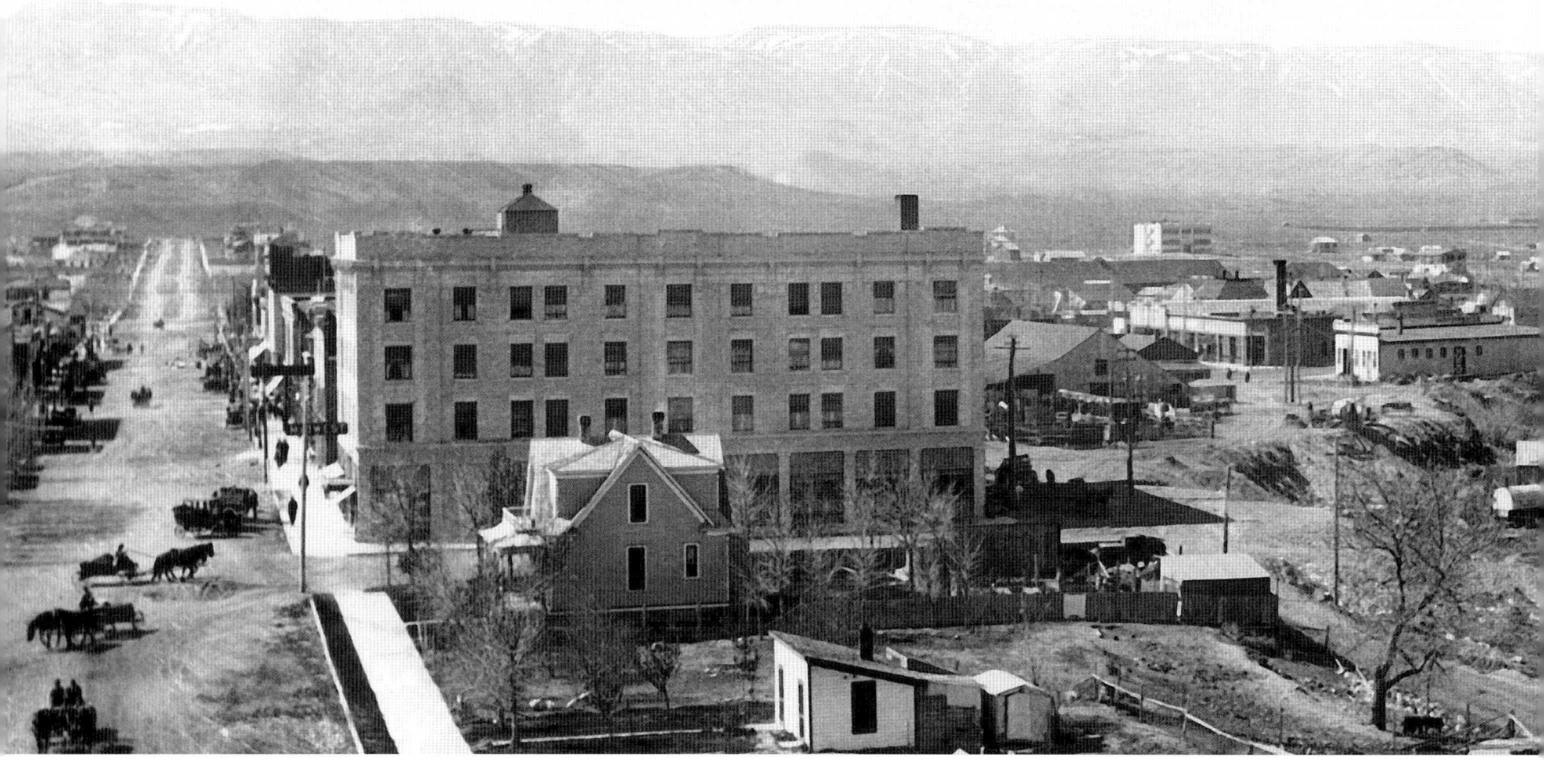

Backyards and streets filled with refuse caused disease and endangered health. *Casper College, Western History Center.*

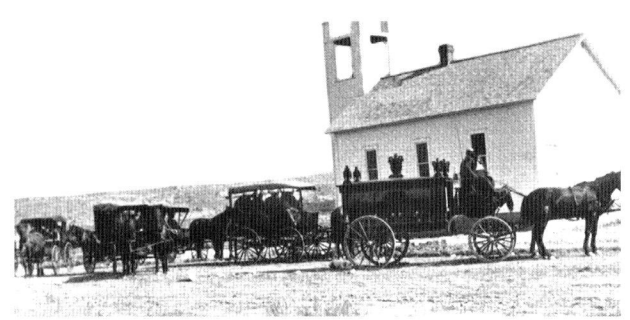

This Casper boy was one of many children lost to disease. *Author's collection.*

During the epidemic, Dr. Leeper set up a system to track the disease by having each case reported to authorities. Believing that the town was exceeding its authority, Dr. J. L. Garner refused to make a report. Dr. Leeper arrested Dr. Garner for not issuing the report but the courts acquitted Garner, and by the next year, he had replaced Dr. Leeper as the city physician.[22]

More serious was an epidemic of cerebrospinal meningitis that hit Casper in May 1898. According to Alfred Mokler, dozens fell ill in one day and those who died often did so in forty-eight hours. So many children caught the disease that town officials once again closed the school and the churches, and quarantined all remaining children. Parents responded on May 10 by taking their children away on the first available train.[23]

The only physicians in town at that time were Dr. Leeper and Dr. W. S. Bennett. They blamed the generally unsanitary conditions such as garbage piles and cow and hog pens within town limits for the outbreak. Dr. Leeper ordered it all cleaned up. By early June, the disease subsided and the families returned later in the summer.[24]

CASPER'S PIONEER PHYSICIANS

Doctors migrating west provided medical care in early Casper. Some were professionally trained and continued to be responsible citizens in the town for many years. Many were well-trained and reliable physicians who spent only a few years in the area and then moved on. Others, often less respectable, fortunately stayed only a short time before seeking other opportunities.

Professional medical schools began to appear in the United States just before the Civil War and the number grew rapidly after the war. There were around ninety in 1880; in 1900, that number grew to 151 schools, although many were not reputable training facilities.²⁵ New technology of the era included stethoscopes, medical thermometers, and X-rays.²⁶ Physicians added to their incomes by producing patent medicines, often alcohol- or opium-based, that they prescribed for their patients.

The uneven training and lack of professional credentialing in the West led to some of Casper's physicians being "quacks," sometimes just one step away from the law. Alfred Mokler reported that one early Casper doctor, Joseph Benson, was a notorious drunk and while incarcerated in 1891 died after setting the city jail on fire. Benson, who was a veteran of the Civil War, county coroner, and a member of the municipal band, lived his entire time in Casper under an assumed name. His real name was Joseph Riley.²⁷

Physicians coming in Casper's early days rarely stayed more than a few years. It was difficult to make a good living in an era when most people cared for their loved ones at home. All physicians made house calls, some even performing simple surgery in the kitchen. Many early physicians held down more than one job. John Leeper took time away from his practice to work his mining claims on Casper Mountain.

Dr. W. S. Bennett followed a pattern common for pioneer physicians. Before coming to Casper he practiced in Cripple Creek, Colorado. He was in Casper during 1895–1896 and sometime after established a permanent practice and a drugstore in Meeteetse, Wyoming.²⁸

> *All physicians made house calls, some even performing simple surgery in the kitchen.*

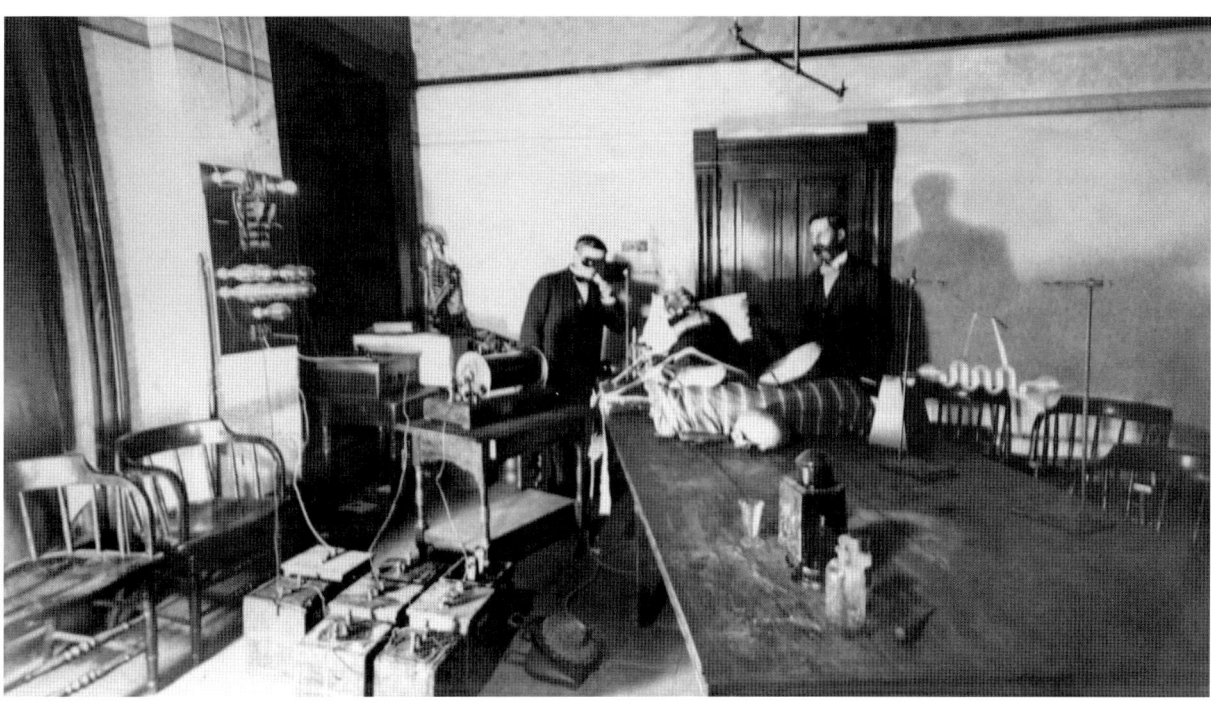

Primitive X-rays were just beginning to be used as a diagnostic tool. The equipment was cumbersome and dangerous. *Presbyterian/St. Luke's Medical Center Archives.*

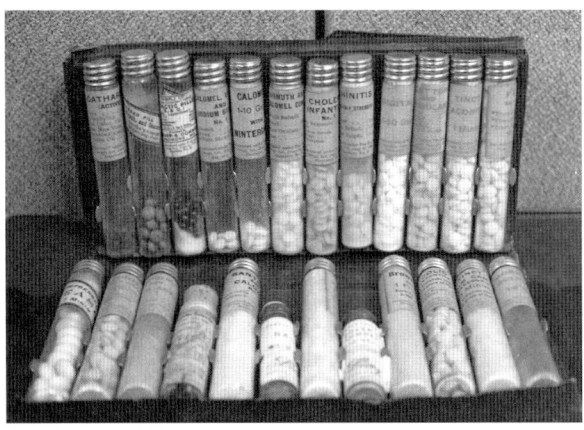

These bottles contain medicines developed to treat an assortment of diseases, often with little effect. *Author's collection*.

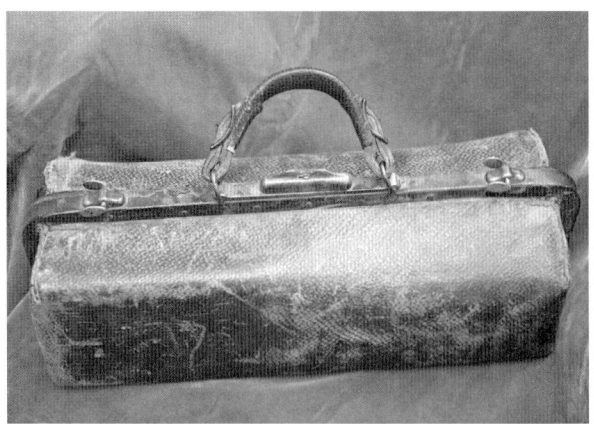

The doctor's bag contained all of his medicines and tools for treating patients. *Author's collection*.

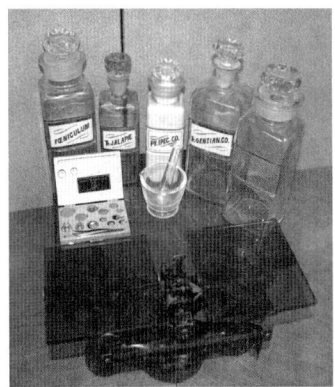

This pharmacy equipment is similar to that used by Wilson Kimball. *Author's collection*.

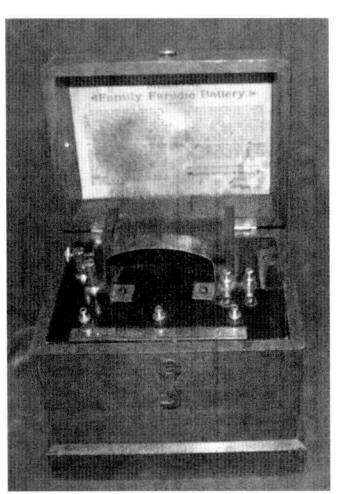

Doctors used electric shock to treat many illnesses and to manage pain. *Author's collection*.

In many ways, John Leeper typified the sort of physician who came, stayed, and became an important part of the early Western town. He came to Casper in the mid-1890s, serving as city physician in 1896 and again in 1898.[29] Later he was an Army medical officer in the Philippines. After his military career, he returned to his Casper practice and continued his involvement in local affairs.[30] By 1917, he was president of the Citizen's National Bank of Casper.[31] He served as mayor from 1918 until his death from cancer in December of 1919.[32]

Physicians such as Dr. Leeper also administered Casper's first private hospitals. Operated out of houses and business blocks, these hospitals served the town until the citizens could find a way to build a public facility. In 1893, reports began to surface of a race to create the first professionally run private hospital in Casper. The *Laramie Daily Boomerang* reported on May 11 that Casper druggist Wilson Kimball and Dr. Leeper had rented a building to create a hospital. The article continued to say that the two men had ordered furniture especially to outfit their hospital and had nurses trained in managing a hospital standing by to tend to patients.[33] Professionally trained nurses began arriving in Casper in the 1890s.

An additional article in the *Casper Derrick* on May 30, 1893, reported that the building stood on the west side of Center Street just north of Kimball's drugstore. The building had been the offices of the *Casper Derrick* newspaper and was next door to what had been Mathew Campfield's barbershop.[34] The article went on to say:

> It contains nine rooms. The first one on the left of the hall is nicely fitted up as Dr. Leeper's office, and opposite is the operating room. Back of these range the patients' apartments. Everything is scrupulously neat, the mattresses are as soft as wool can be made and every facility for rapid recovery seems to be given the patients. Ten or twelve patients can be comfortably cared for at one time. Strangers and others who are taken sick in this section of country with no proper place to be cared for will greatly appreciate the opportunity offered them by the opening of the Casper hospital.[35]

Another *Laramie Daily Boomerang* article, this time on May 31, 1893, said that Dr. L. G. Powell planned to open a hospital that would be two stories high and twenty-four by forty-six feet square.[36] The article did not specify a location other than somewhere in Casper and did not mention an opening date. No further articles mentioned Dr. Powell's facility.

Other newspapers detailed local illnesses and injuries mentioning patients going to Grandma Harrison's house in Casper.[37] It was apparently a convalescent home or another private hospital but not as well known as Dr. Leeper's institution.

Private hospitals in town were not the only medical facilities. In 1885, ranchers in Central Wyoming put together a plan to acquire the hospital at the abandoned Ft. Fetterman army post west of Douglas. They created the Fetterman Hospital Association, a subscription facility available to any ranchers or cowboys who agreed to have a dollar a month deducted from their wages. Cattle companies could also subscribe and the Carey Cattle Company of Natrona County did just that, getting a greatly reduced group rate of one hundred dollars per month.[38]

The Fetterman Hospital Association operations went well for a few years. The first year they had 149 patients, fourteen of whom were not part of the pre-paid system. In the second year, there were 340 patients including three charity patients paid for by Converse County. The disastrous winter of 1886–1887 put many cowboys out of work, cutting their income. Eventually, the corporate members took over and tried to run the hospital on a for-profit basis, but it was too far from population centers to attract patients. Dr. Amos Barber served as the hospital director and sole attending physician from 1885 to 1889. After he left to take up a practice in Douglas, hospital managers failed to find another doctor to take over, so the hospital closed by the early 1890s.[39] Dr. Barber was influential in creating the Converse County Hospital and later became governor of Wyoming.

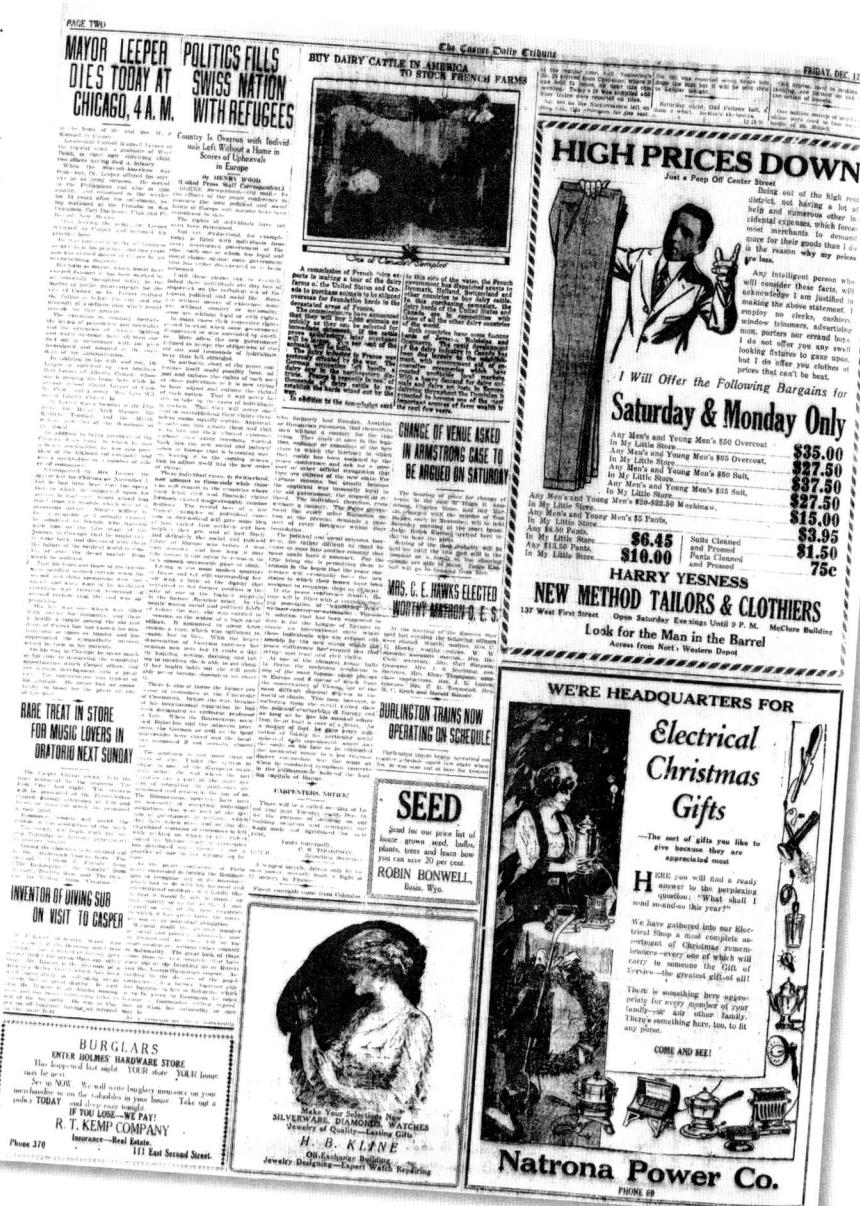

This newspaper carried Dr. John Leeper's 1919 obituary describing his contributions to Casper.

CHAPTER ONE ❖ *Before the Hospital:* UP TO 1909

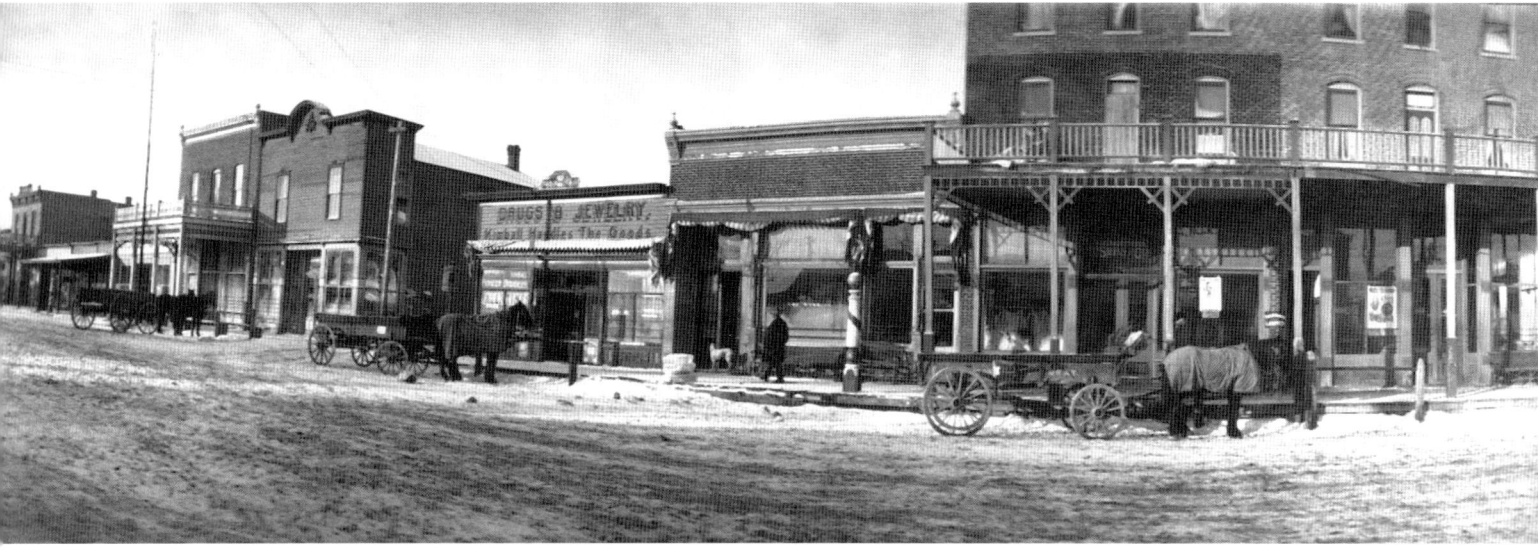

Kimball and Leeper's hospital was in the building that has the barber pole in front of it. *Fort Caspar Museum collection*.

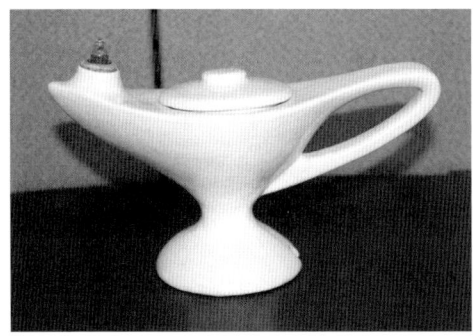

Florence Nightingale lamps were a common gift for new graduate nurses.

After the turn of the twentieth century, Natrona County business leaders realized that Central Wyoming needed a public hospital. On October 29, 1903, concerned citizens gathered for a meeting to look at the possibility of establishing a privately run, non-sectarian hospital, "nonpolitical and in favor of no certain physician."[40] Some town leaders argued that Casper could not support a hospital. The businessmen quoted in the paper noted that people had said the same thing before the town had public water, electricity, and telephones, but now people had a hard time going without these essential services. They cast the hospital in the same light, as an essential service.[41]

This all came at a time when the town was growing, not just as a rail and agricultural center, but also as the focal point of a new oil industry. Casper needed to prove to residents and potential investors alike that it was a good place to bring businesses and raise families. Records do not show that the hospital project actually materialized, but the discussion remained in people's minds.

A March 19, 1906 rail accident reinforced the need for a hospital facility. The Chicago and Northwestern train hit a washed-out culvert west of town during a severe storm. The crash killed ten at the scene and left sixteen injured. Dr. T. A. Dean and Dr. Gilliam soon arrived to aid the survivors. Two doctors from Douglas, as well as Dr. Marshall Keith and Dr. G. T. Morgan, came the next morning. When the patients returned to Casper, physicians treated them in a makeshift hospital set up in the annex of the Episcopal Church.[42] This, added to other needs, planted the seed for what became the Wyoming State Hospital, Casper Branch.

NOTES

1 Elliott West. *Growing Up With the Country: Childhood on the Far Western Frontier*. Albuquerque: University of New Mexico Press, 1989.

2 Alfred J. Mokler. *History of Natrona County, Wyoming, 1888–1922*. Chicago: Lakeside Press, 1923 (reprint Casper, Mountain States Lithography, 1989), pp. 1–2.

3 Mokler, p. 118.

4 Mokler, p. 115.

5 Mokler, p. 117.

6 Mokler, p. 115.

7 Mokler, p. 115.

8 Mokler, p. 116, pp. 117–118.

9 Tom Rea. "Mathew Campfield, Barber and Pioneer Survivor," http://www.tomrea.net/Mathew%20Campfield.html.

10 Irving Garbutt. *I Was There: Recollections of Ten Decades*. Casper: Casper Journal, 2003, p. 21.

11 Mokler, p. 12.

12 *Natrona Tribune*, December 26, 1895, p. 1.

13 Mokler, p. 147.

14 Mokler, p. 124.

15 Mokler, p. 149.

16 Mokler, p. 151.

17 Mokler, p. 167.

18 *Natrona Tribune*, Vol. 3, No. 13, p. 4.

19 Irving Garbutt. *History of Casper and Natrona County, Wyoming, 1889–1989*, Vol. 1. Dallas: Irving Media, 1990, p. 200.

20 *Natrona Tribune*, Vol. 3, No. 15, p. 3.

21 Mokler, p. 126.

22 Mokler, p. 126.

23 Mokler, p. 183.

24 Mokler, p. 184.

25 Duane Smith and Ronald Brown. *No One Ailing Except a Physician*. Boulder: University Press of Colorado, 2001, p. 21.

26 Smith and Brown, pp. 21–22, p. 23.

27 Mokler, p. 10, 65, 167, and 429.

28 Rhonda Schulte. "Centenarian Remembers Childhood Friend, Buffalo Bill Cody," April 6, 2001, http://www.gemstonememoirs.com/4f274ddf-e8b4-4f6e-8e79-335bad8513e3-9.html.

29 Mokler, p. 127.

30 Mokler, p. 63.

31 Mokler, p. 27.

32 Mokler, p. 1.

33 *Laramie Daily Boomerang*, May 11, 1893, p. 1.

34 The buildings in question are just north of the current Ugly Bug Fly Shop on Center Street.

35 *Casper Derrick*, May 30, 1893.

36 *Laramie Daily Boomerang*, May 31, 1893, p. 2.

37 Garbutt, *History of Casper and Natrona County*, p. 185.

38 Phil Roberts. "Greed, Depression and the End of Wyoming's Cowboy Health Cooperative," *Buffalo Bones*, n.d., http://uwacadweb.uwyo.edu/RobertsHistory/buffalobones.htm.

39 Roberts, "Greed, Depression and the End of Wyoming's Cowboy Health Cooperative."

40 *Natrona County Tribune*, October 29, 1903.

41 *Natrona County Tribune*, October 29, 1903.

42 Mokler, pp. 50–52.

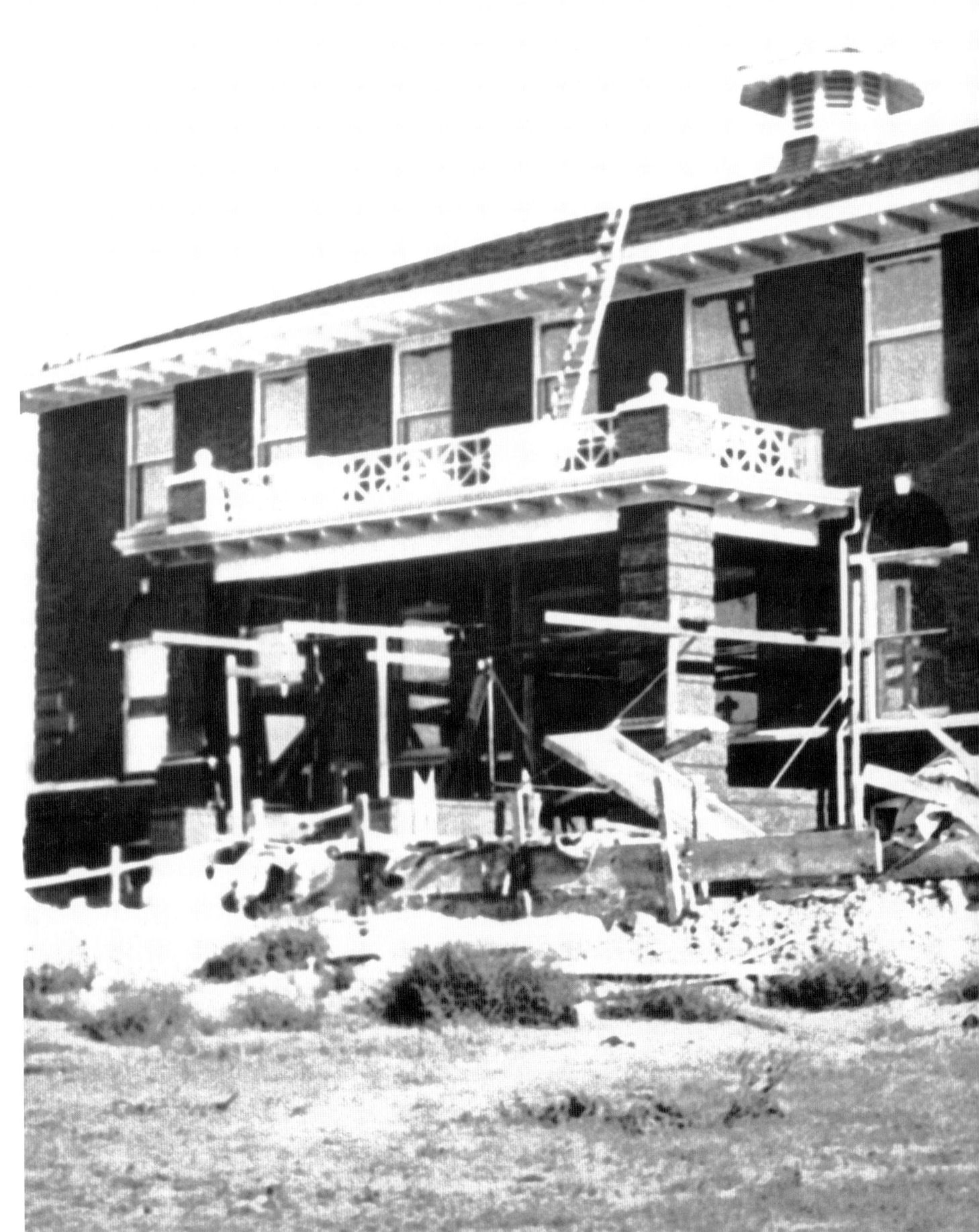

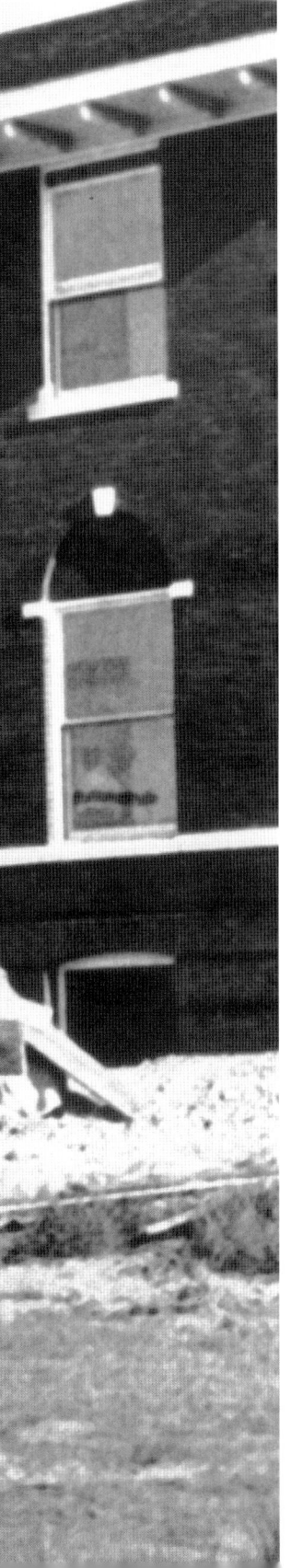

CHAPTER TWO

Casper Gets Her Hospital

1909 TO 1920

Wyoming's enabling documents set aside public lands to sell to fund public institutions. The allotted lands included 75,000 acres to pay for charitable institutions such as prisons, orphanages, and hospitals.[1] The first hospitals served remote areas of Wyoming including Rock Springs and Sheridan. By 1908, Casper's business community, agitating for a Central Wyoming facility, got the state's attention.

In 1909, Governor B. B. Brooks encouraged Natrona County Representative Hugh Patton to submit a bill to appropriate $22,500 to build the Casper branch of the Wyoming State Hospital. Governor Brooks hoped to bring in one of the orders of Catholic sisters who had started many Western hospitals, but legislators opposed his proposal. Governor Brooks later said that he "was accused of trying to establish the Catholic Church here and many other things of like character and in the end the hospital board was obliged to give up the idea of the sisters taking charge and substitute the present system."[2]

Patton's bill passed unanimously with the caveat that Casper provide the land and furnish the building. On April 12, 1909, the State Board of Charities and Reform met with Casper's town council and the hospital committee of the Casper Industrial Club to select a site.[3] The first choice was a property at Center and Eighth streets, recently donated to the city by Joseph Carey to create a park. Initially, Carey agreed to the new use, but on August 26, 1909, his attorney announced that Carey had changed his mind. He was disputing taxes owed the town and felt that at that time use of the land for a hospital was not in his best interest.[4]

Carey also had a philosophical disagreement with the idea of public-run hospitals. He agreed with Governor Brooks that such institutions should be operated

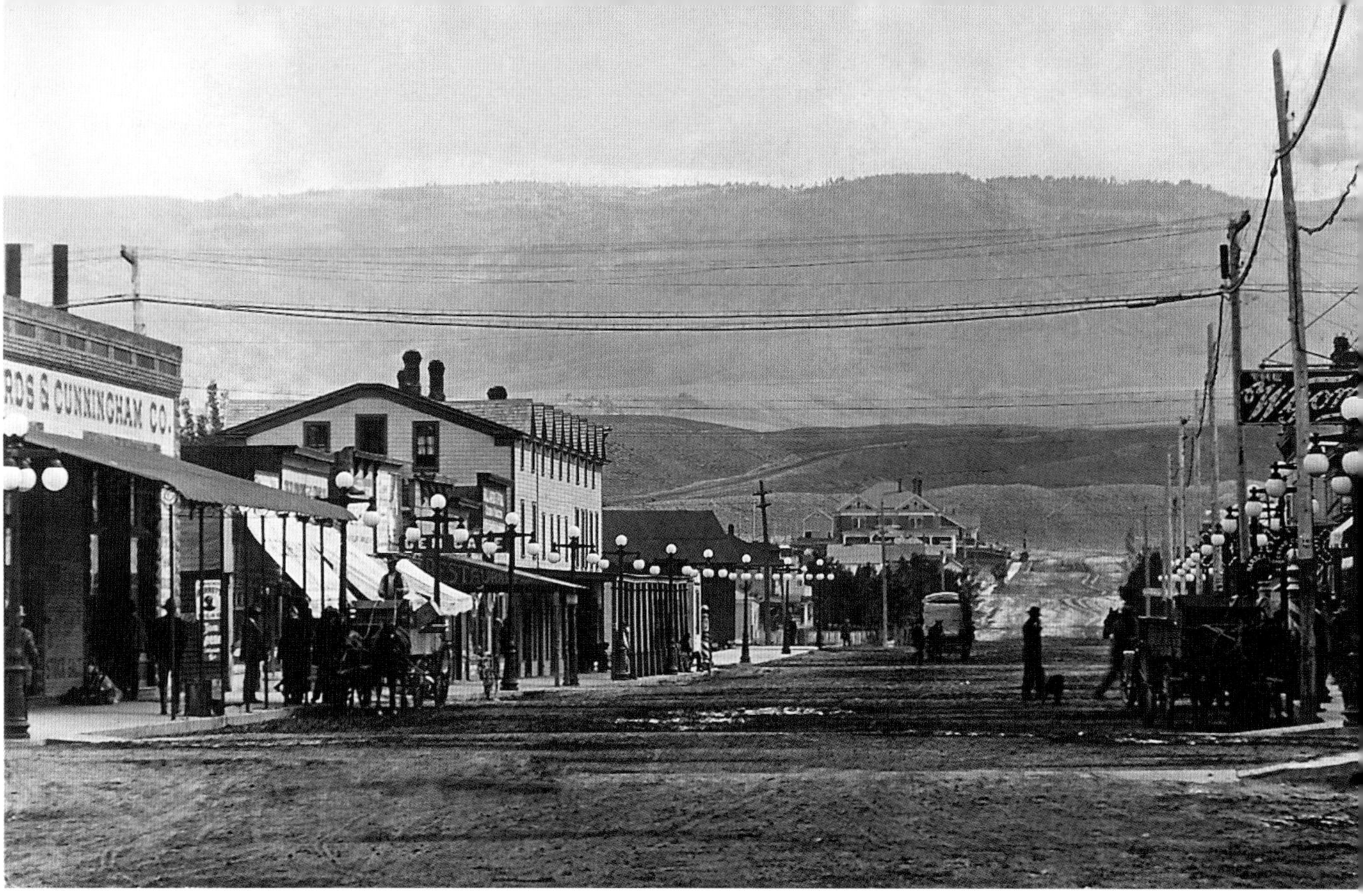

Looking south on Center Street toward Alex Butler's homestead, one possible site of the hospital. *Fort Caspar Museum collection.*

by religious orders rather than by the government. He did not, in fact, believe that the government should be in the business of providing any assistance to the public. Joseph Carey's beliefs would hinder getting the facility operational in a timely manner.[5]

As the town fathers considered other sites for their hospital, two public-spirited men came forward. Alex Butler owned a homestead south of town on the way to Casper Mountain. If the county would put a road out to his land, he could plat it for homes with the idea that the new hospital would draw people to live on the south side of town. Planners rejected Butler's offer because it came with strings attached and it seemed too far out of town.[6]

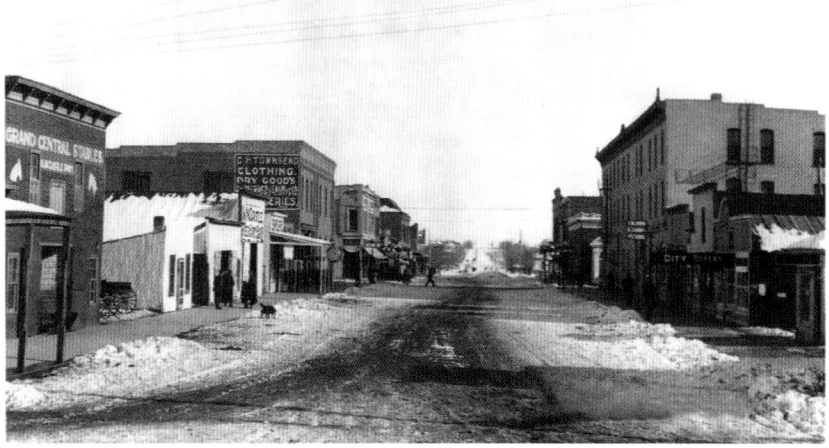

This view looking east on Second Street shows "C" Hill in the distance. This was the site of Henry White's land.

The second piece of land proposed for the new hospital belonged to Henry White. The land was a 300-by-420-foot section on Second Street between Washington and Conwell streets in an area called "C" Hill.[7] This name dated back to the 1890s, when Cheyenne and Casper were in competition for the state capitol. Town leaders designated the hilly portion of East Second Street as the site of the capitol building if Casper won the bid. Townspeople called this "C" Hill.[8] (Note: Readers should not confuse this with the current "C" Hill, the home of

20 *Wyoming Medical Center:* A CENTENNIAL HISTORY

Casper College.) At the time, it too was on the east edge of town with a few scattered houses and Highland Cemetery in the vicinity. Hospital planners accepted White's land and began to look for a suitable builder.

In January 1910, the state let the contract for the new building to Archie Allen of Cheyenne while William Henning of Casper got the heating and plumbing contract.[9] Work began in March 1910, with construction going quickly. The state accepted the completed work on August 31, 1910, when the State Board of Charities and Reform inspected the hospital. An article in the *Natrona County Tribune* noted that the building could not begin to function as a hospital until it had furnishings, nurses, and a superintendent. The next session of the legislature approved the funds.[10]

A disagreement between the state and the town resulted in unnecessary funding delays. When the state allocated the money to build the new hospital, town leaders expected that the cost of the outfitting the building would come out of the original $22,500, but the construction costs ate up all the original money. Casper business leaders resisted putting up any further money for furnishings.

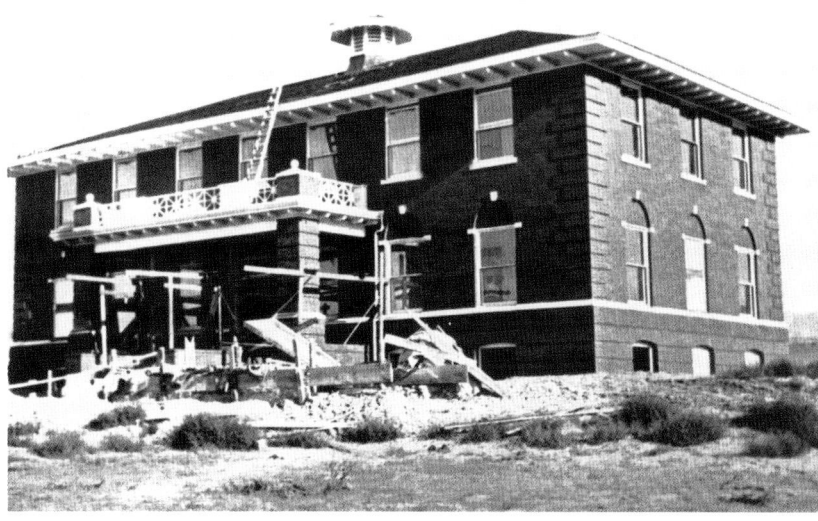

The Wyoming State Hospital, Casper Branch under construction, 1910.

When the state legislature met in January 1911, they produced a bill allocating $12,000 to prepare the building for opening day. New governor Joseph Carey, who was still opposed to the idea of public hospitals, vetoed the appropriation. The legislature then attached the $12,000 to a general appropriation bill for state charitable institutions and Carey had no choice but to sign the bill.[11]

Martha Converse, in her office, was the first superintendent in 1911.

Between January and August of 1911, citizens of Casper waited for workmen to make repairs and for the State Board of Charities and Reform to purchase supplies and equipment. They also waited for the governor to find the time to arrive with the state board to conduct the final inspection. During the interim, the state appointed a watchman who lived in an apartment he created in the basement of the empty building.[12]

On August 3, 1911, the *Natrona County Tribune* reported that State Auditor Robert Forsythe and Martha Converse, R.N. had arrived to take the final steps to get the facility open.[13] With the work done, the doors opened on October 31, 1911, and the first patients arrived on November 1, 1911. The first babies born in the new hospital were Maxine and Murray Sullivan, children of Dan and Ella Sullivan.[14]

Martha Converse, the first superintendent of the Wyoming State Hospital, Casper Branch, had previously been superintendent of the Wyoming State Hospital, Rock Springs, where she worked from 1902

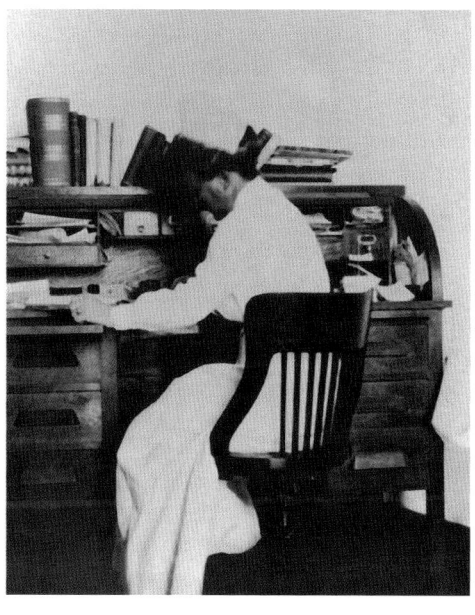

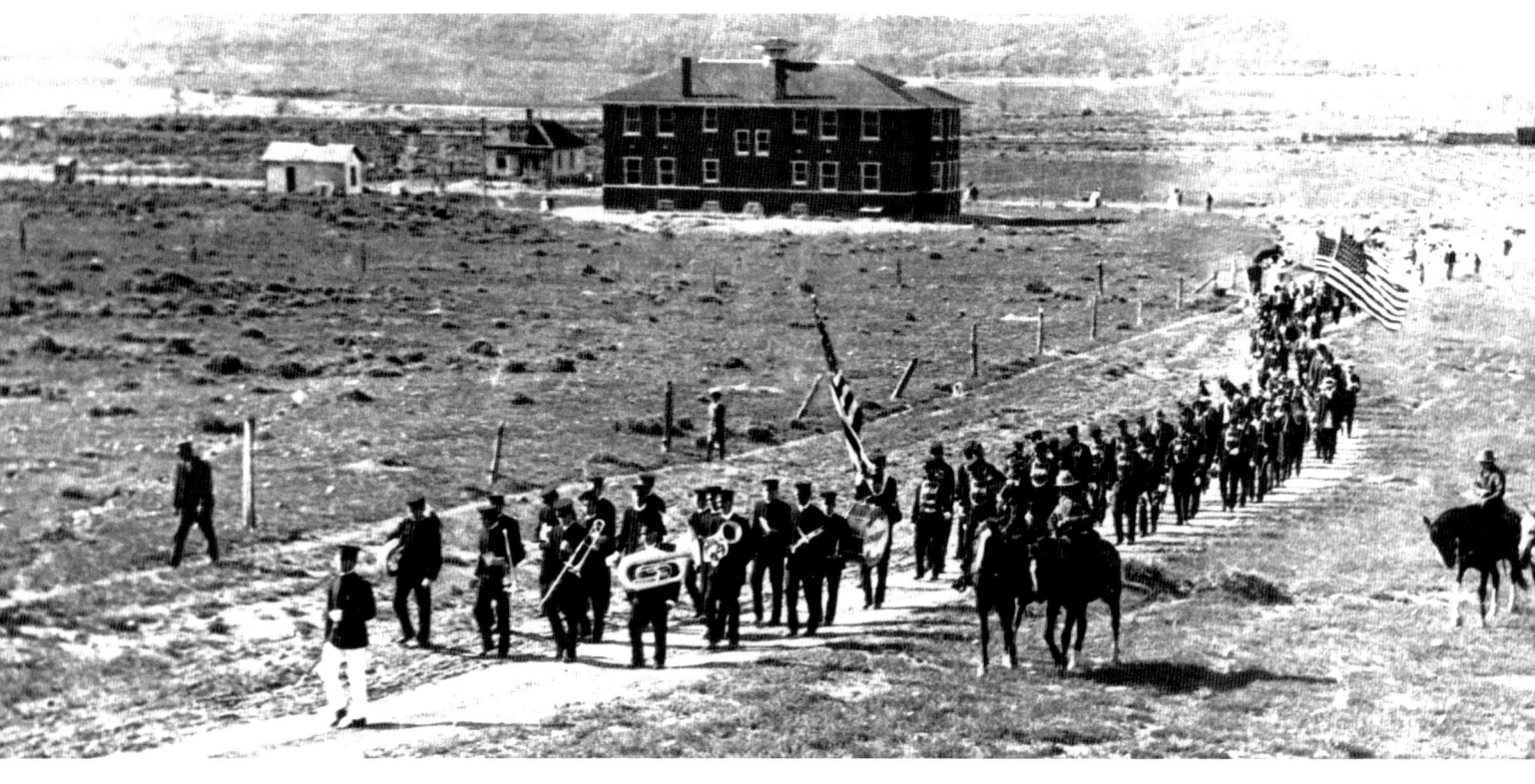

This 1912 Decoration Day photo shows the parade passing the hospital as it winds up Conwell Street to the cemetery.

to 1911. Originally from Mount Victory, Ohio, she graduated from the Columbus, Ohio Protestant Hospital School of Nursing in 1897. Her first hospital superintendent's job was at Grant Hospital in Columbus, Ohio. Converse then cared for Spanish-American War troops in the military hospital in Georgia. A commendation from Clara Barton, founder of the American Red Cross, earned her a position at the U.S. Provisional Hospital for Volunteers in Columbus, Ohio. Her patients were Spanish-American War veterans who were making the transition back to civilian life.[15]

In 1902, ill health due to overwork became the catalyst for Converse's move to Rock Springs, Wyoming. She also served as head of the Sheridan State Hospital, commuting between the two on three-month rotations. Her sterling reputation led to her appointment to the Casper Hospital.[16] Converse served as the head of the Casper Hospital until her marriage to Wilson S. Kimball on December 31, 1916. As an upper-class married woman, she did not work, but she remained active in the nursing field for many years through involvement in the Wyoming State Nurses' Association (WSNA).[17]

The WSNA formed out of a concern that Wyoming patients were not receiving care from trained nurses. The state had passed a law in 1909 requiring nurses to register with the state, but there was an inadequate monitoring of the process.[18] The seven nurses who gathered at a 1909 meeting in Sheridan felt that a professional association might help with the problem. Converse was one of the founding members of the WSNA.[19]

> *The WSNA formed out of a concern that Wyoming patients were not receiving care from trained nurses.*

Over the ensuing years, the WSNA continued to advocate for Wyoming nurses and patients. Nurses at the Casper Hospital formed the Natrona County branch which the association accepted into the state organization in 1925.[20]

Assistant nurses began arriving to help Martha Converse in 1912. Wilhelmina Hamilton, originally of Saratoga, Wyoming, had graduated from the Episcopal hospital in Philadelphia in 1903. She joined the nursing staff in August 1912.[21] Her arrival, according to a newspaper account, allowed Converse to take an extended vacation to see friends in Cheyenne.[22] This was likely the first break Superintendent Converse had taken since she began managing the hospital in 1911.

Casper and Natrona County began to grow rapidly after 1910. Where agriculture, especially cattle and sheep raising, had been at the core of the local economy, now the oil industry brought people to Central Wyoming. The first small oilfield and its refinery built in Casper in 1895 grew to 105,000 acres of producing wells by 1905.[23] Belgo-American Oil began operations in Casper in 1904; Franco-American Oil bought out Belgo-American in 1912.[24] Coloradoans Oliver Shoup and Verner Z. Reed established Midwest Oil Company in 1911 and began operations in Natrona County in 1912. By 1919, Standard Oil and Texas Oil had also established fields around Casper.[25] The big new refineries that went with these projects meant more workers settling in Casper and the surrounding towns.

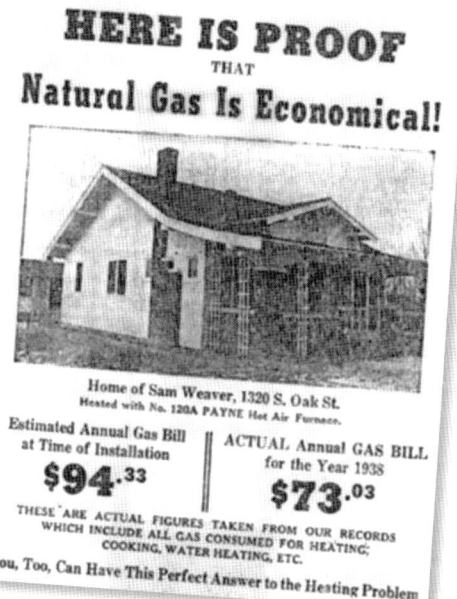

This Casper bungalow house was typical of those built during the boom in the 1920s. *Author's collection*.

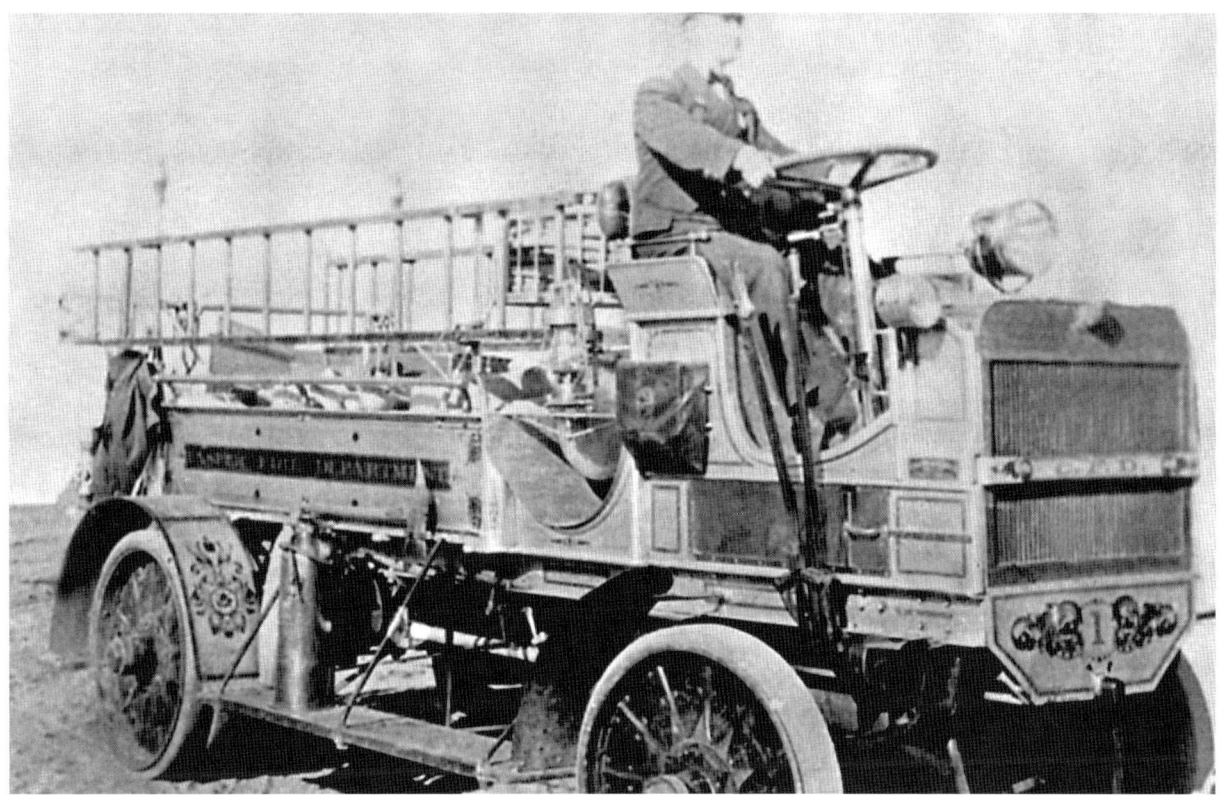

Casper's 1910 motorized fire truck. *Author's collection*.

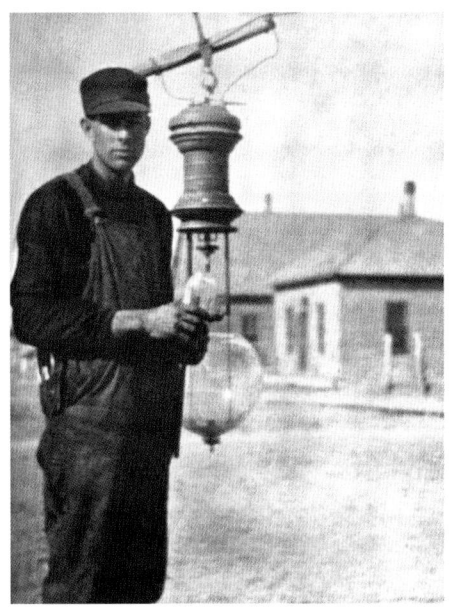

Edgar Davis trims the wick on one of Casper's streetlights. *Author's collection.*

The end of World War I brought veterans and their families to Wyoming looking for work with the oilfields and refineries drawing the bulk of the new residents. As Casper boomed, its population changed. Average wages in Casper in 1920 were one dollar per hour. A share of oil stock also cost one dollar.[26]

The population of the county in 1920 reached 24,272, roughly evenly divided between men and women. One-sixth of residents were between the ages of birth and fourteen. More than half were fifteen to forty-five, prime working and childbearing ages. About one-eighth of the population was over sixty-five.[27]

By 1925, the population had risen to nearly 35,000.[28] English, Irish, Germans, French, Austrians, Hungarians, Italians, Swedes, and Norwegians made up the bulk of the population but smaller groups included Greeks and Jews of various ethnicities. Around half of the population had been born outside of the United States or had at least one parent who was an immigrant.[29] The Abraham Kassis family came from Syria by way of North Dakota and established the Kassis Dry Goods Store in Casper.

Young families with rapidly growing numbers of children also increased the population. One example was the Sam Weaver family, originally from Tennessee. Weaver first came to Casper in 1914 to work for Standard Oil. When World War I began, he enlisted along with other young men from the area. After the war, he came back with a new wife and they settled down. Sam went back to work cleaning oil stills at the

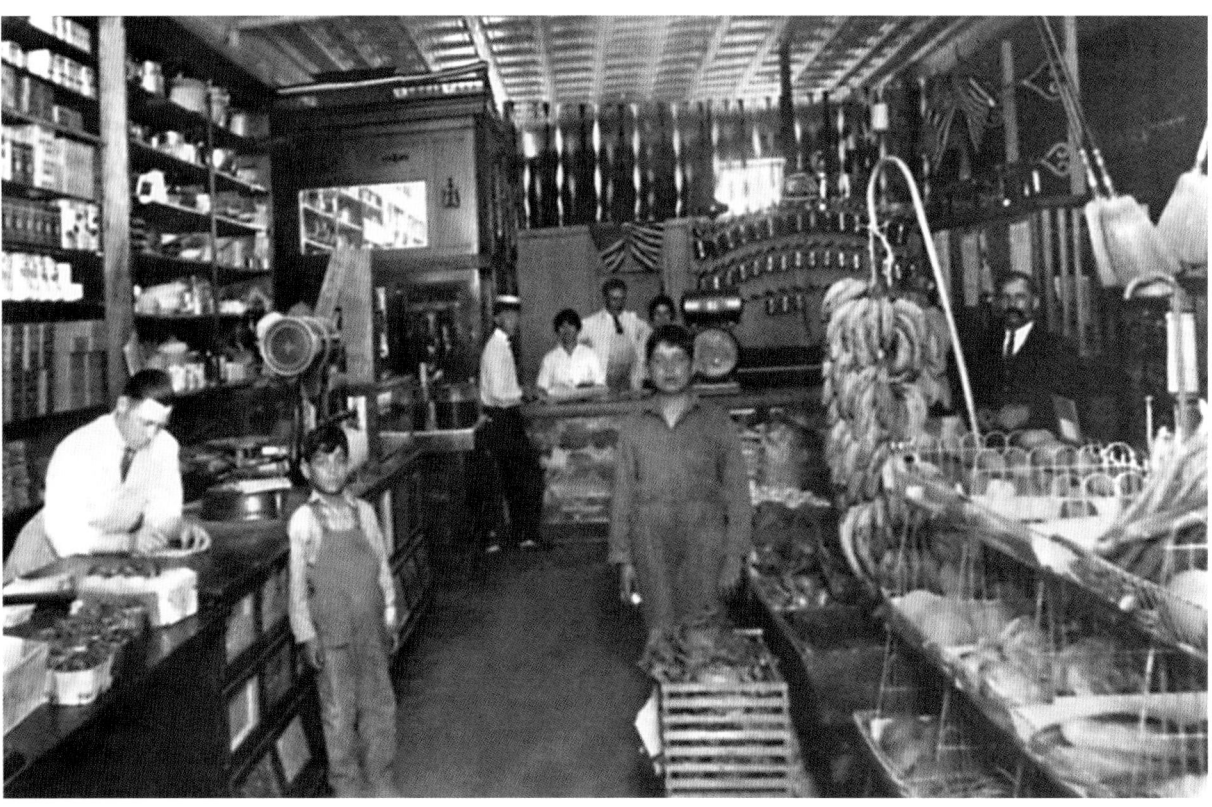

The interior of the Abraham Kassis store in Casper. *Author's collection.*

Standard Oil refinery and Sam's wife Alyce gave birth to four children in three years including a set of twins. They raised all of the children at the new family home at 1320 S. Oak Street.[30]

The population growth led to a housing boom with developments cropping up in all directions from the center of town. To the south, toward the mountain, large gracious homes spoke of the new wealth of the oil men. North, west, and east the homes were smaller, lower middle-class and working-class housing stock. After 1920, all of the area between downtown and the open fields around the hospital filled up with homes.

Services such as electricity and telephones arrived with the beginning of the twentieth century. The first electric lights came on line on June 12, 1900.[31] Telephone service arrived on March 22, 1902, when Mountain Bell installed the first forty-nine phones. By 1910, there were around 300 telephones and in 1925, reflecting the ongoing population boom, there were 5,600.[32] Casper's fire department had a motorized fire truck in 1910.

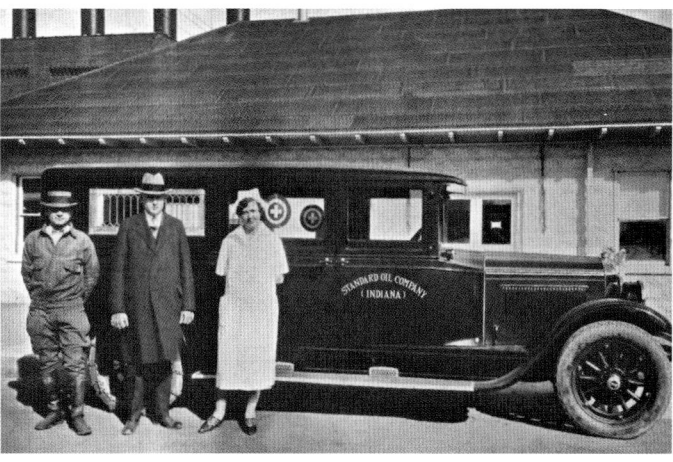

Medical staff and ambulance at the Standard Oil Refinery hospital. *Author's collection.*

This growth tested the limits of the new Casper Hospital, as people began to call it. For many years there was more than one hospital in the county. The Standard Oil refinery had its own medical staff and hospital. The Casper Hospital served the city, the county, and the region around the town. Wolton, west of Casper, had a hospital in a log cabin between 1905 and the mid-1920s.[33] Homer Lathrop, M.D. owned and operated the Casper Private Hospital.

The city and the county allocated money to pay for medical care for indigent patients. As early as the 1890s, part of this went to city and county physicians who earned extra money by tending poor patients. From 1904 to 1907, Dr. E. P. Rohrbaugh was the Casper city physician. Dr. Marshall C. Keith served from 1908 to 1915, Dr. Joseph Kamp from 1918 to 1920, and Dr. G. S. Bawden during 1920 to 1921.[34]

Who was eligible for indigent care sometimes became an issue for the county. In January 1896, William Carter, a worker at the *Casper Derrick* newspaper, lost his job and then fell ill. It cost the county forty-one dollars to help him recover. After he got another job, the County Commissioners sued him to recover costs. His attorney won the case by arguing that he was a pauper when ill and so should not be penalized for that.[35] Free care was and still is a thorny issue.

County physicians in the early part of the century continued to be responsible for dealing with epidemics ranging from influenza to sexually transmitted diseases. They also oversaw cleanup of sewage leaks and garbage dumps. Most of what was in the county physician's job description is now the public health sanitarian's job.

One longstanding Casper county physician was Dr. Homer Lathrop, who came to Wyoming from Colorado in 1901 to work on the Pathfinder Dam project. He practiced in Casper beginning in the early 1900s, although he also ranched east of town.

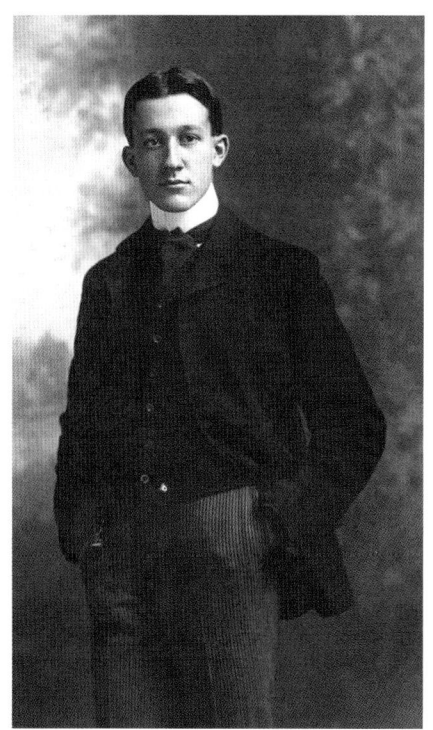

Homer Lathrop, M.D., around 1910. *Fort Caspar Museum collection.*

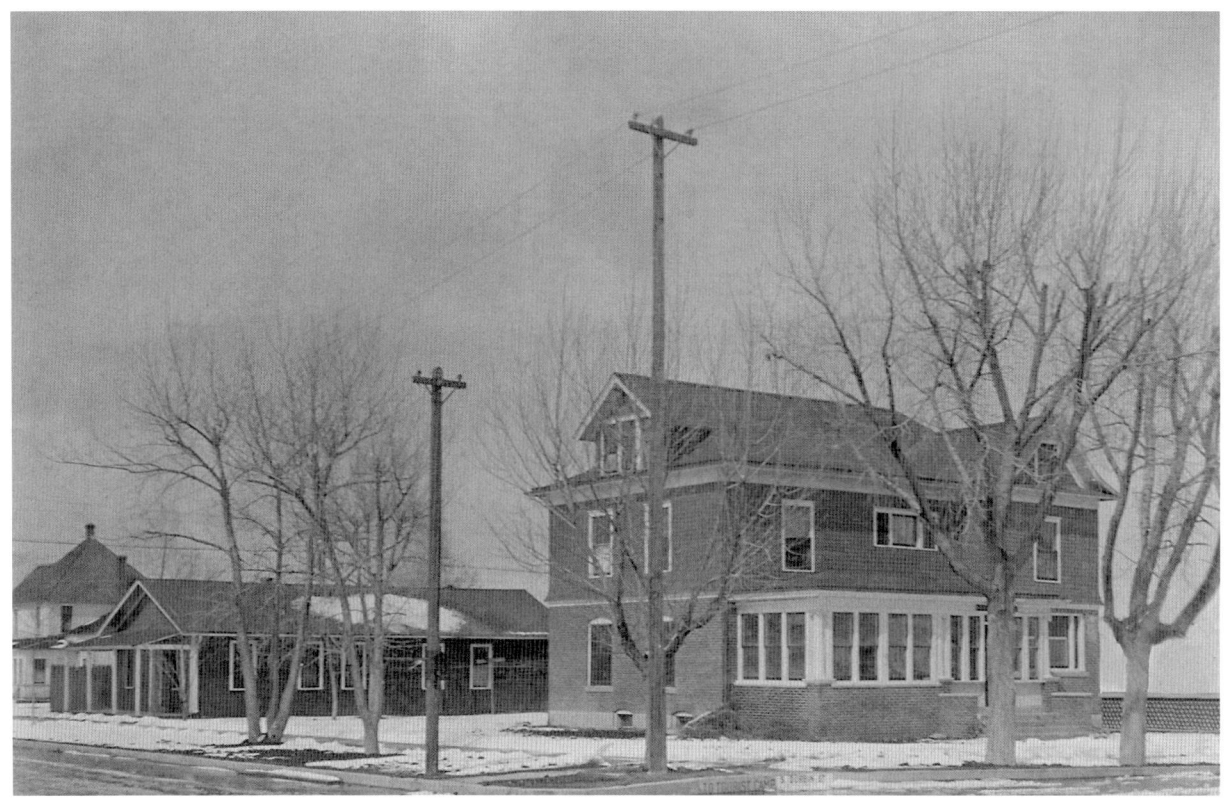

Homer Lathrop's Casper Private Hospital at Tenth and Durbin streets. *Fort Caspar Museum collection.*

According to county records, Dr. Lathrop functioned as the county physician and public health officer for a number of years. During the 1910s and 1920s, expenditures for medicines, house calls, and care in Dr. Lathrop's private hospital were a significant part of the county budget.[36]

By 1915, the Wyoming State Hospital, Casper Branch began running at a deficit. Although the state picked up deficits for the Rock Springs and Sheridan state facilities, it refused to do the same in Casper. An unknown editorial letter-writer in the *Casper Daily Press* noted that the County Commissioners had paid $1,871.50 to Dr. Lathrop and his Casper Private Hospital for the 1914–1915 fiscal year. That was roughly the amount that the state hospital had gone into the red. The writer argued that the Commissioners needed to stop giving their appointed county medical officer preferential treatment at the expense of the taxpayer-supported hospital. He and other Casper progressive citizens favored use of taxpayer money for the hospital as long as the County Commissioners began sending their charity patients where they belonged.[37]

Changing physicians' habits took time. Many physicians preferred to care for patients at home, even performing simple surgery at a patient's house. Irving Garbutt remembered Dr. Joseph Kamp removing his tonsils in the family kitchen. Dr. Kamp strapped young Garbutt to the ironing board.[38] Casper's newspapers provide names and dates that show changes in physician practices and a growing acceptance of the hospital. Articles give a detailed look at the general impact of the new hospital in its first decade.

The November 11, 1913 issue of the *Natrona County Tribune* reported that Doctors Kamp and Gilliam performed three abdominal surgeries at the hospital.

They operated on two women and an infant.³⁹ Another article in the *Casper Daily Tribune* on March 11, 1922 reported that O. J. Cacharelis was recovering at his home after successful surgery at the hospital.⁴⁰ Both indicate that doctors were increasingly sending their patients to the hospital, at least for major surgeries.

Apparently local residents, as well as their doctors, took some time to get accustomed to the presence of the state hospital. In 1912, the Scherck family, unwilling to do a home birth and not sure of the care available at the new state hospital, went to Douglas to have their daughter Bernadine at the Converse County Hospital.⁴¹

The 1918 influenza epidemic tested the mettle of all medical personnel in Casper. Each day during October 1918, the *Casper Daily Tribune* and the *Casper Daily Press* advertised for nurses to help care for the multitude of people falling ill from the flu. Isabella Nelson, R.N., representing the Casper Red Cross, was accepting applications from anyone who had received any level of nurses' training. Doctors also worked around the clock trying to save lives during the epidemic. The hospitals, public and private alike, were full. Eventually, quarantines closed churches, schools, and other places where people gathered before the epidemic gradually wore itself out in early winter of 1919.⁴²

In an interview, Casper author Frances Seely Webb reported that when she gave birth to her daughter Ann, so many nurses were either ill or away serving in World War I that there was not one qualified person available to care for her in the hospital.

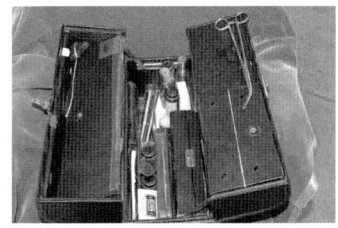

Doctors of the 1920s and 1930s carried this type of medical bag. *Author's collection.*

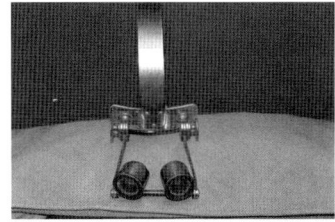

This head-mounted magnifying device allowed a doctor to get a closer view during surgery. *Author's collection.*

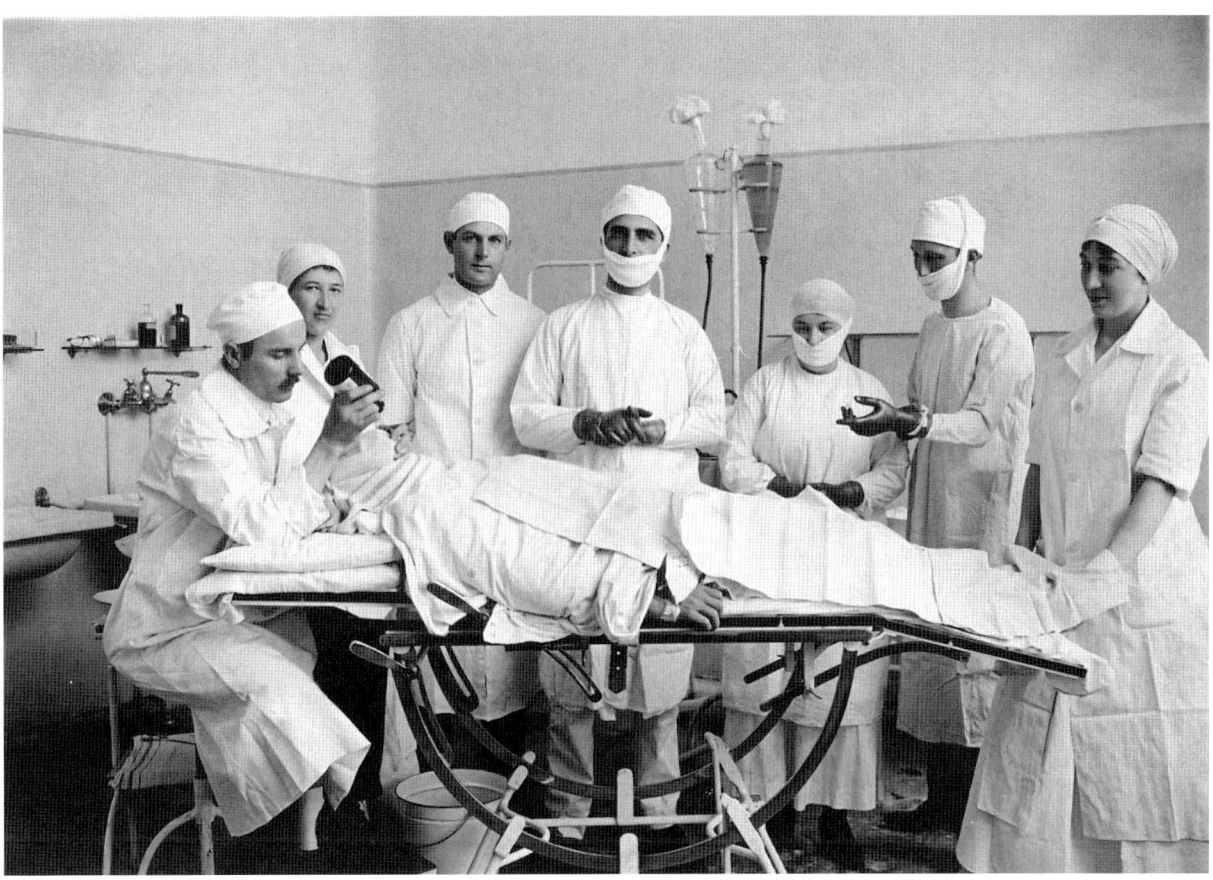

Hospital operating room, around 1910. *Fort Caspar Museum collection.*

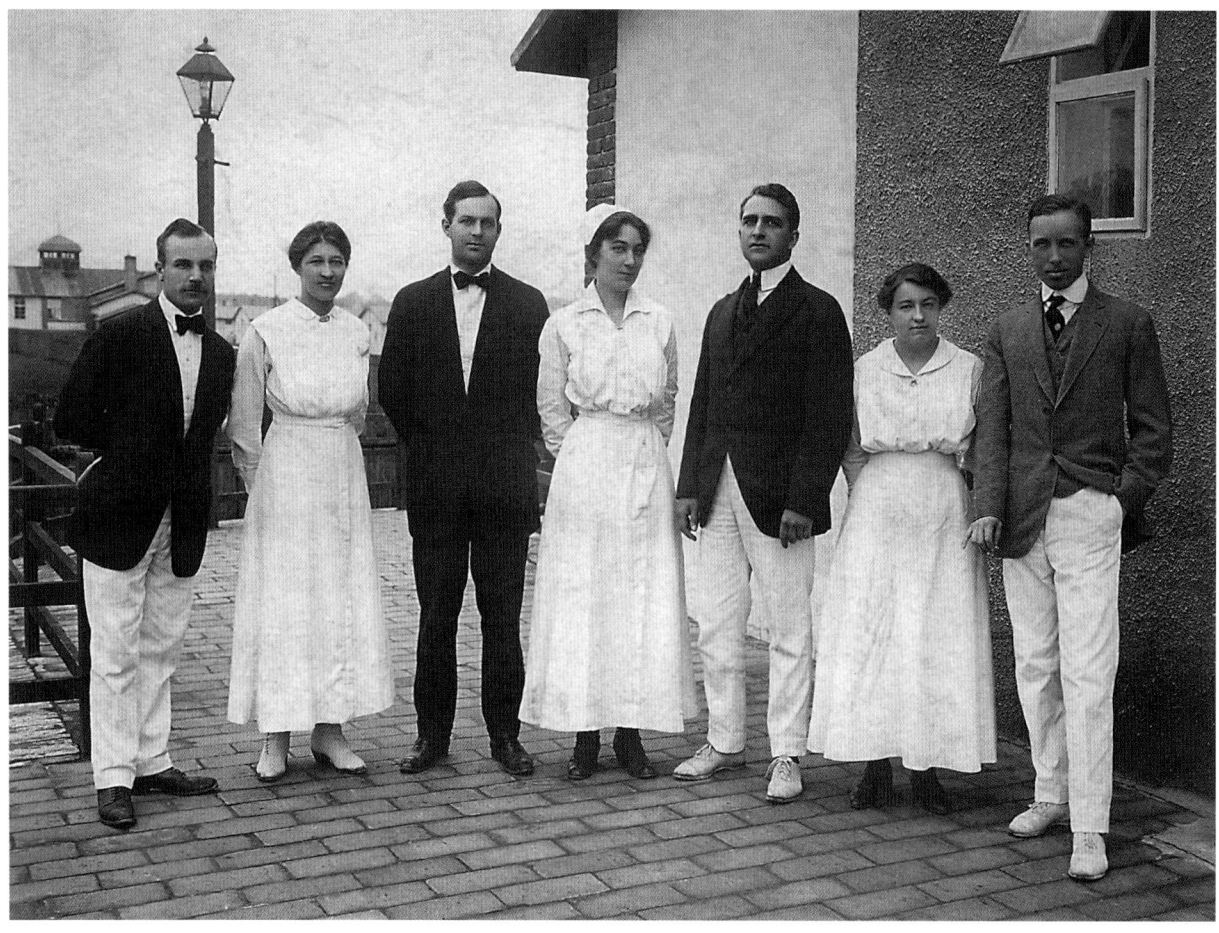

Doctors and nurses, around 1910. *Fort Caspar Museum collection.*

Her caregiver was the daughter of the hospital cook. Virtually all of the new mothers and their babies were ill from the influenza, with a number eventually dying. In response, her doctor, Joseph Kamp, removed her from the hospital and had her finish her ten-day recuperation at home.[43]

According to newspaper reports, many accident victims ended up at Dr. Lathrop's private hospital, continuing the tension around the number of patients treated by Dr. Lathrop as opposed to those who went to the new hospital. Since Dr. Lathrop was the county physician, he decided where he cared for charity cases and accident victims.

Dr. Kamp and others slowly began to support the state hospital by becoming staff physicians. The hospital did not adopt a formal medical staff structure until after it became the Memorial Hospital of Natrona County in the mid-1920s. That change would wait for further enabling legislation from the state of Wyoming.

NOTES

1 Alfred J. Mokler. *History of Natrona County, Wyoming, 1888–1922*. Chicago: Lakeside Press, 1923 (reprint Casper, Mountain States Lithography, 1989), p. 3.

2 "Local Endorsement of Law Enforcement Bill Rejected by Chamber," *Casper Daily Tribune*, February 1, 1921.

3 Mokler, p. 44.

4 Mokler, pp. 44–45.

5 *Natrona County Tribune*, August 25, 1909, p. 1.

6 *Natrona County Tribune*, August 25, 1909, p. 1.

7 *Natrona County Tribune*, August 25, 1909, p. 1.

8 Mokler, p. 45.

9 *Natrona County Tribune*, September 7, 1910, p. 4.

10 Mokler, pp. 45–46.

11 Mokler, p. 46.

12 *Natrona County Tribune*, Vol. 21, No. 13, August 9, 1911, p. 1.

13 Mokler, p. 46.

14 Henry Ward. *The Story of Casper's Irish*. Plainfield, IL: Bantry Publications, n.d., www.casperirish.com. The Natrona County Memorial Hospital, 1941 Hospital Day scrapbook mentioned Murray Sullivan as the first baby and first twin born in the new hospital.

15 Martha Kimball obituary, *Casper Tribune-Herald*, March 23, 1947, pp. 1–2.

16 Martha Kimball obituary, *Casper Tribune-Herald*, March 23, 1947, pp. 1–2.

17 *Rock Springs Rocket*, Vol. 9, No. 7, January 7, 1916, p. 1.

18 T. A. Larson. "Highlights of the Wyoming Nurses' Association's First Half Century," typescript, 1959, pp. 2–3.

19 T. A. Larson, p. 10.

20 Historical notes on the WSNA, 1908–1928, typescript, p. 3.

21 *Natrona County Tribune*, Vol. 22, No. 12, August 7, 1912, p. 1.

22 *Natrona County Tribune*, Vol. 22, No. 13, August 14, 1912, p. 1.

23 Joseph Orr. "Anatomy of a Western Town," WPA, Wyoming Writers' Project, typescript, March 10, 1940, pp. 9–10.

24 BP Amoco Timeline, http://trib.com/news/local/article_95dec472-b119-5f7d-8be3-740c6deaf8a1.html.

25 Orr, p. 13.

26 Orr, p. 12.

27 Charline Sackett. "Casper, Wyoming," WPA, Wyoming Writers' Project, typescript, 1936, p. 1.

28 Orr, p. 13.

29 Sackett, p. 1.

30 Rebecca Hunt. Weaver Family history, typescript, 2005.

31 2009 Calendar, Wyoming Heritage Center, Cheyenne: WHC, 2009.

32 Nancy Stebbins. "Casper's Telephone Exchange," WPA, Federal Writers' Project, field editor, Platte River Empire District, Casper, typescript, 1936, p. 36.

33 Irving Garbutt. *History of Casper and Natrona County, Wyoming, 1889–1989*, Vol. 1. Dallas: Irving Media, 1990, p. 107.

34 Mokler, p. 129.

35 *Casper Tribune*, January 31, 1896.

36 Natrona County records, facsimile copies of typescript, December 8, 1921 to January 5, 1926.

37 "Casper's Hospital," *Natrona County Tribune*, August 25, 1909, p. 1.

38 Irving Garbutt. *I Was There: Recollections of Ten Decades*. Casper: Casper Journal, 2003, p. 15.

39 *Natrona County Tribune*, November 20, 1913, p. 1.

40 *Casper Daily Tribune*, March 11, 1922, p. 3, c. 3.

41 *Casper Daily Tribune*, October 13, 1918.

42 Elaine Hough, interview with Frances Seely Webb.

43 Garbutt, *History of Casper and Natrona County*, p. 260.

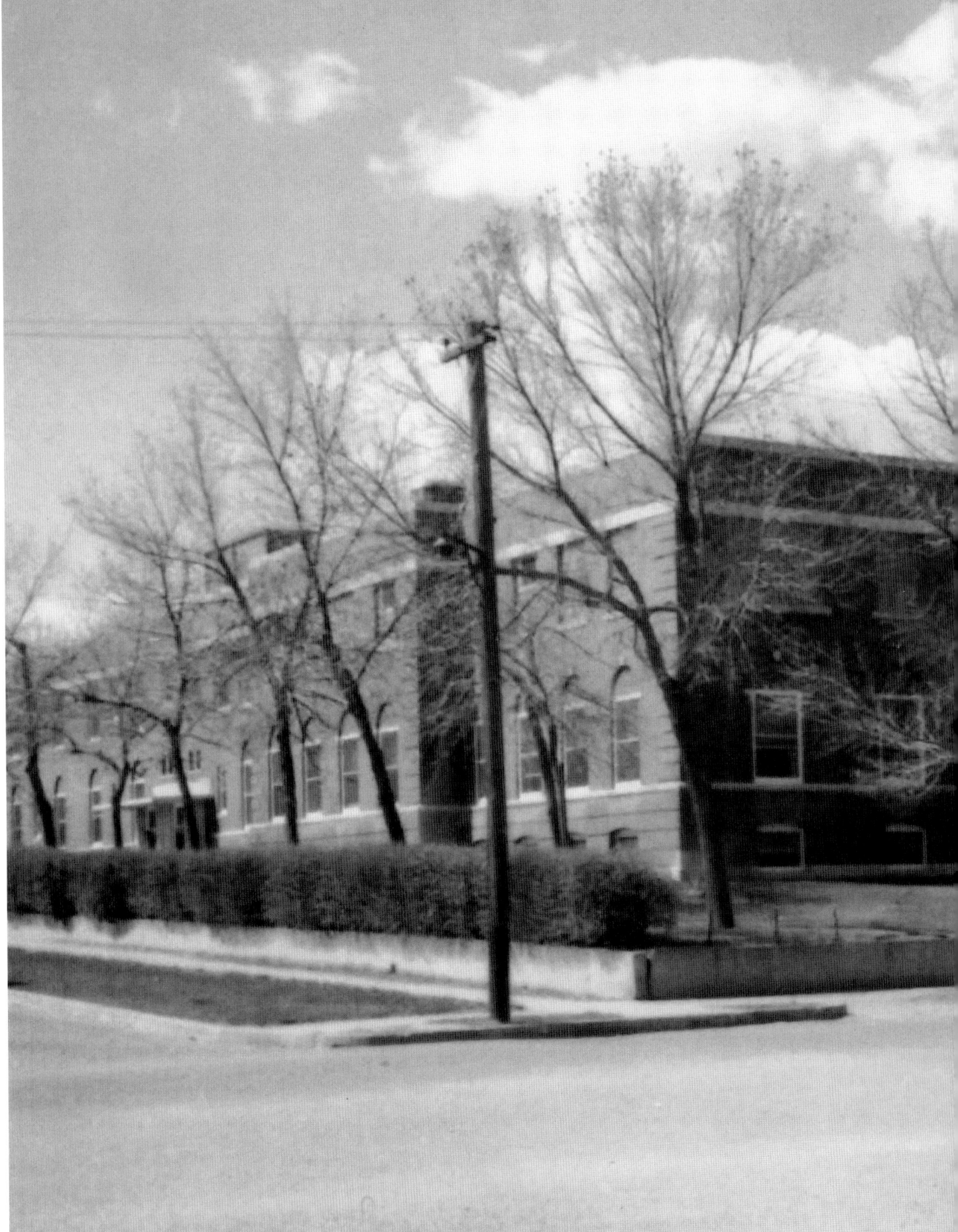

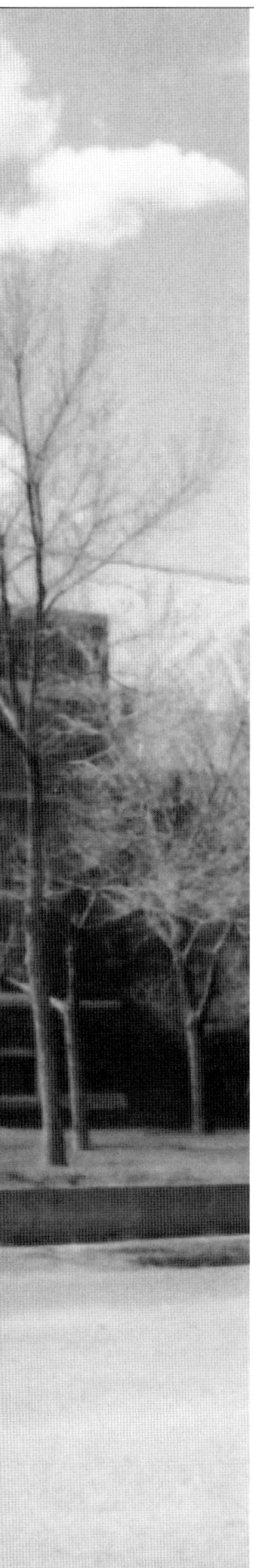

CHAPTER THREE

The Hospital Grows
1921 TO 1940

In 1921, the Wyoming Legislature decided to get out of the business of running community hospitals in Casper, Sheridan, and Rock Springs. They passed legislation allowing the counties to purchase their local facility for a dollar. Natrona County agreed to the deal and became the new owner of the Wyoming State Hospital, Casper Branch on January 1, 1922. The new name was the Natrona County Hospital.[1]

When Natrona County took over the hospital they allocated $15,000 for its operation. At the same time they had approved $20,000 for the Poor and Pauper Fund, $2,500 for the salary for the county physician, and $4,000 for a county health officer. A yearly total of $5,000 combated the spread of infectious diseases and $4,000 maintained the venereal disease clinic.[2] The clinic treated men who had visited the prostitutes in the Sand Bar and in other red light districts near the oilfields.

In February, the hospital fund had a reserve of $292,542.88 that included the market value of the building and equipment. That month the operating budget got a boost of $9,877.32 to pay for poor and pauper services.[3]

BUILDING BOOM

In 1921, the state legislature, in response to concerns voiced by the Wyoming State Nurses' Association, passed a law requiring all hospitals in Wyoming to provide a training program for nurses.[4] The Commissioners decided to construct a new residential building since state law required them to add the nursing school to the hospital operations. This nursing program helped deal with the nursing shortage created by losing nurses to World War I and the flu epidemic. In August 1922, the county let the contract to begin construction of the nurses' residence on the hospital

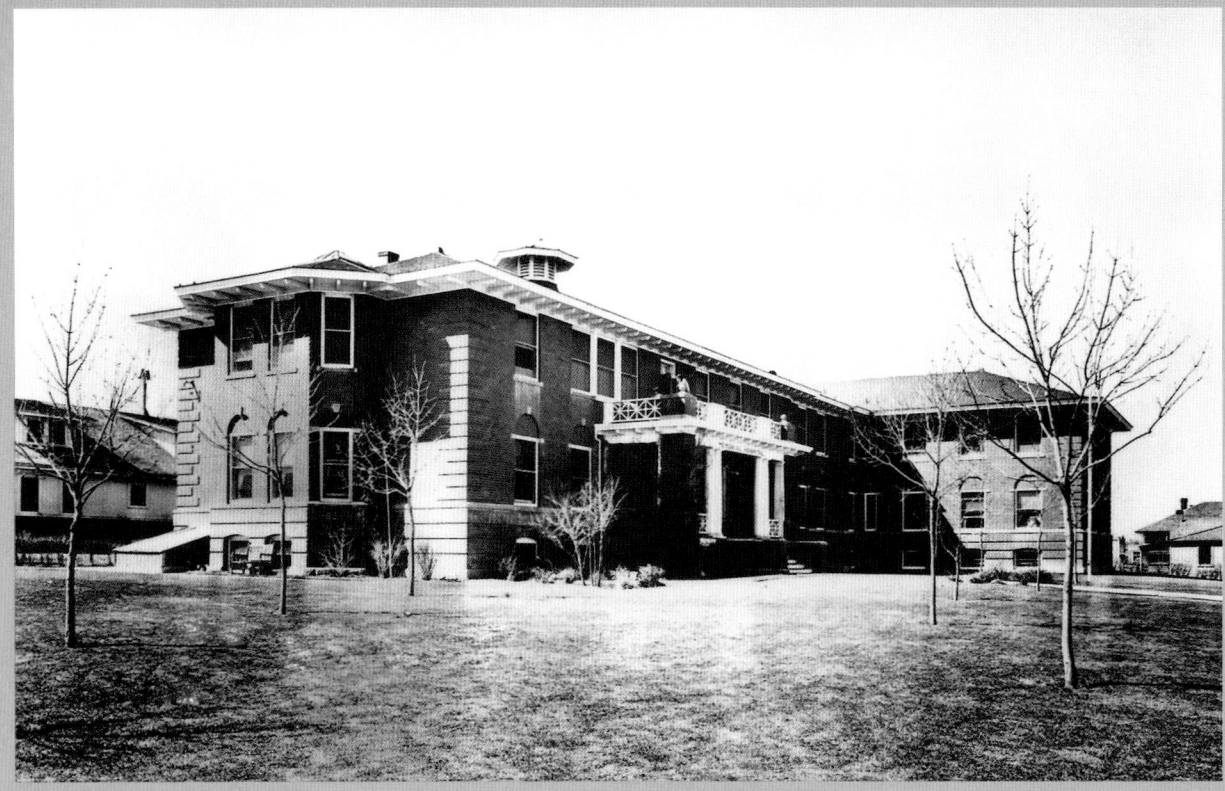

The nurses' residence is visible on the left, around 1925.

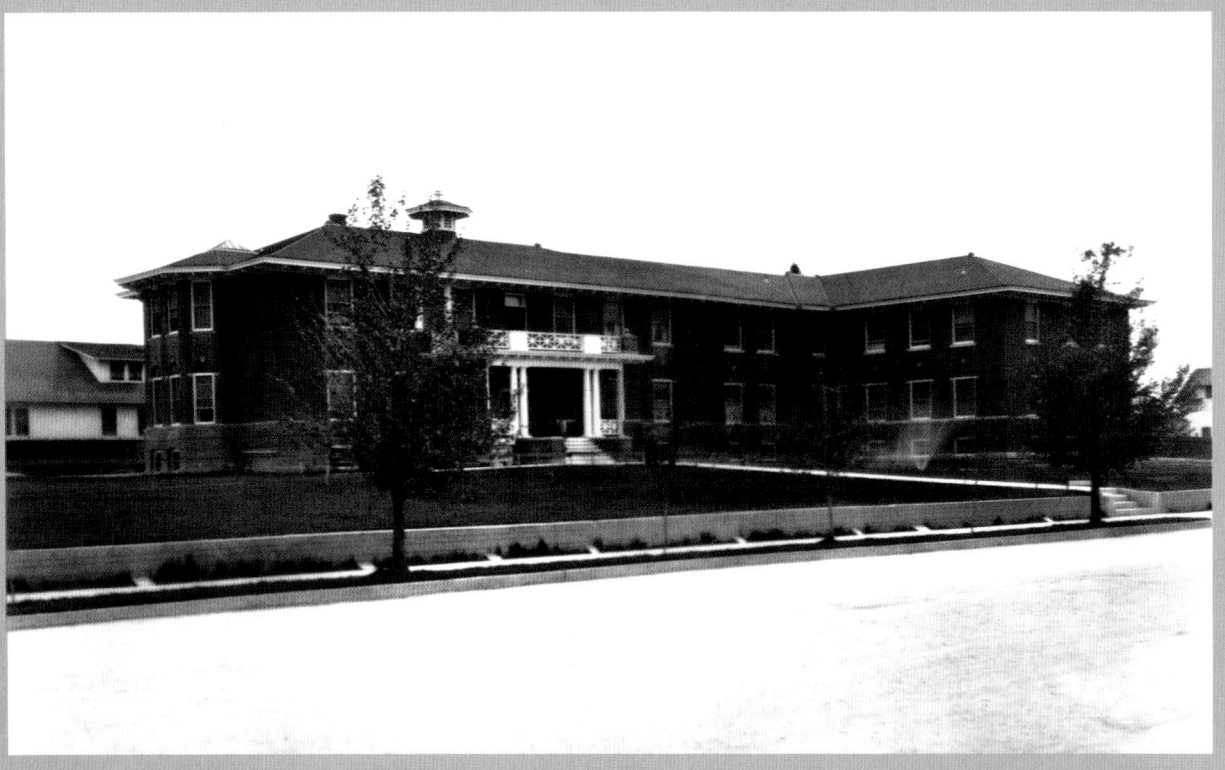

The two-story west addition is visible on the right.

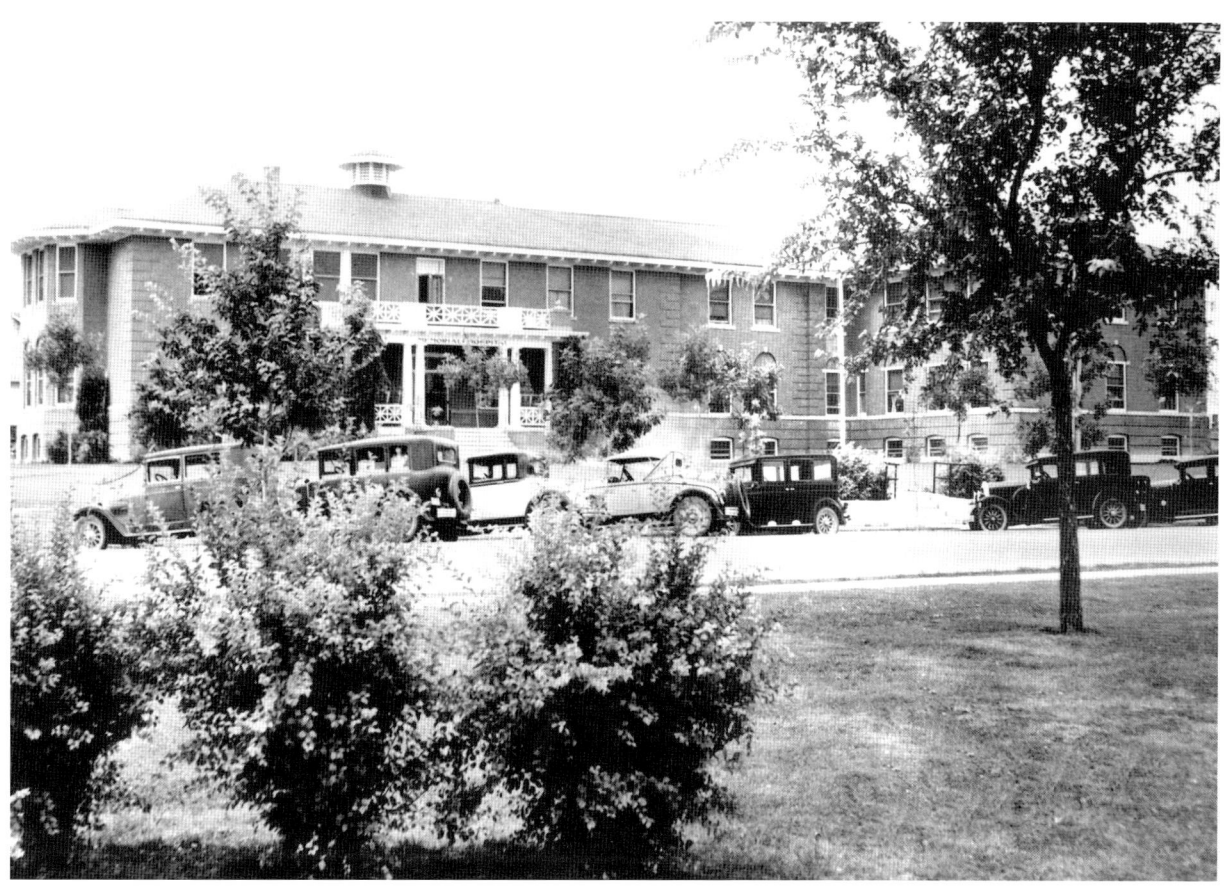

Landscaping efforts began to pay off in the mid-1920s.

grounds, just behind the main building.[5] The nurses' home had nine rooms, two bathrooms, and would house up to eighteen nurses.[6] There also was a kitchen, laundry, and sun room that served as a recreation room.[7] The $14,000 building opened in November of 1922.[8]

The next building campaign began in May 1923 to add an isolation building. This building grew out of two realities. The influenza epidemic had convinced physicians that there needed to be a place to house severely contagious patients. There was also an increase in tuberculosis patients, mostly troops who had gotten the disease in Europe.[9] The bid went to Larson and Jorgenson, who broke ground on May 9, 1924.[10] On June 4, 1924, the county opened bids for a two-story addition and a basement for the 1911 building. The bid also went to Larson and Jorgenson for $41,460.[11] This addition opened in 1925. The new additions brought the total number of beds to sixty-five, requiring a nursing staff of twelve.[12]

While much of the focus was on new buildings, there was an additional push to beautify the grounds. Since the original grounds were open prairie, trees were the first greenery added. On May 5, 1924, the hospital paid $130.65 for trees and in June hired G. M. Penley to plant them and do other work on the grounds. That same month the county hired A. J. Thomas to create a garden around the hospital. In July 1925, Nils Fougstadt, a trained forester from Sweden, began additional work on the trees and grounds.[13]

CHAPTER THREE *The Hospital Grows:* 1921 TO 1940   33

DAILY OPERATIONS

The County Commission minutes of the 1920s record salaries paid to all hospital workers. Isabella Nelson, the superintendent, received $150 per month. Other nurses received between ninety dollars and $112. They included Mrs. Katherine DeClue, who earned $112. WSNA membership records documented Casper nurses who were members and indicated who worked at the hospital. Names of longstanding nurses included Mary Anne Eschwig, who became superintendent in 1926. Throughout the period of 1923 to 1926, women who were probably student nurses received fifteen dollars per month for their work.[14] An average of eleven young women being paid each month during 1924 indicated a class of eleven student nurses in the early 1920s.[15]

Superintendent Isabella Nelson appeared in the county records on November 13, 1923, as receiving an additional duty. The Eighteenth Amendment to the U.S. Constitution had banned sale of all alcoholic beverages except those used for religious or medical purposes. However, federal laws required hospital officials to account for any purchases of whiskey for medicinal use. This had fallen, as an extra duty, to the County Commission's staff. The Commissioners authorized Superintendent Nelson to sign the monthly whiskey allotment reports for the hospital.[16]

On January 6, 1923, the Commissioners began work on setting up a medical staff system at the hospital. Because there had been so many complaints about Dr. Lathrop's monopoly over the poor and pauper care, the Commissioners decided that in addition to having privileges at the hospital, each physician must take turns caring for charity patients, with each doctor taking a six weeks' rotation. The doctors would provide the care without pay and could not turn away any patients during their duty period. They also had to be available seven days a week. Each physician guaranteed to tend the sickest patients at the county hospital unless the chief of staff approved an outside consultation. Outside consultants received five dollars per case. Staff physicians attended a weekly meeting with the chief of staff to review charity cases. The chief of staff also granted admission privileges to the town's doctors.[17]

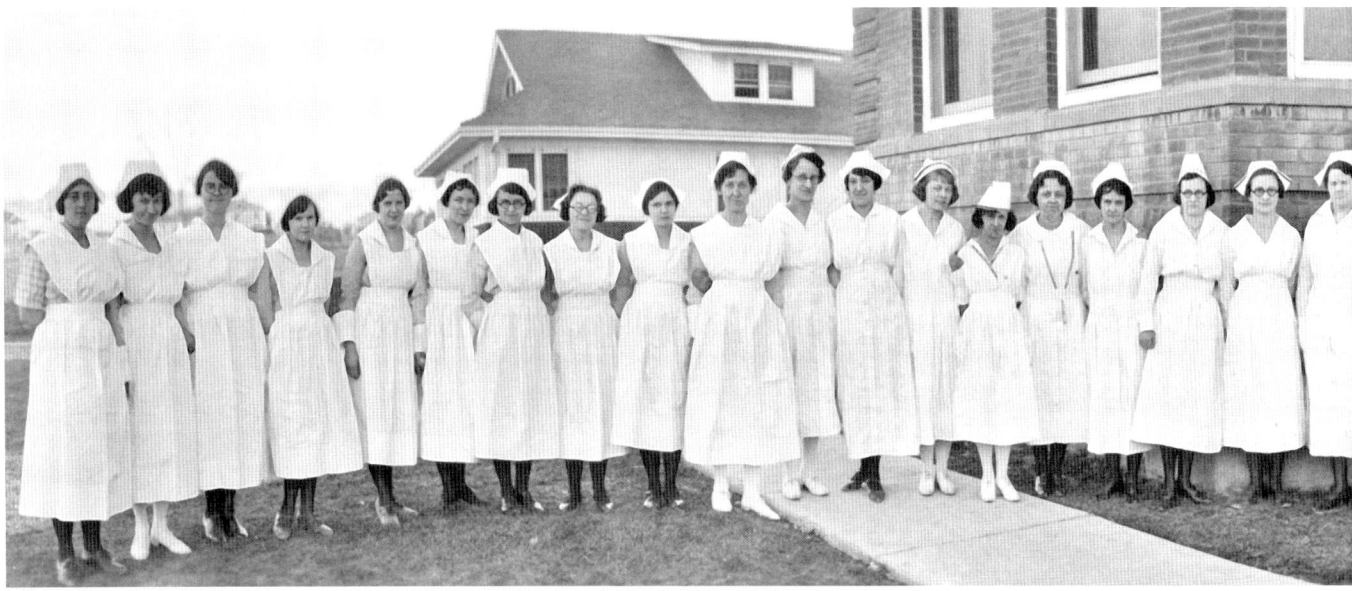

Doctors and nurses posed outside of the east end of the hospital. The ten on the left were students.

The first chief of staff appointed by the county was Dr. T. A. Dean, an obstetrician who had been practicing medicine in Casper since the 1890s.[18] As the records show, most early prominent physicians served as chief of staff at some point in their careers.

The doctors also taught the classes for the nursing students. They included Dr. Allen McLellan, Anatomy; Dr. A. P. Kimball, Physiology; Dr. A. L. Willis, Materia Medica; Dr. N. C. Geis, Surgery; Dr. I. N. Frost, Gynecology; Dr. H. A. Reichenbach, Obstetrics; Dr. Marshall C. Keith, Pediatrics; and Dr. T. A. Riach, who taught Histology, Bacteriology, Neurology, and Psychiatry.[19]

In December 1923, the Commissioners once again reorganized the medical staff. The new president of the medical staff was Dr. Joseph C. Kamp. The medical departments now had chairmen, members, and consultants. Dr. N. C. Geis chaired Surgery; Dr. H. A. Reichenbach chaired Medicine; Dr. Marshall Keith chaired Obstetrics; Dr. George Smith chaired Ear, Nose, and Throat; and Dr. T. A. Riach chaired Neurology. New physicians in town, who also served as departmental chairs, were Dr. M. J. Nolan in Anesthesiology; Dr. Wynn in X-ray; and Dr. Walott in Pathology, Bacteriology, and Sanitation.[20]

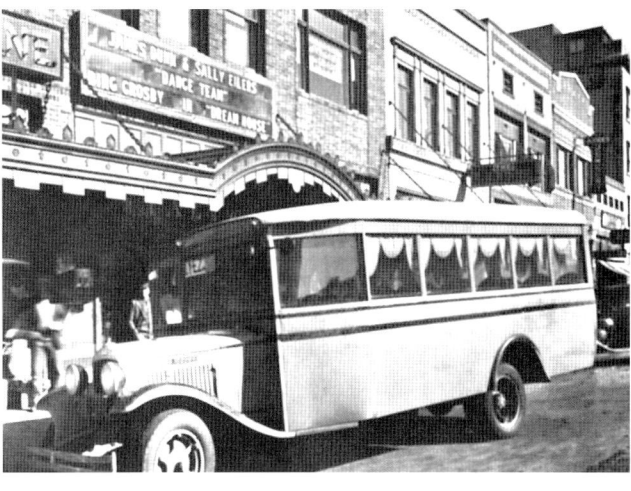

This bus brought people to Casper to work in the 1930s. *Author's collection.*

Dr. Kamp was one of the leaders of the newer generation of physicians in town. He had graduated from the Denver and Gross College of Medicine in Denver in 1908. One of the school's two top students, he set up shop in Casper soon after.[21] By 1922, he not only was the staff president but also head of the Natrona County Medical Society.[22]

County Commission minutes from 1921 to 1926 also provided insight into many operating costs of the hospital. The national and local economic impact of a county hospital was clear in the reports. In 1924, the cost of surgical supplies paid to Johnson and Johnson totaled $156.75. There were other bills paid locally for

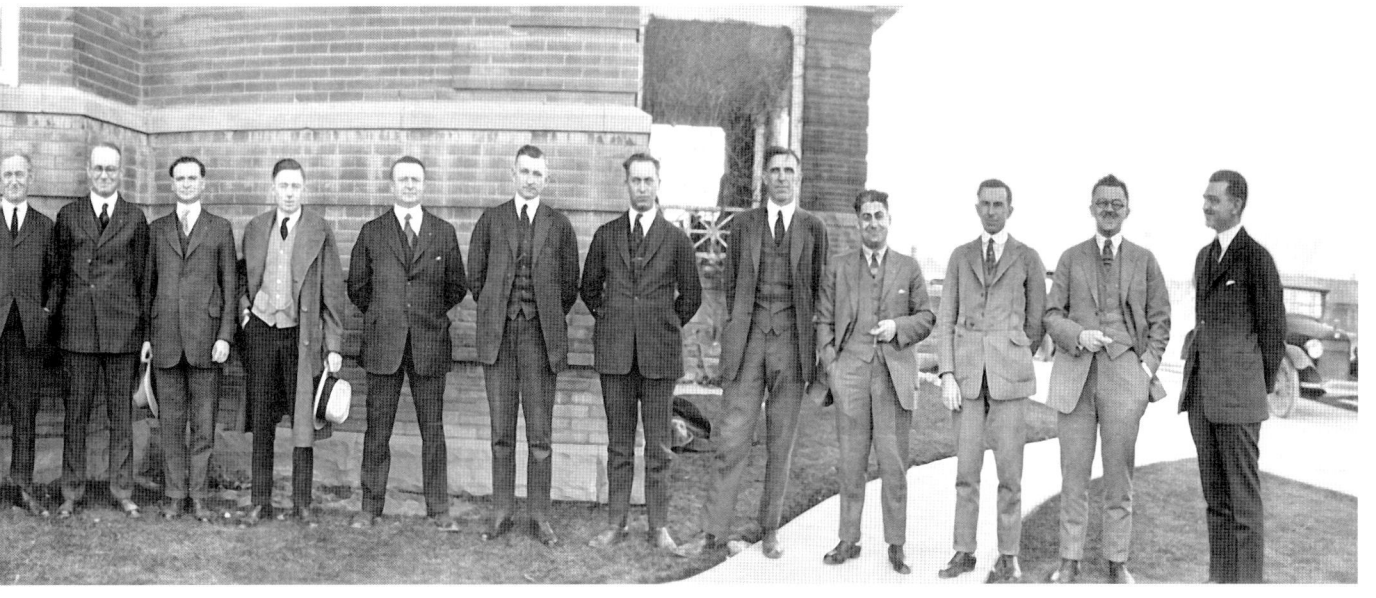

ice, food, and about $218 to four pharmacists for medicines. Laundry, at $545.82 for the month of March, was a big expense. Later in March, $2,065.92 went to Victor X-ray and $1,414.03 to J. Durbin Surgical Supply. Other receipts in May 1924 accounted for purchases of rubber sheeting, ice bags, medical books, and chart papers.[23]

THE TRANSITION TO MEMORIAL HOSPITAL OF NATRONA COUNTY

Although the Great Depression hit most of the nation in 1929, it began in Natrona County between 1925 and 1926. The cause in Wyoming was the precipitous drop of oil prices after World War I. In one week alone in late 1925, oil production dropped 40 percent.

In 1925, Casper had about 25,000 residents. Property values declined about $2 million per year in the late twenties and payrolls dropped by about $1 million per year. Casper's tax base dropped as businesses closed and residents lost jobs and moved away.[24]

As the Depression began, the state forced Natrona County to manage the hospital in a new way. The hospital became a separate unit of the county government with the County Commission having indirect control of the operations through a Board of Trustees. Among other things, this required Isabella Nelson to reapply for her job as superintendent. She did and was rehired.[25]

The Commissioners moved quickly to appoint a Board of Trustees to perform the actual oversight, reporting their actions to the county. The first Trustees were P. J. O'Connor, W. M. Holland, M. J. Foley, H. H. Schwartz, and R. S. Ellison.[26] Beginning with the change over to the new structure in January 1925, the County Commission monthly reports no longer included hospital salaries. They did, however, report expenses such as food, medicines, and utilities for running the hospital.

On October 8, 1925, the Trustees officially changed the institution's name. The Natrona County Hospital became the Memorial Hospital of Natrona County.[27]

In 1926, Mary Anne Eschwig, R.N. took over as superintendent of Memorial Hospital of Natrona County. Mary Anne Eschwig was born Mary Ann Craig in Broxburn, Scotland, on January 13, 1895. After her family immigrated to British Columbia, Canada, she married Frederick Eschwig and they had a daughter, Violet. She nursed in Nordegg, Alberta, until her husband, a fireman on the Great Northern Railroad, died in an accident. She left her daughter with her parents and moved to Denver, where she trained at St. Anthony Hospital School of Nursing, graduating in 1922.[28] Eschwig came to Casper in 1922 to work for Dr. Homer Lathrop, then began her career at Memorial Hospital in August 1922, when she became a charge nurse there. By January 1923, Superintendent Nelson promoted her to surgical supervisor and then the Trustees hired her to be the superintendent in 1926. She held that job until 1939, when she left to marry G. O. Wiley in 1940.[29]

As the Depression began, the state forced Natrona County to manage the hospital in a new way.

MEMORIAL HOSPITAL OF NATRONA COUNTY IN THE GREAT DEPRESSION: 1930 TO 1940

When the 1930s opened, Casper was a much smaller town, struggling along with the rest of the country. Unemployment was growing, nationally reaching a high of 25 percent by 1934. Natrona County was not hit as hard as the rest of the country but people still struggled throughout the decade.

Much changed when Franklin Roosevelt became president and instituted his New Deal programs to provide relief and reform to a country wracked by economic depression. Casper and Natrona County benefited from the money and jobs programs of the New Deal. The Civilian Conservation Corps maintained forests and developed roads, trails, and ski facilities on Casper Mountain. Works Progress Administration and Public Works Administration projects built roads and bridges. Alcova Dam, designed to supply electricity to rural residents, was a Bureau of Reclamation project funded by the PWA. Construction began in 1935. The dam began generating electricity in 1938.[30]

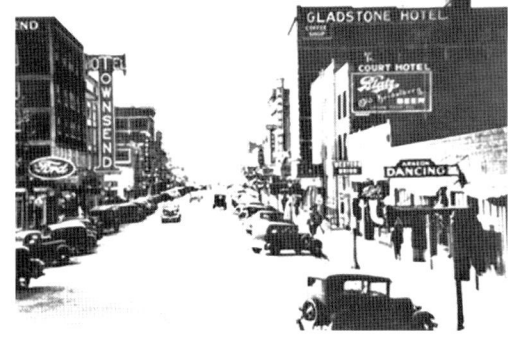

The Federal Writers' Project hired writers to work with noted Casper newspaperman and historian Alfred J. Mokler to produce reports on the region they called the Platte River Empire. One report documented the businesses in the county in 1935.[31]

In the 1930s, Casper's downtown drew people from the region who also received medical care at the Memorial Hospital of Natrona County.

One of the regional assets mentioned in the FWP reports was Wardwell Field, the municipal airport. The airport was a Civilian Works Administration project.[32] Located one and a half miles north of town, in the early 1930s it became home to Wyoming Air Service. The first passenger flight was Billings, Montana, to Casper to Pueblo, Colorado, in 1931. It supplied mail and cargo flights to Denver in 1936.[33]

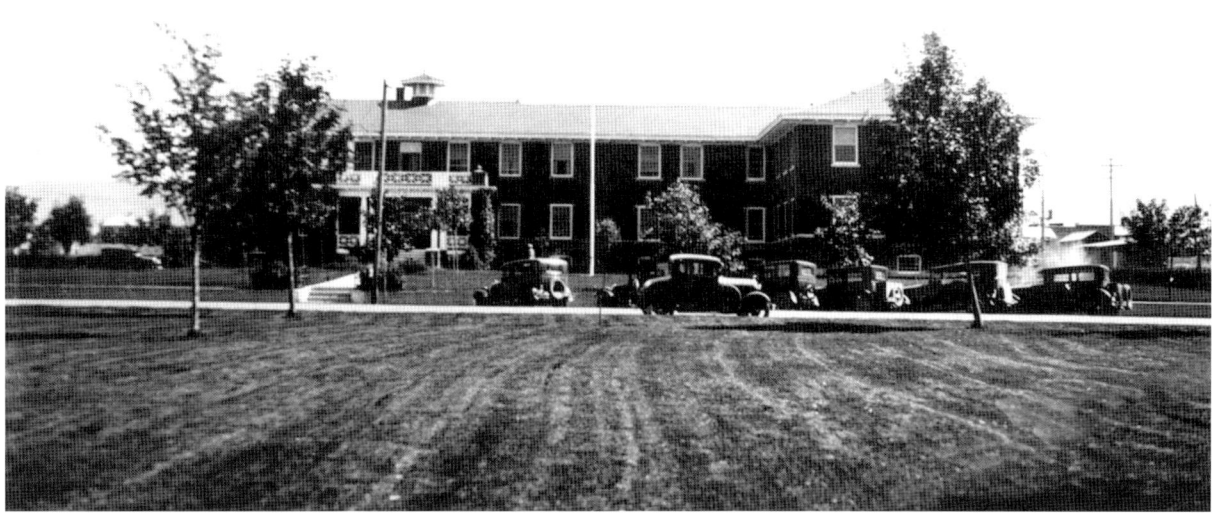

This exterior view of the Memorial Hospital of Natrona County does not reveal the busy hive of activity that went on inside its walls.

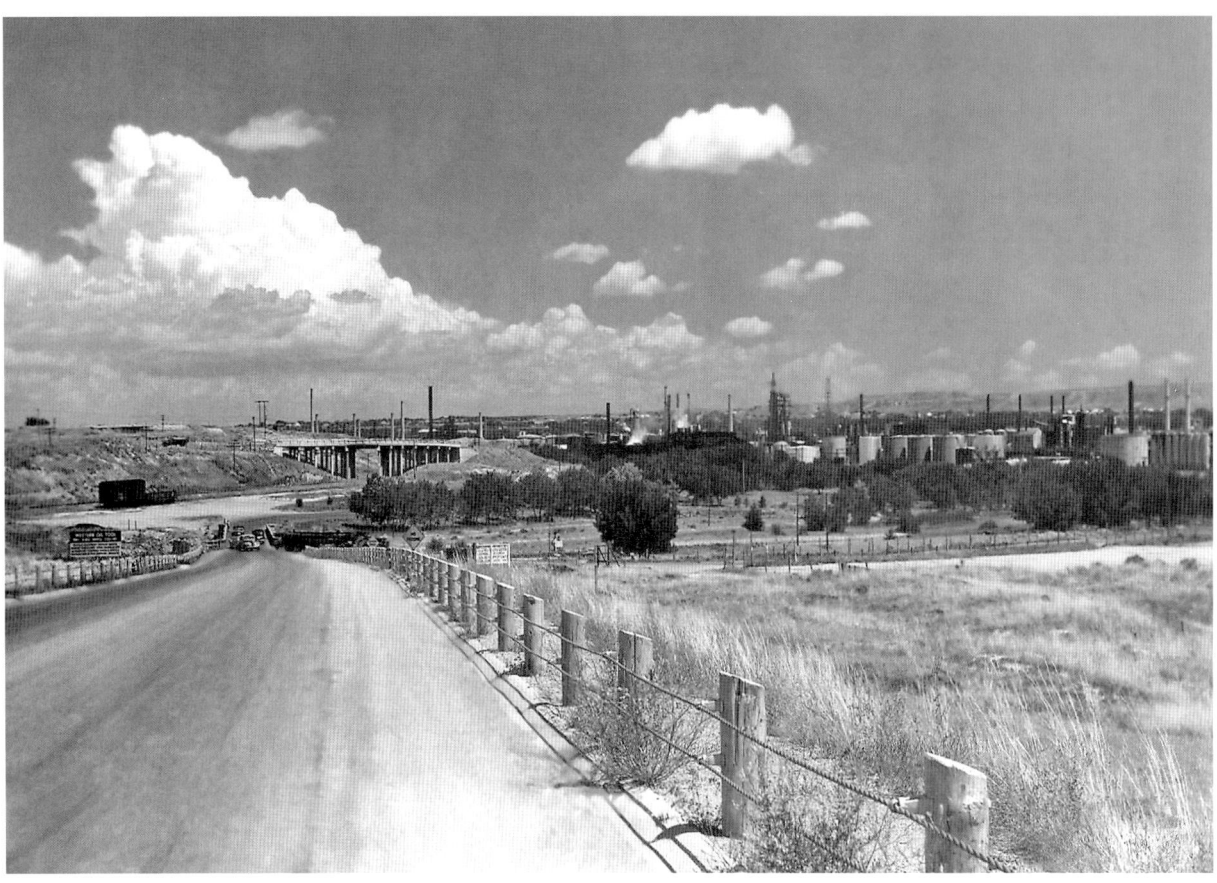

The Yellowstone Highway took travelers past the refineries on their way to the national park. *Author's collection.*

Casper now had three highways coming through town although the most important was Highway 20.

A new federal building, including a post office and courthouse, rose at First and Wolcott streets in downtown Casper as federal money funded construction of new public buildings.[34] Paved roads were another New Deal benefit. Casper now had three highways coming through town although the most important was Highway 20. The Yellowstone Highway carried travelers to Yellowstone Park, necessitating stops for food, lodging, and other services in Casper.[35]

On January 1, 1930, Casper's first local radio station went on the air. KDFN, owned and operated by Don Hathaway, began as a one-hundred-watt station that became 200 watts in 1932. In November 1933, Hathaway opened a new station building at First and Lennox streets. The station broadcast every day from 7:30 a.m. to 9:00 p.m.[36] In an era when only major metropolitan areas had clear channel radio, a local station was a very progressive luxury. KDFN was one of only a handful of radio stations in Wyoming.

In 1936, the state opened its Home for Dependent Children on Twelfth Street southeast of Highland Cemetery. Another PWA project, it housed seventy-five children. Some were orphans while others were displaced children whose families could not care for them. The home included an infirmary, kitchen, dormitories, and sufficient grounds to allow growing children room to run.[37]

Another Federal Writers' Project interview with Superintendent Minnie Retzloff, R.N. provided a snapshot of the history and status of the Memorial Hospital as of the late 1930s. The first level housed public areas, laboratories, a small distribution kitchen, and administrative offices. There and on the second floor were patient rooms and wards. Most days patients filled all of the beds and the reception area had more than once been pressed into service as a temporary patient ward. The basement held all of the behind-the-scenes functions including the main kitchen. A dumbwaiter took food to the first-floor kitchen for distribution to patients. Storage for supplies and the main drug room were also in the basement. Dining rooms for nurses and other staff filled out the space.[38]

By 1936, the hospital had sixty-nine beds and a ten-patient capacity in the isolation wing. The two operating rooms contained the latest in equipment and lighting. There was one room set aside for dealing with fractures. The obstetrical wing included one birthing room and a nursery with ten cribs for normal deliveries. Premature babies had a special room with two incubators.[39]

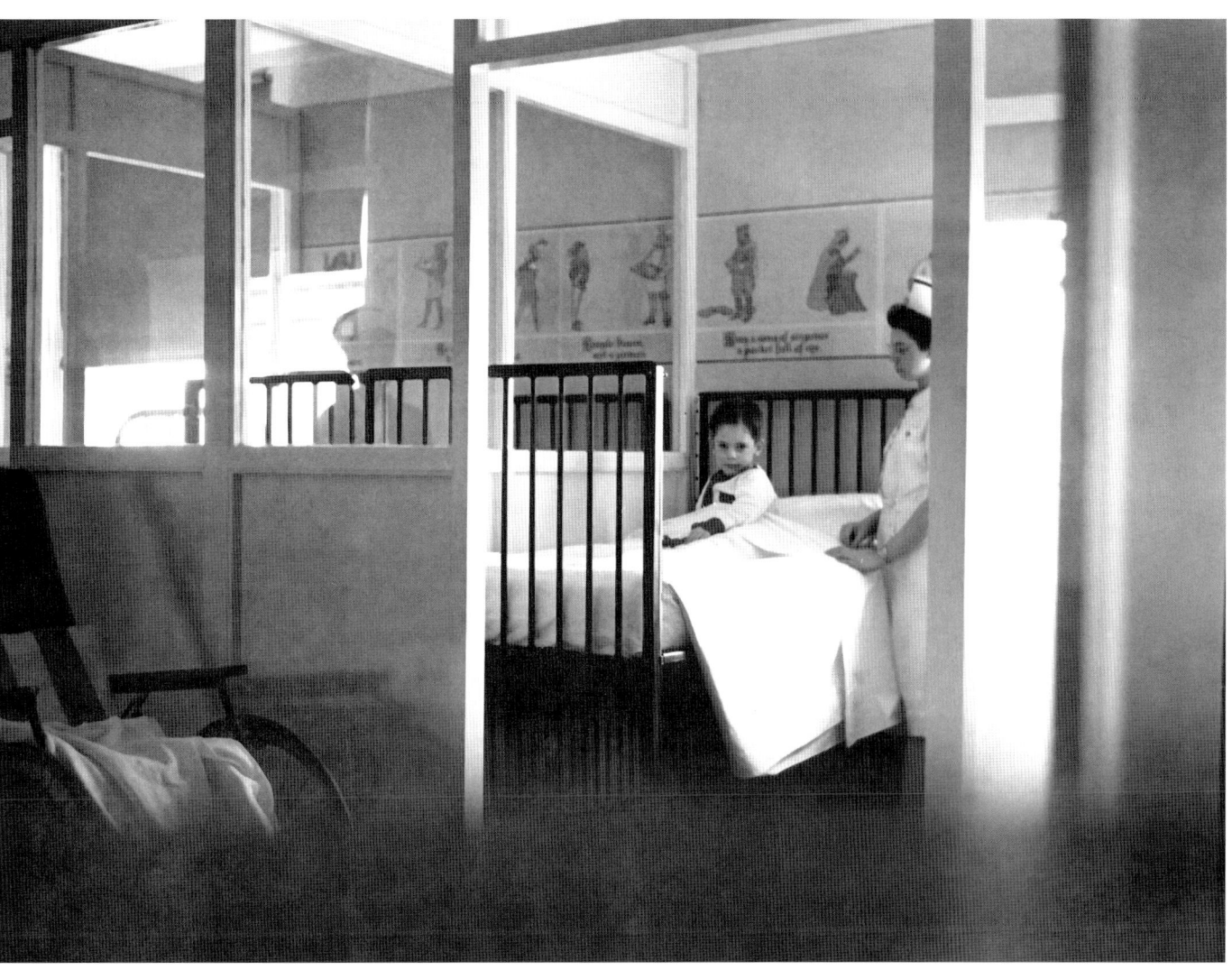

Wall decorations in the pediatric ward featured pictures and phrases from nursery rhymes.

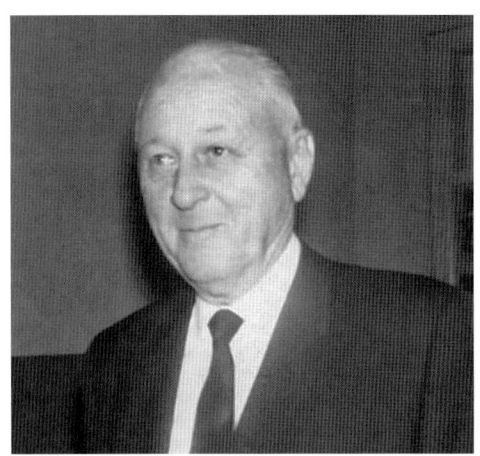

Dr. Harry Stuckenoff joined the Memorial Hospital of Natrona County staff in 1930. *Wyoming Medical Center collection.*

The hospital had cared for 493 patients and delivered 205 babies in 1935. Staffing included thirty registered nurses, a pathologist, and an X-ray specialist as well as the seventeen appointed staff physicians. Technicians worked in radiology and in the fully equipped laboratory. Thirty-nine other employees rounded out the numbers of those working there. One of the employees cared for the guinea pigs and rabbits kept in hutches at the rear of the hospital grounds. Staff used these animals for pathology and pregnancy tests.[40]

Other examples of modern equipment in 1936 included two Heidbrink oxygen tents, a stationary Victor X-ray machine, and a portable X-ray machine. A fireproof vault built outside of the hospital stored the nitrate X-ray films.[41] This was an innovation prompted by devastating fires in other parts of the country caused by burning film stock.

By 1936, there were twenty-one physicians in Casper.[42] The staff physicians included a number who arrived in the 1930s. Dr. Harry Stuckenoff trained at Creighton University in Omaha, Nebraska. He arrived in 1930, attracted by an offer of partnership with Dr. N. E. Morad. When he arrived he lived for four years at the Gladstone Hotel, serving as the hotel physician. Eventually Dr. Stuckenoff and Jack Perry bought the hotel. Stuckenoff married Mary Tobin, daughter of one of Casper's oldest Irish-American families, who was the society editor of the *Casper Tribune-Herald*. In the 1950s, Stuckenoff bought the Brooks ranch east of town and used income from his practice to subsidize his ranch.[43]

Another physician arriving in the 1930s was Dr. George James, an eye specialist. He established his partnership with Dr. John Nelson, ear, nose, and throat doctor, in 1933.[44] Casper prematurely lost one of its established physicians when Dr. Joseph Kamp died on May 13, 1939, at age fifty-eight.[45]

The 1930s marked a turning point in nurses' training. The state took control of all of the nurse-training programs to insure a standardized curriculum and clinical experience. All graduate nurses entered training for three years. Trainees had to be more than nineteen years old and have a high school diploma. They needed to be vaccinated against smallpox, diphtheria, typhoid, and be tuberculosis-free. The cost included a twenty-dollar application fee, a ten-dollar breakage fee, and all students paid for their own books. They had to provide a fountain pen, a watch with a second hand, uniforms, and a wool school cape. They could only live in approved housing, either in town or at the hospital.[46] At Casper, the students lived in the nurses' quarters built in 1922 and expanded in the 1930s.

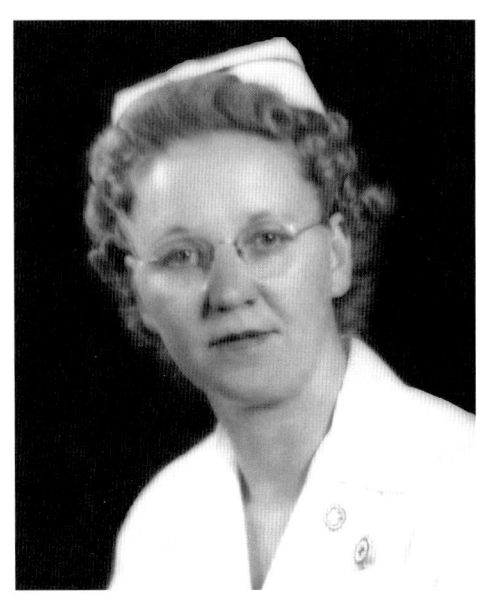

Louise Becker graduated from the Memorial Hospital of Natrona County nursing program in the 1930s and then worked for many years at the hospital.

Memorial Hospital of Natrona County revamped its nursing school in 1936, opening with a new class in 1937. Superintendent Mary Anne Eschwig hired Winifred Koontz to run the school. A number of problems led to Koontz's replacement in the first year. Her successor was Leona Mohr, R.N.[47] The budget for the program for 1938 was $9,202.78, including a four-month salary of $1,820 for the program director and $120.42 for a skeleton and case for teaching. Department heads supervised clinical training.[48]

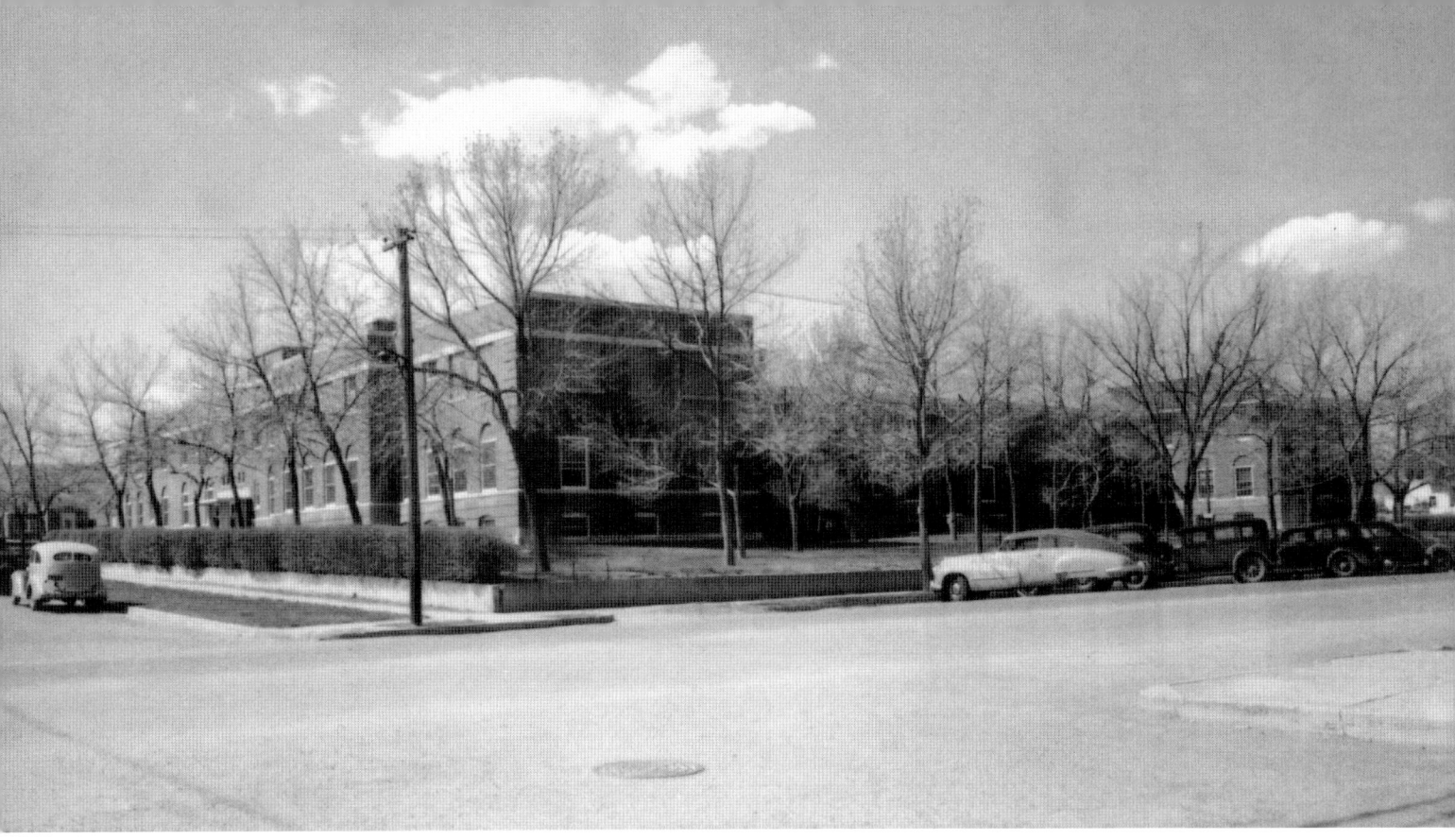

The new east wing of the hospital went up in time for the World War II population boom.

Individual hospitals provided basic coursework but physicians read and marked all examinations. The doctors reported back to the program directors on scores as well as their feelings about the student's probability of success as future nurses. A report from Dr. W. W. Arrasmith to Leona Mohr in 1940 was quite scathing, practically ordering her to send certain girls packing when their work did not measure up.[49] Mary Anne Eschwig reported that in the 1938, the first year of the newly opened program, they expelled five of thirteen students.[50]

In 1938, the County Commission asked the citizens of the county to approve a bond issue to match federal funds to build an addition to the east side of the hospital. They approved $208,000 as a 55-percent match.[51] The hospital opened its new wing as the Depression decade ended and World War II approached.

NOTES

1 *Casper Daily Tribune*, Vol. 4, No. 71, December 31, 1921, p. 1.

2 Natrona County Commission records, January 6, 1921.

3 Natrona County Commission records, February 8, 1921.

4 *The American Journal of Nursing*, Vol. 21, No. 11, 1921.

5 Natrona County Commission records, August 23, 1922.

6 Alfred J. Mokler. *History of Natrona County, Wyoming, 1888–1922*. Chicago: Lakeside Press, 1923 (reprint Casper, Mountain States Lithography, 1989), p. 47.

7 Nancy Stebbins. "The Natrona County Memorial Hospital," WPA, Federal Writers' Project field editor, Platte River Empire District, Casper, typescript, 1936, p. 3.

8 Mokler, p. 47.

9 Rebecca Hunt and Sandy Durkin. *A Century of Healing: The History of Swedish Medical Center, 1905–2005*. Englewood, CO: Swedish Medical Center, 2005, p. 21.

10 Natrona County Commission records, May 4, 1923–May 9, 1924.

11 Natrona County Commission records, June 4, 1923–June 25, 1924.

12 Scrapbook, National Hospital Day at Memorial Hospital of Natrona County, Casper, Wyoming, May 11, 1941.

13 Natrona County Commission records, July 7, 1925.

14 Natrona County Commission records, March 4, 1924–July 1, 1924.

15 Natrona County Commission records, February 5, 1924–May 6, 1924.

16 Natrona County Commission records, November 13, 1924.

17 Natrona County Commission records, January 6, 1923.

18 Natrona County Commission records, January 6, 1923.

19 Natrona County Commission records, January 6, 1923.

20 Natrona County Commission records, December 6, 1923.

21 *Denver Medical Times*, Vol. 28, No. 1, July 1908.

22 *Casper Daily Tribune*, January 5, 1922, p. 5.

23 Natrona County Commission records, March 6, 1924–May 5, 1924.

24 Joseph Orr. "Anatomy of a Western Town," WPA, Wyoming Writers' Project, typescript, March 10, 1940, pp. 14–16.

25 Natrona County Commission records, January 7, 1925–March 11, 1925.

26 Natrona County Commission records, April 8, 1925.

27 Natrona County Commission records, October 8, 1925.

28 Christopher Craig. Mary Ann Craig, Craig Family genealogy. http://familytreemaker.genealogy.com/users/c/r/a/Christopher-J-Craig/WEBSITE-0001/UHP-0057.html.

29 Special interest gift, *Casper Star-Tribune*, c. 1977.

30 Alcova Dam, "Reclamation: Managing Water in the West," http://www.usbr.gov/projects/Facility.jsp?fac_Name=Alcova+Dam&groupName=General.

31 Nancy Stebbins. "Casper's Assets," Federal Writers' Project, typescript, 1936, p. 6-e.

32 Nancy Stebbins. "Wyoming Air Service," WPA, Federal Writers' Project field editor, Platte River Empire District, Casper, typescript, 1936, p. 16.

33 Stebbins, "Wyoming Air Service," p. 16.

34 Alfred J. Mokler. "Casper's Post Offices and Postmasters," WPA, Wyoming Writers' Project, typescript, 1936, p. 7.

35 Orr, p. 14.

36 Nancy Stebbins. "KDFN Broadcasting Station," WPA, Federal Writers' Project field editor, Platte River Empire District, Casper, typescript, 1936, p. 1.

37 Charline Sackett. "Casper, Wyoming," WPA, Wyoming Writers' Project, typescript, 1936, p. 18; Nancy Stebbins. "State Home for Dependent Children," WPA, Federal Writers' Project field editor, Platte River Empire District, Casper, typescript, 1936, p. 25.

38 Nancy Stebbins. "The Natrona County Memorial Hospital," WPA, Federal Writers' Project field editor, Platte River Empire District, Casper, typescript, 1936, p. 3–4.

39 Stebbins, "The Natrona County Memorial Hospital," p. 2.

40 Stebbins, "The Natrona County Memorial Hospital," p. 3.

41 Stebbins, "The Natrona County Memorial Hospital," p. 3.

42 Stebbins, "Casper's Assets," p. 3-e.

43 Irving Garbutt. *History of Casper and Natrona County, Wyoming, 1889–1989*, Vol. 1. Dallas: Irving Media, 1990, pp. 38–39.

44 Garbutt, *History of Casper and Natrona County*, p. 193.

45 Polk's City and County Directory, Casper, Wyoming, 1941, p. 112.

46 Bulletin of the School of Nursing, Memorial Hospital of Natrona County, 1937–1938, p. 1.

47 Mary Anne Eschwig. "Yearly Report of Training School," to the Board of Trustees, MHNC, typescript, 1938, p. 1.

48 Eschwig, pp. 2–3.

49 W. W. Arrasmith, M.D. Letter to Miss Leona Mohr, R.N., February 15, 1940.

50 Eschwig, p. 1.

51 Elaine Hough, "History of the Hospital, 1911–2001," typescript outline, p. 1.

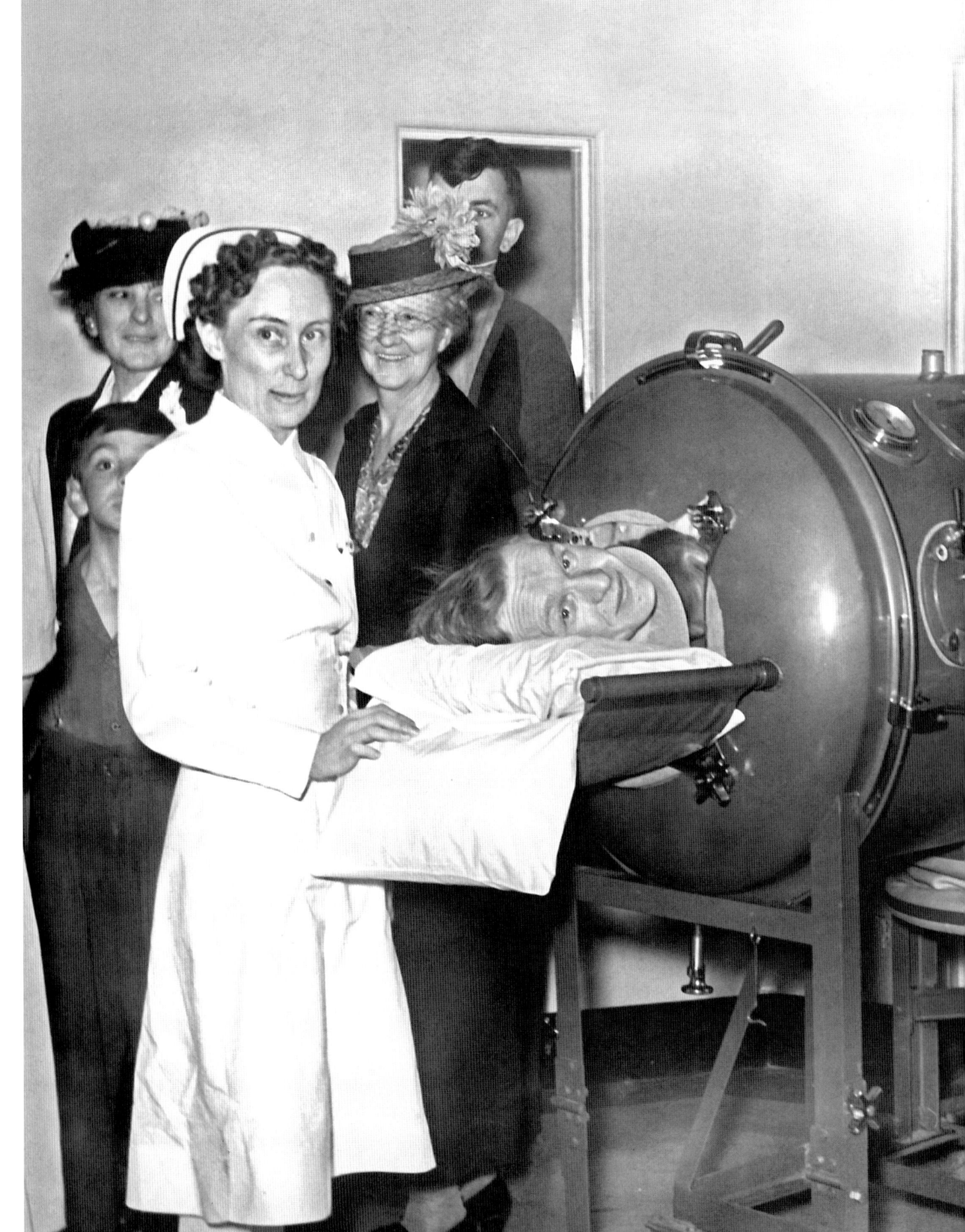

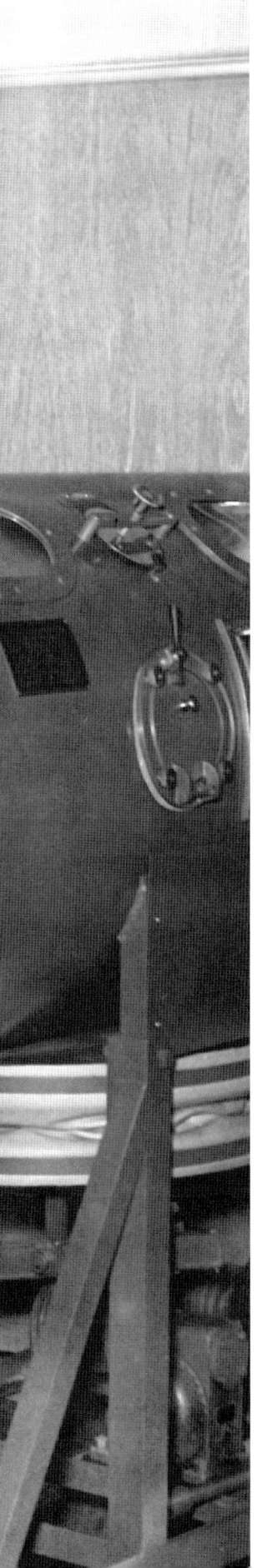

CHAPTER FOUR

The War Years and Beyond

1941 TO 1959

Casper's economy and population picked up as early as the late 1930s when the war created a greater need for petroleum products. This brought workers back to the county, helping push the region into another boom.[1] Casper's demographics continued to reflect the fact that the primary jobs were industrial. Seventy percent of the population was blue-collar. The other 30 percent was a mix of middle-class community and business people, educators, and those involved in the health care field. Ninety-five percent of the population was native-born.[2]

Hospital leadership changed in 1940 when Minnie Retzloff left and Martha Partridge took over. Partridge had worked as a staff nurse for Memorial Hospital through the 1930s. As the new superintendent she dealt with the challenges of staffing a hospital in a time of rationing, supply shortages, and the constant search for more staff.

In May 1941, Partridge arranged a very special Hospital Day celebration. She used the thirtieth anniversary of the hospital's founding to honor the past and the institution's continuing leadership in the region. The celebration brought the community into the hospital as well as took the hospital out into the community.

Partridge kept a scrapbook of the event, providing much of what we know about the state of the hospital at the onset of the 1940s. Partridge organized coverage on the radio stations and many downtown businesses had displays in their windows highlighting some aspect of hospital operations.[3]

The official celebration began with a receiving line. Dignitaries included Jean Lathrop of the Board of Trustees, Martha Partridge, Martha Converse Kimball, and Murray Sullivan, one of the first twins.[4]

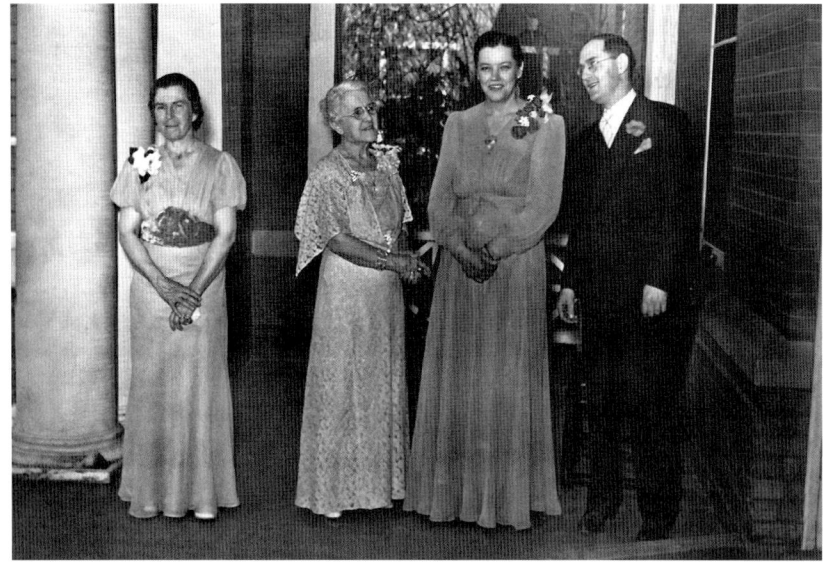
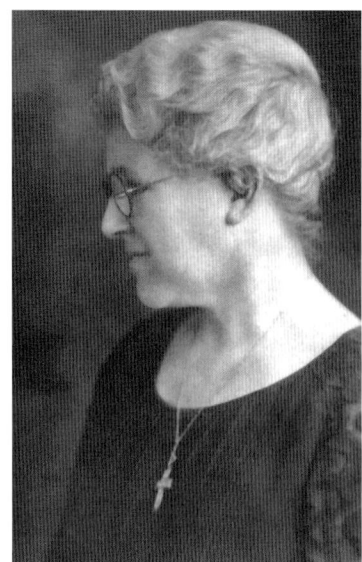

In the receiving line on May 11, 1941, are (from the left) Jean Lathrop, Martha Kimball, Martha Partridge, and Murray Sullivan.

Martha Converse Kimball in 1947.

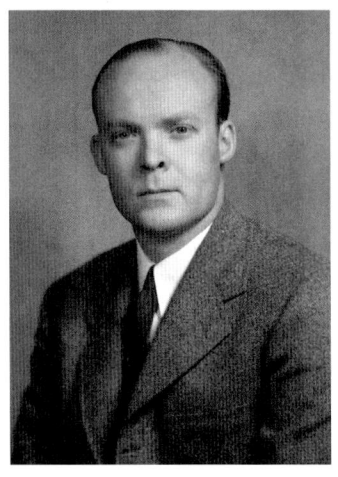

Dr. George Baker was chief of staff at Memorial Hospital of Natrona County in 1941.

Staff offered hospital tours but the highlight of the day was a reunion in Conwell Park for children born in the hospital in the past several years. Photographers documented the hospital departments and staff as well as provided images of the outside of the facility. The North Casper Junior Orchestra played on the hospital steps.[5]

WARTIME

The Japanese attack on the U.S. base at Pearl Harbor, Hawaii, on December 7, 1941, changed life in Casper. Young men and women signed up for the military or for civilian jobs to help the war effort. Eighteen-year-old Warren Weaver joined the Navy. His twin brother Wayne signed up for the Tenth Mountain Division, an elite Army ski and mountaineering unit. Sara Bowron, with training in drafting, went to Hawaii as a civilian, designing parts for damaged airplanes.[6]

The war effort also affected Casper when on September 1, 1942, the Army opened the Casper Army Air Base eight miles west of town. The Army built 200 buildings and four runways, providing construction jobs. The base trained B-17 and B-24 heavy bomber crews and also housed a repair facility for airplanes, employing women as "Rosie the Riveters." After her husband's death in March 1942, Casper Mountain resident and artist Neal Forsling took a job as a welder at the base.[7]

One contractor who helped build the air base structures was Whitey Pursel. During summers in 1943 and 1944 his daughter Shirley visited him in Casper and worked as a nurses' aide at Memorial Hospital. Shirley married Louis Carubie in 1945 and following the custom of the day, stayed home as a wife and mother.[8]

Through the end of the war more than 16,000 troops and civilians lived and worked at the base and passed through Casper.[9] They ate in restaurants, drank in bars, and patronized local businesses. Some also spent time at the local red light district.

Sexually transmitted diseases had been a problem in the county for decades. Cowboys, oilfield workers, and in the 1940s, flyboys visited the bordellos and cribs of the Sand Bar. Public health officials along with the military came up with a plan to close down the Sand Bar area, dispersing the prostitutes. The women merely moved into the Townsend Hotel on Center Street and into the Van Rooms on First Street.[10] The hospital and the county's communicable disease clinic continued to see young men and women suffering from sexually transmitted diseases.

World War II also brought an increased patient load to the hospital. Staffing shortages became a problem as doctors, nurses, and support staff all joined the war effort. Older physicians and nurses did their part, staying behind as their younger colleagues departed for the war zones. Young women flocked to nursing training programs partly because the U.S. government paid for their training if they agreed to enter the Women's Army Medical Corps. This influx of students helped supplement the group of nurses remaining on duty.

Some military personnel arrived with their families who needed medical services including obstetrical care. Injuries of all kinds taxed surgical services. Occasional bouts of influenza, childhood diseases such as measles, mumps, and chicken pox, and waterborne intestinal problems put pressure on the understaffed hospital. Penicillin was the sole antibiotic available until after the war so older remedies and good nursing were often the only recourse.

The war finally ended with victory in Europe in May 1945 and victory in Japan in August. The warriors could now come home. Casper journalist Irving Garbutt described Casper in the post-war era as "all cautious businessmen and young military folks returning to civilian life."[11] This meant the return of young men and women who had put aside their dreams of a college education and family as they served their

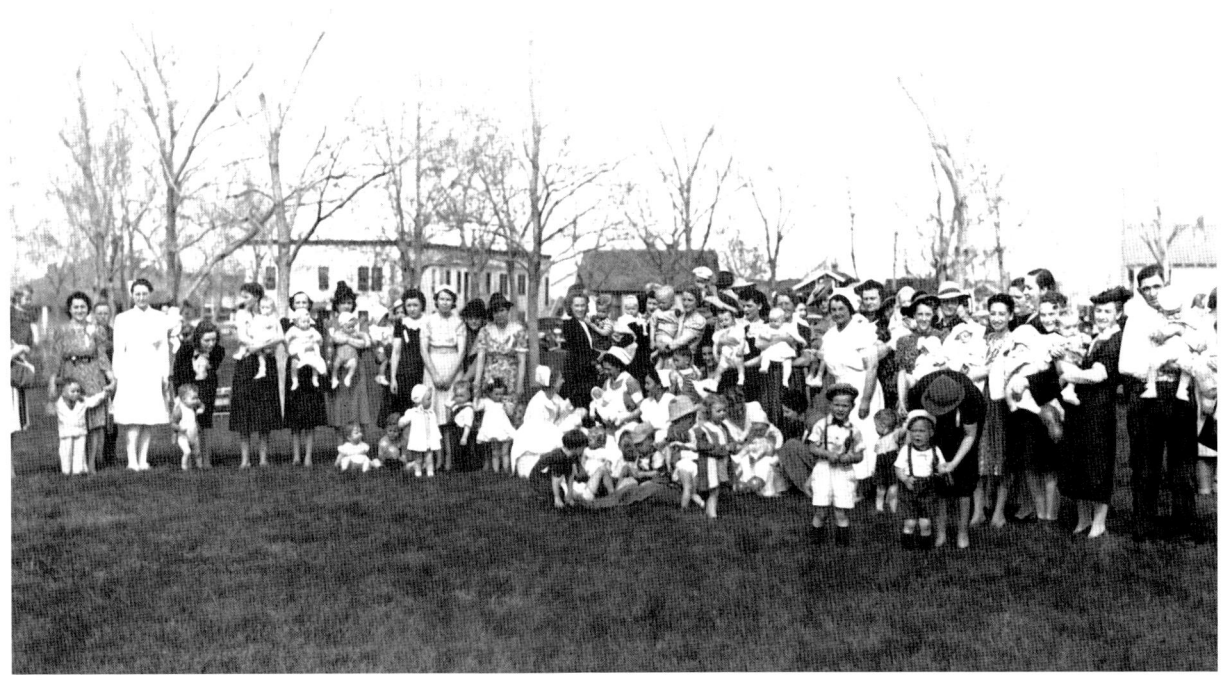

Mothers, children, and nurses posed for this photo at the baby reunion in Conwell Park in May 1941.

country. The G.I. Bill of Rights helped many veterans get that education and helped young families get a start in home ownership. What this meant to Casper was new homes funded by Veterans Administration home loans. What it meant to the Memorial Hospital was a space shortage and the need for a major facilities overhaul.[12]

Between 1940 and 1950, Wyoming's population grew by 39,887 people. Natrona County alone had an increase of 7,529. During the decade of 1950–1960, 8,186 more people joined those already in the county.[13] Much of the increase was births in the era called the Baby Boom. One example of this was in the Warren Weaver family. When Weaver returned from the Navy he married Sara Bowron, who had returned from her duties in Hawaii. Between 1952 and 1960, the Weavers had four children all born at Memorial Hospital. Most of their relatives and friends also returned and had their children at the hospital.[14]

Leadership at the hospital changed rapidly after the war. Superintendent Partridge left in 1946 then a series of short-term administrators followed. Ralph Steen served during 1947–1948, Genevieve Greene, R.N. from 1948 to 1950, and then W. B. Haselmire from 1950 to 1953.[15] Community members felt that the hospital managers came and went too quickly, interfering with the efficient operation of the hospital.

Finally, James G. Carr, Jr. took the reins in March 1953.[16] Carr had the responsibility for bringing the organization's operations up to a standard that would encourage community support. Among Carr's duties were figuring out better ways to use the building and reorganization of the hospital departments.[17]

James Carr brought new ideas to the hospital. Perhaps one of the most significant was creating the Women's Auxiliary on May 13, 1953. This group of volunteers became a crucial part of hospital operations. Their first service was staffing the information desk in the main lobby of the hospital. Eventually they also ran the library and hospitality carts, delivered flowers to rooms, served as hostesses on the surgical floor, and escorted patients around the hospital. In May 1955, they approved their charter and bylaws. One original member was Kathleen Hemry, a Wyoming pioneer and high school teacher.[18]

Medical personnel were dealing with changing medical conditions in this era. Infections, especially staphylococcus, were a severe problem in many hospitals including Memorial Hospital. With few antibiotics available for treating the infection, the primary preventive measure was frequent hand-washing. In the 1940s and early 1950s, staph especially attacked new mothers. Nurse Helen Ideen came to the hospital in 1954 and was head of the Newborn Nursery for the next twenty-eight years. When she retired in 1997, she had worked at the hospital for forty-three years, and trained several generations of nurses about the importance of hygiene.[19]

This nurse posed with a boy who had been her special charge after his birth.

Poliomyelitis was a major health issue between the late 1940s and the mid-1950s. While many of those diagnosed with the disease were children between the ages of five and nine, it hit adults as well. The largest polio epidemic with 58,000 cases hit the United States in 1952. The death toll reached 3,145 and 21,269 suffered from paralysis ranging from mild to disabling.[20]

Twenty-nine-year-old Eleanor Carrigen contracted polio in 1952. She spent weeks in the iron lung at the hospital, hovering between life and death. Eventually, through physical therapy, she regained a measure of independence although she walked with crutches for the rest of her life.[21]

After the war, physical therapists treated disabled veterans returning to civilian life. When the polio epidemic hit, victims benefited from the therapists' training, prompting the growth of physical therapy as an important specialty within the hospital.

There were also other treatments for polio. In 1949, after staying home with her son, Shirley Carubie went back to work, this time for Dr. Gordon Whiston, Dr. Robert Carnahan, and Dr. Harlan Anderson. They were orthopedic surgeons who brought Sister Kenney's pioneering treatments for polio to Casper. Carubie helped them treat patients at the hospital, where she soaked blankets in hot water in a wringer washer. The physicians then wrapped the patients with them to relax the muscles in their limbs and aid recovery. Carubie remembered that after the Salk polio vaccine came out in 1954, she helped administer thousands of doses that the children took in sugar cubes.[22]

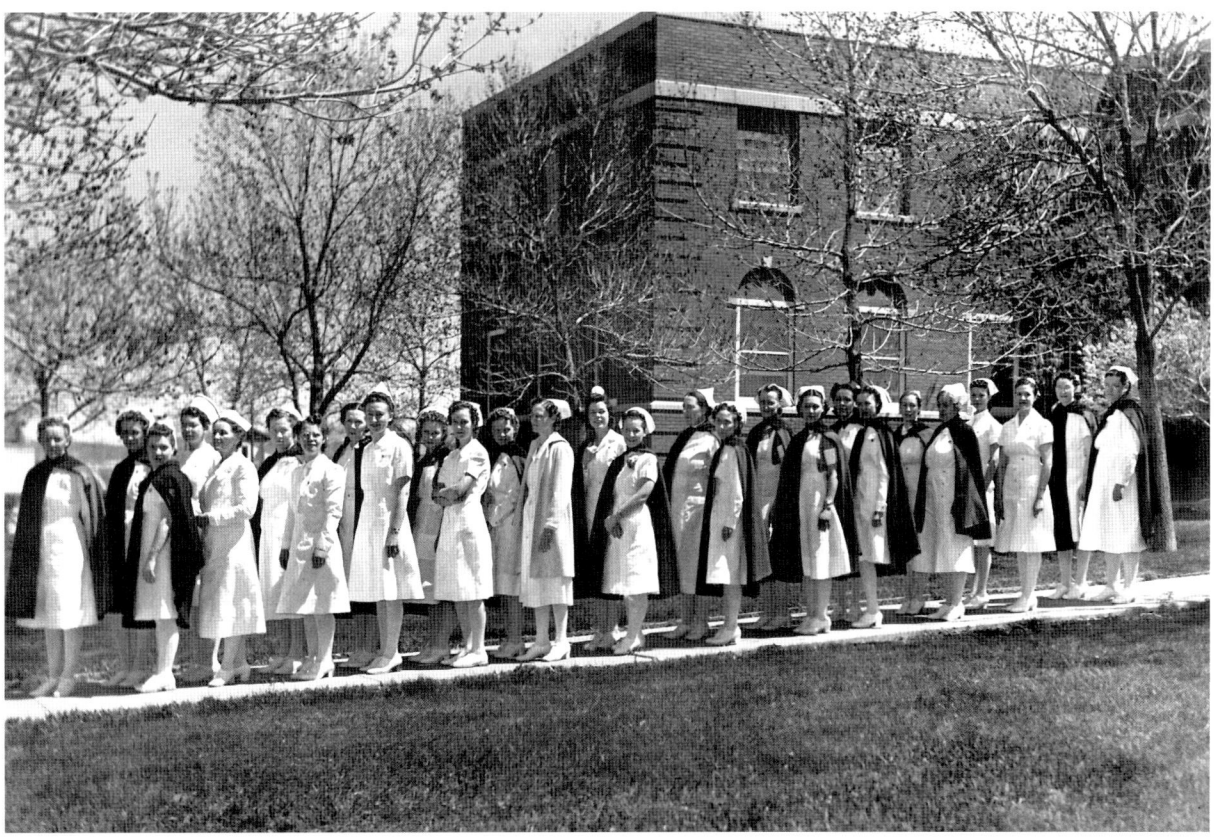

Memorial Hospital's nurses and nursing students marched across the hospital grounds at the Hospital Day celebration.

By 1950, the original hospital building was out of date and needed repairs. Other issues also required urgent attention. More patients wanted semi-private or private rooms, so general wards were a bit archaic. Equipment purchased in the 1940s needed replacement. Throughout the 1950s, maintenance staff struggled to keep the central heating boiler in running condition. Everything from the elevators to the parking areas needed updating. Things got more complicated when in 1953 the Casper Fire Department condemned the second floor of the 1911 building, requiring its closure.[23]

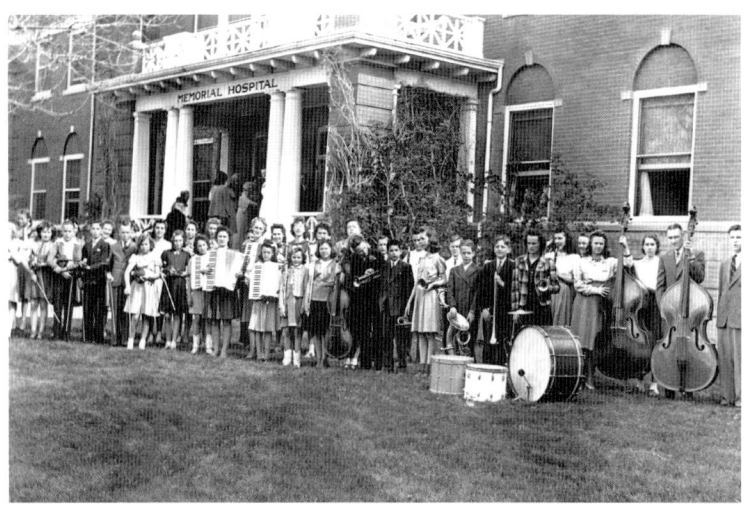

The North Casper Junior Orchestra entertained the guests on Hospital Day, 1941.

In February 1953, Chief Dietician Dorothy Quinlan reported to the Trustees that the kitchen needed new equipment. These included a new range, a new icemaker, and a steam table for keeping food warm as kitchen staff packaged it for the patients. Mr. Carr made a trip to Denver to investigate a patient meal service system called Meal-Pac, which the hospital purchased.[24]

Back in 1951, the Natrona County Commissioners and the hospital Trustees had put a capital bond measure on the ballot. The community was divided on whether the hospital was properly managed, leading to the bond's defeat. The Trustees voted to resubmit the building proposal to the voters and after the measure passed, the Trustees began the long process of hiring an architect and contractor and getting the building built and open. In the meantime, they considered reopening the second floor of the center wing, but determined that they could not justify the potential danger to patients.[25]

In October 1953, the Trustees signed a contract with Fisher and Fisher Architects of Denver to design the new wing of the hospital. Part of the contract included extensive remodeling of the older sections including the surgical areas. The general contractor was the Rediesel-Lowe Construction Company.[26] Construction began in 1954 and continued into 1955.

While the construction project progressed there were internal issues going on as well. There was a shortage of trained graduate nurses because many nurses, upon returning from the war, did not go back to work but joined the legions of women who decided to marry, stay at home, and raise their children. Young women who in past years might have gone into the field either became full-time mothers or trained for other types of professions.

When Barbara Goetz, the director of nursing, and Eleanor Walters, assistant director, reported to the Trustees in September 1953, they noted that although their department was running well their nurses needed a raise to keep the hospital competitive with other institutions. This prompted a salary survey that was the first of many conducted through the 1950s.[27]

The study showed that a forty-four-hour-per-week graduate nurse received $3,010 per year. A licensed practical nurse (L.P.N.) earned $2,100, and a ward attendant earned $1,920 per year. Student nurses received from ninety cents to one dollar per hour for working during the three-month clinical period. The nursing director recommended merit raises on a monthly basis. She asked for a new wage scale based on training and job description. New salaries would range from $3,240 for a recovery room graduate nurse to $4,980 for an associate director of nurses. Nurses would be evaluated for a merit raise at six-month intervals.[28]

At the same time the Trustees were restructuring nursing salaries, they were working with the physicians to revise the medical staff bylaws. The main body of the bylaws did not change much from those established in the 1920s, but other parts reflected changes in the Casper medical population. An increase in the number of physicians practicing in Casper meant that there were more doctors than slots for attending staff. Under the revised plan, new doctors received associate status as they waited for a vacancy on the regular medical staff. Regular staff separated into medical, surgical, obstetrical, and specialty divisions.

The bylaws also laid out the requirements for keeping patient medical histories. Physicians had to write up all new admissions' histories within forty-eight hours of a patient's entry into the hospital. No surgeon could undertake a procedure without the full written record and they had to send the pathologist a written report that accompanied any tissues removed during surgery. This section was a response to increased governmental recordkeeping requirements and to occasional lapses by attending physicians.[29]

In January 1954, of the 252 employees at Memorial Hospital of Natrona County, sixty-six were nurses and another sixty-six were nurses' aides. The Dietary Department had the equivalent of twenty-nine and one-quarter workers. The laundry, maids, and janitors comprised another forty-five employees while twenty people worked in administration. The labs had the equivalent of twelve and three-quarters workers. Other areas included Physical Therapy (four), Anesthetics (three), and Central Services (six). This reflected an increase of ten employees over 1953 numbers.[30]

A post-war recession hit as the economy resettled into peace-time status. This meant that bonds were not returning as much interest as the board had expected, causing financial concerns through late 1953 and into early 1954. A February 1954 report indicated that the patient count had dropped and the Trustees began to have serious concerns about maintaining income in the face of the ongoing building project. During much of the year, discussion centered on cost-cutting measures for the new building. Trustees began to balance the budget by scaling back on the project, buying standard rather than specialized products, or cutting special features. They also instructed Administrator Carr to cut the operating budget by $2,000, bringing cuts for the fiscal year to $6,000. While the nurses got their March raises, any additional merit increases were subject to an improved financial condition.[31]

By August 1954, budget cuts had reduced staffing levels in surgery and obstetrics. Layoffs of nurses led to frequent rotations and fewer nurses on night duty, leading to patient care concerns. The Trustees feared that there was now too much use of ward clerks and wanted more nurses on duty. They were attempting to decrease nursing issues and to increase patient satisfaction, so they requested a report from Barbara Goetz, director of nursing.[32]

> *Layoffs of nurses led to frequent rotations and fewer nurses on night duty, leading to patient care concerns.*

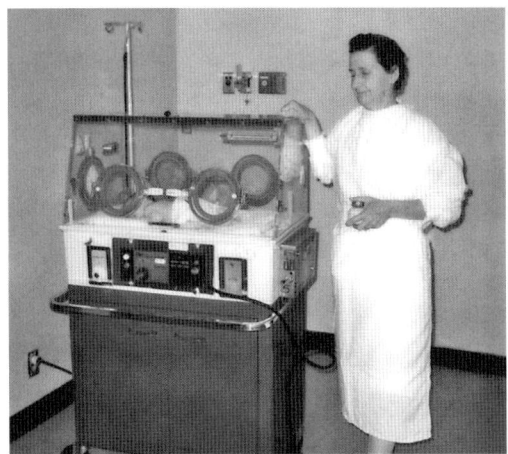

Helen Ideen was a Memorial Hospital of Natrona County Labor and Delivery nurse from 1954 to 1997.

Nurse Goetz's October 28 report pointed to the changes she had instituted at the hospital since she arrived in 1952. She had been concerned about lax attitudes among the nurses toward doctors, patients, and other hospital personnel and had worked to change this. One example she cited was that Western nurses did not always remember to offer a doctor a chair when he came to the nurses' station. She felt she brought high standards of ethics and decorum to the hospital so she regularly lectured her staff about their behavior. She felt that her department was running well even with budget cuts but her major concern was that the doctors were not appreciative of her improvements. Physicians had charged her with overstepping her duties as a nurse, a charge that she was attempting to refute. While the report cleared her with the Trustees, it probably did not improve her standing with the medical staff.[33]

Times were changing; not just in staff relations, but in technology as well. In October, the employees received the right to participate in the new county credit

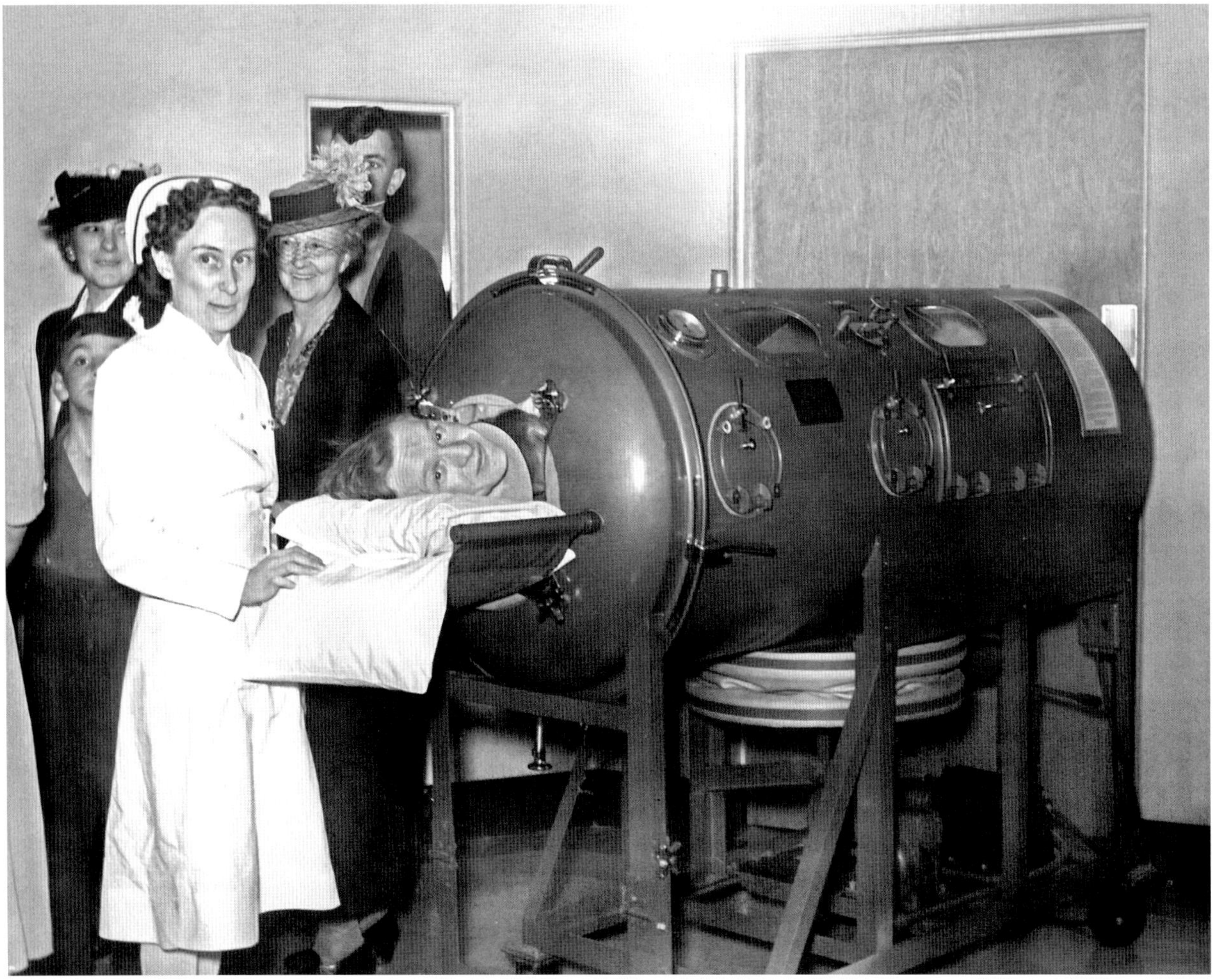

This iron lung was a life-saving device for those who had contracted polio.

52 *Wyoming Medical Center:* A CENTENNIAL HISTORY

union. Also in October, the hospital got a new oxygen machine and a laundry tumbler.[34] For the first time wiring for telephones to patient rooms was part of the new building. The administration negotiated a contract with Mountain States Telephone and Telegraph in December 1954 to set up a private exchange in the hospital.[35]

In May 1955, Donald Becker, M.D. renegotiated his contract as pathologist at Memorial Hospital of Natrona County. Rather than working for a salary, most physicians negotiated contracts that gave them a share of the revenues in their department in exchange for them managing expenses. His contract granted him "28% of the gross laboratory income less welfare laboratory income and less 7% for bad debts."[36] When needed he and other doctors renegotiated their contracts, often to allow them to purchase equipment for their labs.

Dr. Becker was part of a team that in 1954 established an innovative mandatory Strep Throat Culture Program in the Natrona County public schools. Called the Casper Project, it helped reduce cases of rheumatic fever brought on by undiagnosed strep throat. The program trained nurses and lay people to culture children's throats in clinics set up in the public schools. Many mothers, including Sara Weaver, volunteered to receive the training and took turns helping out in the program. By the time Dr. Becker and his associates Brendan Phibbs, M.D., Charles R. Lowe, M.D., Roy Holmes, M.D., Robert Fowler, M.D., Oliver K. Scott, M.D., Kenneth Roberts, M.D., Walter Watson, M.D., and Ralph Malott, M.D. wrote of their project in the *Journal of the American Medical Society* in 1958, it had proved its effectiveness and became a model around the world.[37]

One of the unintended consequences of the strep program was that doctors saw children with sore throats who did not have strep throat but instead had tonsillitis. This led to a boom in tonsillectomies beginning in the mid-1950s. Dr. Charles Kudolla and Dr. Fred Haigler performed many of these surgeries. Donna Yount, an aide at Wyoming Medical Center, remembered her experience more than fifty years later.

Patient transport had evolved over the years. In the 1930s, a local mortuary maintained a hearse that it used as an ambulance to move patients to the hospital.[38] Later the hospital set up its own ambulance service, using a variety of leased vehicles. In May 1955, Ambulance Services, run by Stanley Jourgensen, leased a Pontiac station wagon-style ambulance for the hospital. Although they really needed two vehicles, they were trying to keep costs down so instead leased one. By July, James Carr had recommended and the board had approved the purchase of the ambulance. It cost $1,950 but was cheaper in the long run than the lease.[39] As the number of calls increased, Ambulance Services worked to increase its staff to seven employees.[40]

Another innovation was building linkages with the burgeoning health insurance industry. In 1929, Justin Kimball of Baylor University in Texas created a health insurance program for teachers which he called Blue Cross. Over time it expanded to other parts of the country. It came to Wyoming in 1945 when a group of women approached the Wyoming Farm Bureau to see if it was possible to open a Blue Cross in Wyoming. A $5,000 no-interest loan paid the expenses for starting the non-profit Wyoming Hospital Service.[41] By 1955, 70 percent of Americans had health insurance coverage and Wyoming's Blue Cross program contributed to this growth.[42]

On June 18, 1955, the Memorial Hospital of Natrona County signed an agreement to affiliate with Blue Cross.[43] This allowed individuals and companies to purchase

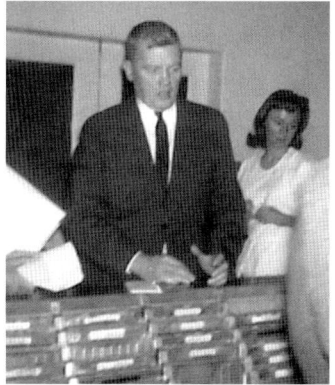

Dr. Brendan Phibbs (center) was the physician who spearheaded the Casper strep throat culture project.

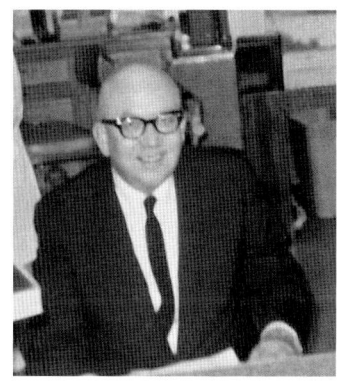

Dr. Charles Kudolla was an ear, nose, and throat physician who performed many tonsillectomies on Casper children. *Wyoming Medical Center collection.*

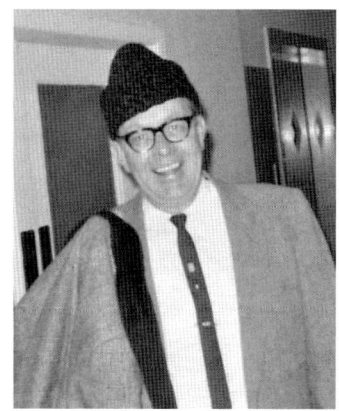

Dr. Fred Haigler was a physician in Casper who took care of children with tonsillitis. *Wyoming Medical Center collection.*

insurance by becoming part of the non-profit network. It also gave the hospital the ability to take patients who carried the insurance, increasing patient load and decreasing bad debt load. It was socially responsible and good business.

All of this was going on amid the chaos of a building program. On December 15, 1955, the new wing opened facing Second Street. Ceremonies included tours of the new facilities for the public as well as a gala with local leaders. Tours highlighted the ground-floor kitchen and the surgical areas on the third floor of the new wing. Completion of the new building meant the start of remodeling projects, although funding did not allow all to proceed at once. Air conditioning, piped oxygen, and a pneumatic tube system all improved basic infrastructure. The old operating rooms and nurses' stations needed upgrades, as did the doctors' lounge and medical record room. During planning, the administration and board took physicians' advice on changes in the surgical areas and in their lounge.

> *Completely separate from the Cold War preparations was concern about dealing with a bus or plane crash that could flood the hospital with mass casualties.*

Some services simply moved. The laundry went to part of the old kitchen space once the kitchen moved to the new wing.[44] Radiology moved into part of the laboratory, the laboratory moved into the physical therapy rooms, and physical therapy moved into the remainder of the old kitchen. Determining the most pressing projects and finding the funds to complete them took the board well into 1956.

In early 1956, the $137,000 price tag came in for all of the most important work. Remodeling the operating rooms and installing air conditioning cost $50,000. The new laundry with updated equipment was another $12,000. Most changes, including nurses' stations and the doctors' lounge, ranged from $1,000 to $4,000.[45]

Other areas of operations changed as well. When patients complained, informally and on surveys, that the food was cold when it arrived in their rooms, kitchen management revamped the Meal-Pac system to better heat the food. Administration produced an ongoing survey that patients filled out with each meal detailing their feelings about their dietary experience.[46]

As internal changes continued, an unsettled world led to a new concept; disaster planning. The 1950s was the era of the Cold War with its accompanying fear of nuclear war. While Wyoming seemed far away from the rest of the world, it was in fact integrally involved in Cold War preparations. Shirley Basin uranium became fuel for nuclear electric power plants and enriched nuclear weapon trigger material. Intercontinental ballistic missiles sat in underground bunkers along what is now the I-25 corridor. Completely separate from the Cold War preparations was concern about dealing with a bus or plane crash that could flood the hospital with mass casualties.

The disaster plan created in 1956 set up a chain of command for major disasters and described how the hospital could use personnel and resources during the emergency. Details included which areas of the hospital would become assembly, triage, and care centers. It also laid out a plan for releasing patients who were not too ill, to clear beds for the incoming injured. The National Guard and nurses in Casper who were not currently employed in their field could supply additional personnel. The Women's Auxiliary took up many non-medical tasks.[47] Knowing that the hospital was prepared for emergencies reassured the public.

As public regard for the hospital increased, so did donations from outside organizations. In February 1956, the Natrona County Chapter of the American Cancer Society offered $2,000 toward creation of a radioisotope laboratory to provide radiation treatments for cancer. The Trustees accepted the donation and pledged the extra money needed to establish the lab.[48] Additional donations provided cribs for the new pediatric ward. The Women's Auxiliary gave $300 for a pediatric playroom.[49]

In October, the Wyoming Tuberculosis Association offered $6,000 to help purchase an X-ray machine to screen patients for tuberculosis. The idea was to take a miniature X-ray of each patient as they entered the hospital. This required the medical staff to issue standing orders for the procedure so the Trustees deferred their decision until a future meeting with medical staff.[50] In late April 1957, the board finally accepted the donation for the X-ray machine, setting the stage for the universal screening of new patients.

Employee numbers continued to climb in 1956. To help manage the increasingly complex hospital, James Carr needed an assistant administrator. On August 21, he

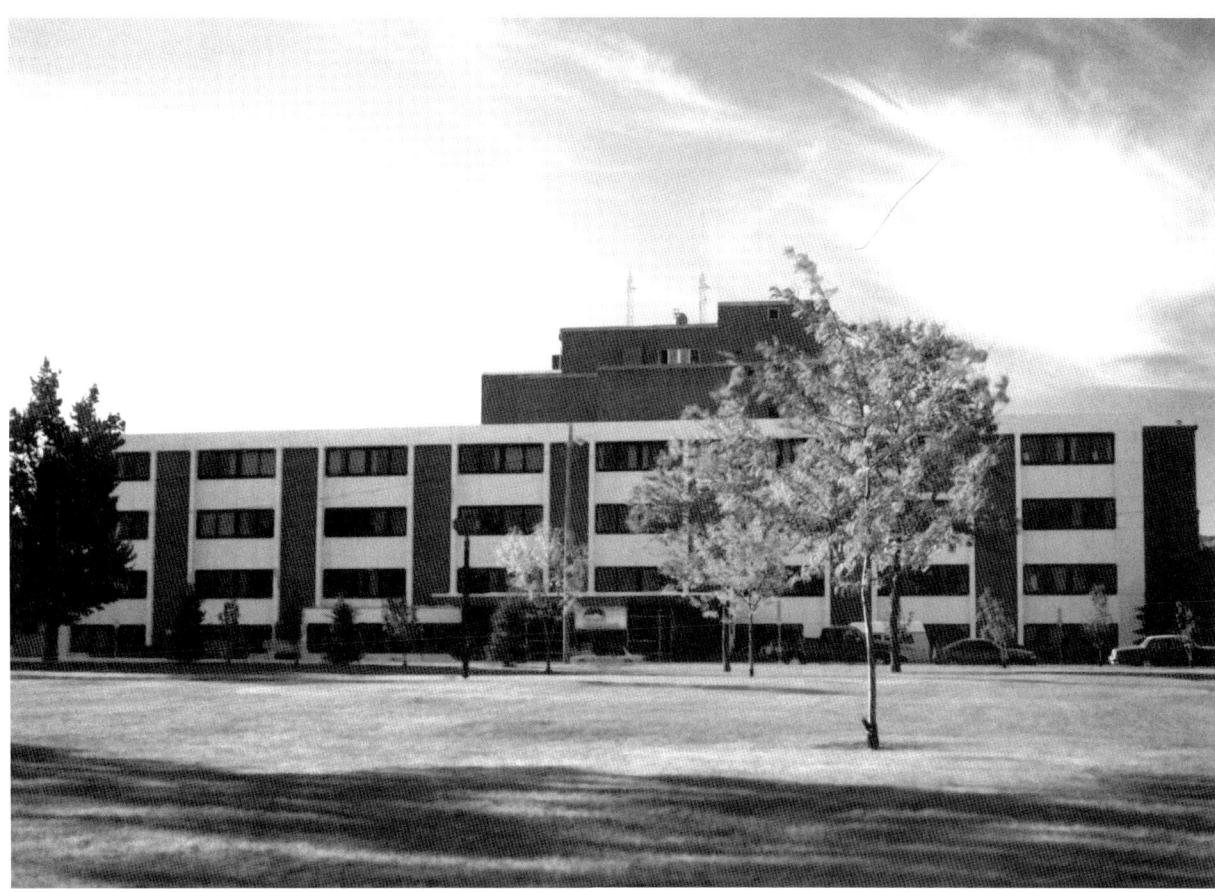

The new addition facing Second Street opened in December 1955.

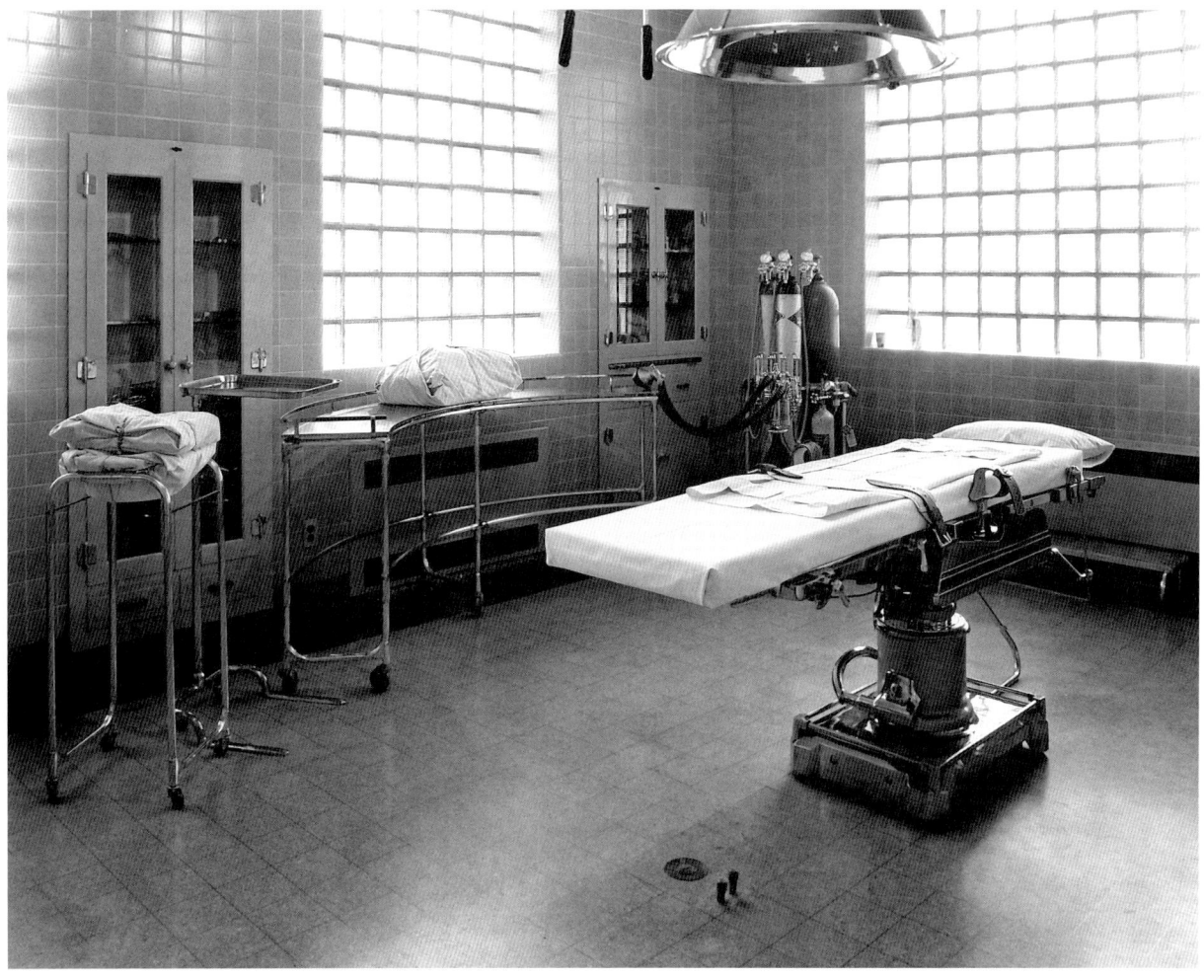

The remodeled operating room was part of the 1955 building project.

presented Robert Manville's name to the Trustees for that position. Manville, who had effectively been the second in command for some time, accepted the promotion and the twenty-five-dollar-a-month raise that it brought.[51]

Physicians had long been critical of the lack of parking for them around the hospital. In September, the issue came to a head. Physicians now demanded that the hospital pay more attention to their needs. Dr. Bowden, secretary of the medical staff, relayed the "request that immediate action be taken."[52] The Trustees said they would give the matter due consideration.

In 1956, televisions were a new but increasingly popular phenomenon. The Casper Rental TV Company proposed to rent televisions to the hospital patients at a rate of ten dollars per week or two dollars per day. The rental company would get 80 percent and the hospital would get 20 percent of the fee. The black-and-white televisions were the latest design with remote controls and bedside speakers. Hospital management decided to consider the program but not take immediate action.[53]

Although many women who had trained as nurses were still staying home in 1956, there was a temporary end to the nursing shortage. This reflected a new generation of young women who wanted to make a difference in society by becoming nurses. The popularity of the Cherry Ames nursing books for girls and the presence of future nurses programs in high schools attested to the return of nursing as a desirable career option.

In September 1956, the Natrona County Heart Association offered to pay for the services of Lois Wheeler, R.N. to supervise the growing rheumatic fever prevention program. Dr. Brendan Phibbs sent a letter to the hospital with a check from the association telling them that she was an employee of the strep throat program but asking the hospital to handle her payroll of one hundred dollars per month.[54] This came as the rheumatic fever program increasingly became a focus for community effort and fundraising activities.

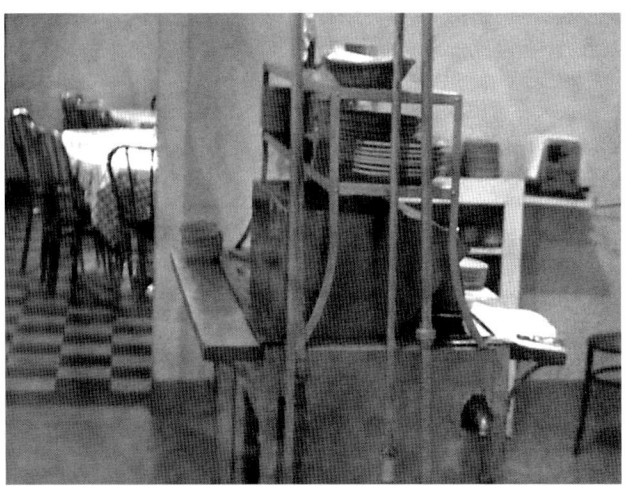

Food service workers placed food on this steam table for those eating in the new cafeteria in the hospital.

In early 1957, Memorial Hospital of Natrona County hired a new director of nurses when Nona Pair, R.N. joined the institution at a salary of $6,000 per year.[55] This came at a time when the administration and Trustees were considering a new salary scale for nurses that included not only raises but also increased vacation time.[56]

One way to offset salary increases and new equipment was to raise the rates for patient stays in the hospital. In January 1958, the board instituted the following changes. Pediatric stays went from $8.50 to $11 per day. The east wing, general medical, and obstetrics room rates went up depending on where a patient stayed. Wards became $11.50, up from $10; semi-private rooms went to $13.50; and the rate for private rooms became $17.50. The new building had the best facilities and so cost the most. Semi-private rooms rose to $16 and private rooms ranged from $22 to $23.[57]

Each year since 1953 the monthly patient day count had increased by about thirty patients per month. By 1958, that growing patient load was causing concern. Construction undertaken just a few years earlier was proving inadequate and remodeling was helping but not solving the problem. Elderly patients, who often needed extended care, accounted for a large part of that growth. National studies showed that about 5 percent of Casper's population was over the age of sixty-five, a percentage decrease from 1950 but an increase in actual numbers to 2,010. The state of Wyoming was conducting a study to see if there needed to be more nursing and convalescent homes. Memorial Hospital was helping to plan for those facilities.

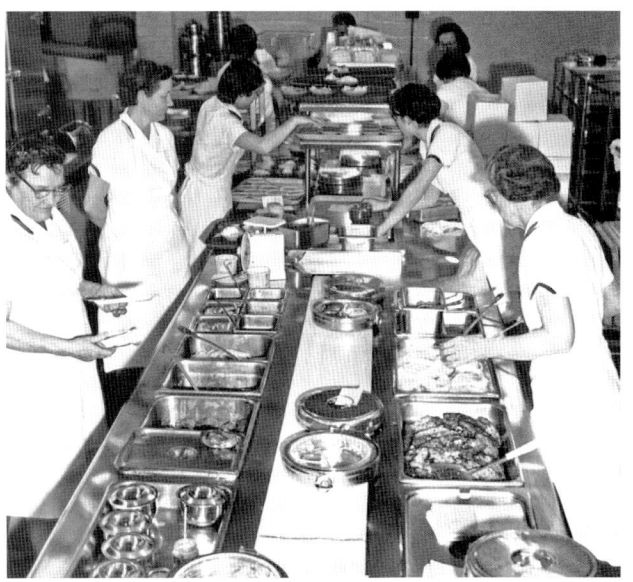

Food service workers prepared food for patients using this assembly line to work faster and keep food hot.

By September 1958, the Trustees received a report that there was once again a shortage of trained nurses. The Personnel Department had posted a number of job openings but few qualified candidates had applied.[58] One solution was to train additional licensed practical nurses. This led the hospital to begin collaboration with Casper College in an L.P.N. training program.[59]

CHAPTER FOUR ❖ *The War Years and Beyond:* 1941 TO 1959   57

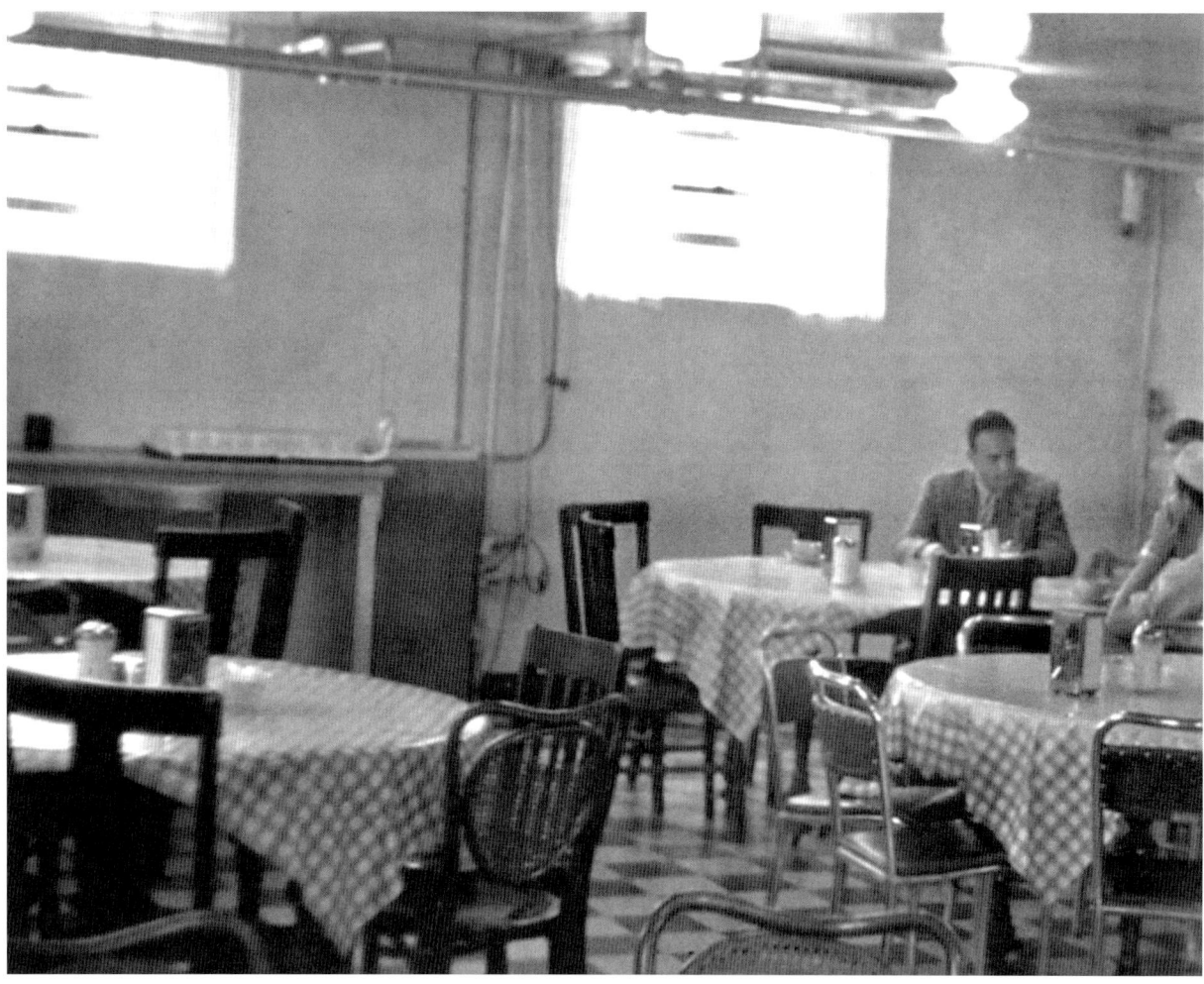

The basement dining room in the hospital had a café feel.

A major milestone for health care in Casper was the 1958 formation of the Natrona County Voluntary Health Council, eventually called the Blue Envelope Health Fund. This organization was a collaboration of community leaders and physicians who were unhappy with the high level of administrative costs of other programs. The founders focused on three types of programs. The first was donations for research and treatment of heart disease, especially supporting the strep throat program. The second focus was cancer research and treatment. The third was raising money for mental health services. The Blue Envelope Health Drive elected John Tripeny, Jr. as its first president. Ironically, Tripeny died in 1971 at age forty of complications of open-heart surgery performed to deal with rheumatic fever damage to his heart.[60] Tripeny oversaw a corps of community volunteers who canvassed the county, raising money for the three programs. Because this was an all-volunteer group, more than 95 percent of the money raised went to the three target areas.

The 1950s was the decade that saw a renewed interest in definition and treatment of mental illness. Psychiatry was an old field, dating back to Dr. Sigmund Freud in the late nineteenth century, but was slow in coming to the Western United States. In 1958, Dr. Mark Farrell moved to Casper to become its first psychiatrist. The mental health focus of the United Health Drive and Dr. Farrell's arrival allowed the hospital board to consider development of an in-house psychiatric program at the hospital.[61]

The hospital was changing rapidly and sometimes the public had trouble keeping up. To clarify changes, in the fall of 1958, the hospital published a flyer for patients and visitors that presented some facts about the Memorial Hospital of Natrona County. It had 242 beds and over 10,000 in-patients per year as well as almost 9,000 outpatients. It was the largest general hospital in Wyoming with 350 employees working in many areas including special services such as physical therapy, pathology, and radiology. Nearly half of the employees were nurses. Forty-six physicians and seventeen dentists served as the medical staff. Over 300 women volunteered through the Women's Auxiliary.[62]

The document also clarified the hospital's relationship to the county. Natrona County owned the buildings but the hospital was an independent non-profit that received money for building maintenance but had to rely on patient fees for all operating costs. The County Commissioners appointed the five-person Board of Trustees that oversaw all operations and building campaigns. The operating budget for 1957–1958 was $1.7 million, which came to twenty-eight dollars per patient per day.[63]

During 1958, the Trustees created a long-range plan for the hospital that served as a guide into the 1960s. The report called for replacing the old boiler system that for years had given the maintenance staff headaches, with a central heating plant. It also noted the quarters, dating from 1953, that housed the Laboratory and X-ray departments. This space was now inadequate for the volume of work the departments took on. They either needed to be moved to a floor of the new building or to their own building on the site of the old nurses' quarters, which had been unsafe for some time and needed to come down. The report noted that if the surgical suites moved, then the nursery could go into the old operating room space and move out of the 1911 building. Finally, there needed to be a provision for additional beds for psychiatric and general nursing care. Although the report called for additional space for tuberculosis patients, advances in the antibiotic treatment of TB reduced patient load in that area.

Options the report considered included building two new floors on the 1955 wing of the building or even the creation of a second hospital in town, perhaps by a church group. However, no one seemed interested in creating a second hospital, so expansion of Memorial Hospital was the best option. Purchasing the entire block that the hospital stood on would be a good start to the process.

The New Year began with continuing concerns about nursing staff. The average length of employment was about two years. It was true that some nurses came to Casper and to the hospital and worked there for their whole careers, but the population was fluid

> *It was the largest general hospital in Wyoming with 350 employees working in many areas including special services such as physical therapy, pathology, and radiology.*

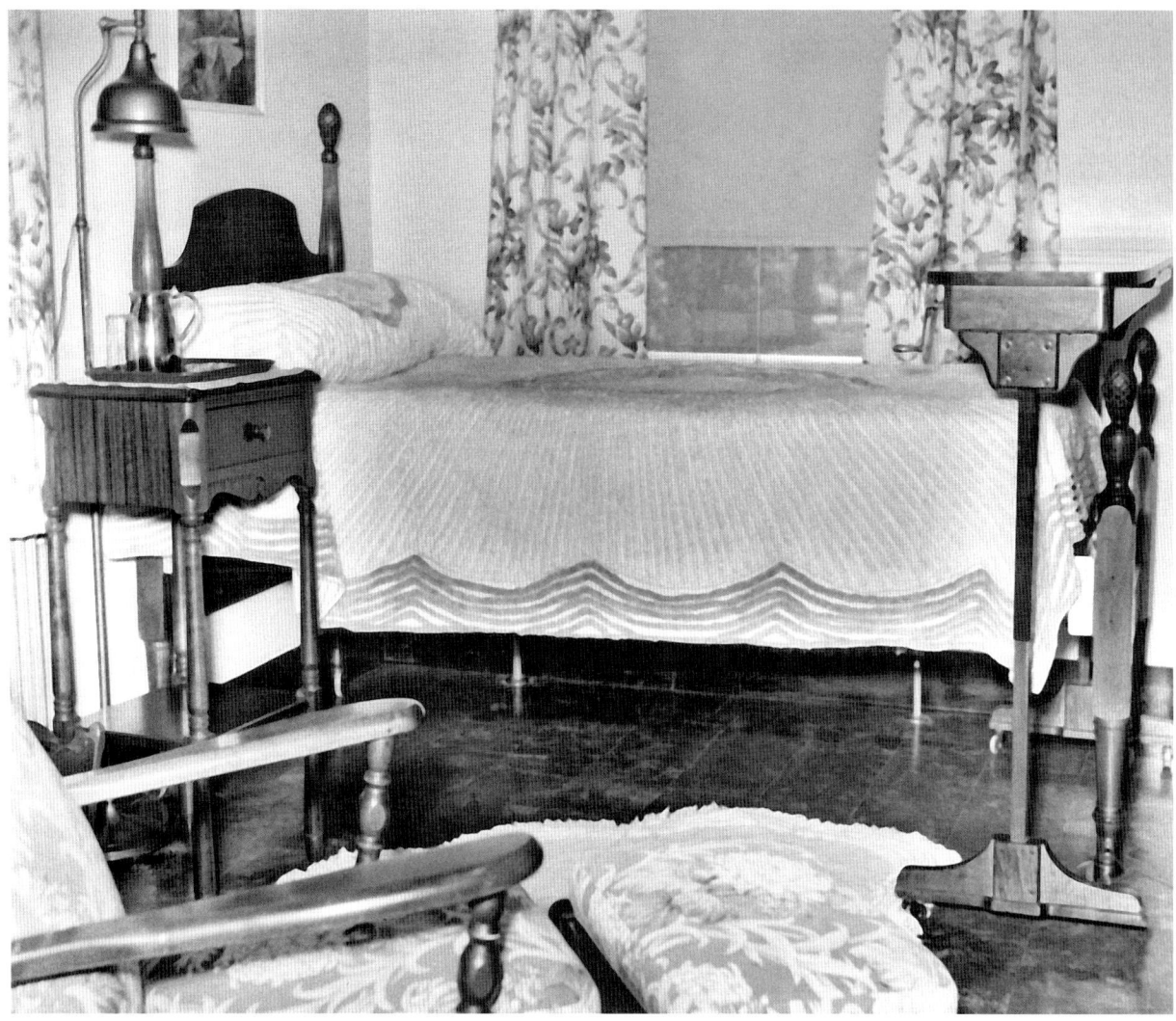

The rate for this private room was twenty-two dollars in 1958.

and many factors led to turnover. Many young nurses left the field when they married and had children. While they might return when the children were in school or grown, they were still out of the workforce for many years. Some nurses got valuable experience at Memorial Hospital then moved on either to hospitals in larger cities or to small towns that needed their services. Training and keeping good nurses was a constant battle.

In May 1959, Memorial Hospital of Natrona County and Casper College finally drew up the formal agreement to run the licensed practical nurses' training program at the college. The program followed the state guidelines for technical education which had grown out of the rules set up for nursing students in the 1930s. The first class of twenty-five students would receive both classroom and clinical training for one year. Students received a stipend if they completed the first two months. This started at forty dollars and rose to eighty dollars in the eighth month in the program. Each student also got food coupons for the hospital cafeteria. Instructors worked for the college but they had access to all hospital departments when functioning as clinical teaching supervisors.[64] The students supplemented the graduate nursing staff and ideally stayed on to work at the hospital after they graduated. Many used this as a first step toward becoming registered nurses.

Casper College also collaborated with the University of Wyoming to provide R.N. training. Shirley Carubie became a registered nurse after she got her degree through that program. That led her back to the hospital where she worked in the Obstetrics Department.[65]

Even as the hospital struggled to keep enough nurses, the welfare patient load increased each year between 1956 and 1959. There had been 543 free care patients in 1956, 675 in 1957, and 690 in 1958. The first two months of 1959 had eighty-one and ninety-seven patients. In 1958, the total represented 9,288 patient days, averaging thirteen days per welfare patient.[66] While the county repaid the hospital for much of the cost, it was still a financial burden that management accepted as part of the role of the hospital in its community.

The hospital finally began the parking lot paving project. The plan called for blacktopping the whole northwest corner of the lot adjoining Second and Washington streets as well as paving the northeast corner of Conwell and Third streets.[67] This would ideally allow for sufficient physician, employee, and visitor parking well into the future.

In early November 1959, Fisher and Davis Architects recommended that the hospital tear down the nurses' home and begin buying up surrounding houses to provide land to expand the building. The Natrona County Commission agreed to a meeting in early 1960 to discuss the next round of expansion.

NOTES

1 Joseph Orr. "Anatomy of a Western Town," WPA, Wyoming Writers' Project, typescript, March 10, 1940, p. 11.

2 Orr, pp. 21–22.

3 Scrapbook, National Hospital Day at Memorial Hospital of Natrona County, Casper, Wyoming, May 11, 1941.

4 Scrapbook, National Hospital Day, May 11, 1941.

5 Scrapbook, National Hospital Day, May 11, 1941.

6 Rebecca Hunt. Weaver Family history, typescript, 2005.

7 Neal Forsling memoirs, typescript, 1964.

8 Carol Crump. "Registered Nurse Shirley Carubie still at work at 85," *Casper Journal*, October 4, 2009, pp. 11–12.

9 "West Across the Skies: Wyoming's Aviation History," online exhibit, http://wyomuseum.state.us/Exhibits/Aviation.asp.

10 Irving Garbutt. *I Was There: Recollections of Ten Decades*. Casper: Casper Journal, 2003, p. 45.

11 Garbutt, p. 45.

12 Garbutt, p. 45.

13 Population of Counties by Decennial Census: 1900 to 1990, http://www.census.gov/population/cencounts/wy190090.txt, 3/27/1995.

14 Hunt, Weaver Family history, 2005.

15 Elaine Hough, Memorial Hospital of Natrona County History notes, typescript, p. 4.

16 Board of Trustees Minutes, April 20, 1953, p. 1.

17 Board of Trustees Minutes, February 11, 1953, p. 2.

18 Elaine Hough, ed. *MHNC Outreach*, Vol. 1, No. 2 (Spring/Summer 1978), p. 5.

19 Patti Legler, R.N. "Farewell, gentle lady," *Wyoming Medical Center Highlights*, February 2006, p. 2.

20 Evelyn Zamula. "A New Challenge for Former Polio Patients." *FDA Consumer* 25 (5), 1991, http://www.questia.com/googleScholar.qst?docId=5002167868.

21 Mark Junge. *A View from Center Street: Tom Carrigen's Casper*. Casper, WY: McMurray Foundation, 2003.

22 Crump, pp. 11–12.

23 Board of Trustees Minutes, August 24, 1953, p. 1.

24 Board of Trustees Minutes, February 11, 1953, p. 2.

25 Board of Trustees Minutes, August 14, 1953, p. 1.

26 Contract, MHNC and Fisher and Fisher, dated October 1953, p. 1; Board of Trustees Minutes, October 28, 1954, p. 1.

27 Board of Trustees Minutes, September 22, 1953, p. 1.

28 Board of Trustees Minutes, October 1, 1953, pp. 1–2.

29 MHNC, Medical Staff Bylaws, revised, 1953, pp. 10–11.

30 Board of Trustees Minutes, January 1954, p. 1.

31 Board of Trustees Minutes, February 25, 1954, p. 1.

32 Board of Trustees Minutes, August 28, 1954, p. 1.

33 Board of Trustees Minutes, October 28, 1954, p. 1.

34 Board of Trustees Minutes, October 28, 1954, p. 1.

35 Contract, Mountain States Telephone and Telegraph with MHNC, December 3, 1954.

36 Board of Trustees Minutes, May 3, 1955, p. 1.

37 Brendan Phibbs, M.D., Donald Becker, M.D., Charles R. Lowe, M.D., Roy Holmes, M.D., Robert Fowler, M.D., Oliver K. Scott, M.D., Kenneth Roberts, M.D., Walter Watson, M.D., and Ralph Malott, M.D. "The Casper Project—An Enforced Mass-Culture Streptococcic Control Program," *Journal of the American Medical Association,* 1958:166 (10):1113-1119.

38 Garbutt, *I Was There*.

39 Board of Trustees Minutes, July 8, 1955, p. 1.

40 Board of Trustees Minutes, May 26, 1955, p. 1.

41 History of Blue Cross Blue Shield Wyoming, https://www.bcbswy.com/about/timeline.html.

42 Blue Cross Blue Shield Association, http://www.bcbs.com/about/history/1920s.html.

43 Agreement, MHNC and Wyoming Blue Cross, June 14, 1955.

44 Board of Trustees Minutes, August 18, 1955.

45 Board of Trustees Minutes, February 23, 1956.

46 Board of Trustees Minutes, March 22, 1956.

47 Natrona County Memorial Hospital Board, Disaster Planning document, Spring 1956.

48 Board of Trustees Minutes, February 10, 1956.

50 Board of Trustees Minutes, August 21, 1956.

51 Board of Trustees Minutes, August 21, 1956.

52 MHNC Medical Staff letter, September 11, 1956.

53 Proposal from the Casper Rental TV Company, 1956.

54 Brendan Phibbs, M.D. Letter to MHNC regarding Lois Wheeler, R.N., September 29, 1956.

55 Board of Trustees Minutes, January 3, 1957, p. 1.

56 Board of Trustees Minutes, January 3, 1957, p. 2.

57 Board of Trustees Minutes, January 23, 1958.

58 Board of Trustees Minutes, September 23, 1958.

59 Board of Trustees Minutes, December 30, 1958, p. 1.

60 "Lab Named for Tripeny," *Casper Star-Tribune*, March 21, 1971.

61 Board of Trustees Minutes, January 23, 1958.

62 Facts About Memorial Hospital, September 1958.

63 Facts About Memorial Hospital, September 1958.

64 Contract, MHNC and Casper College, May 11, 1959.

65 Crump, pp. 11–12.

66 Board of Trustees Minutes, February 19, 1959, pp. 2–3.

67 MHNC parking lot paving maps, March 19, 1959.

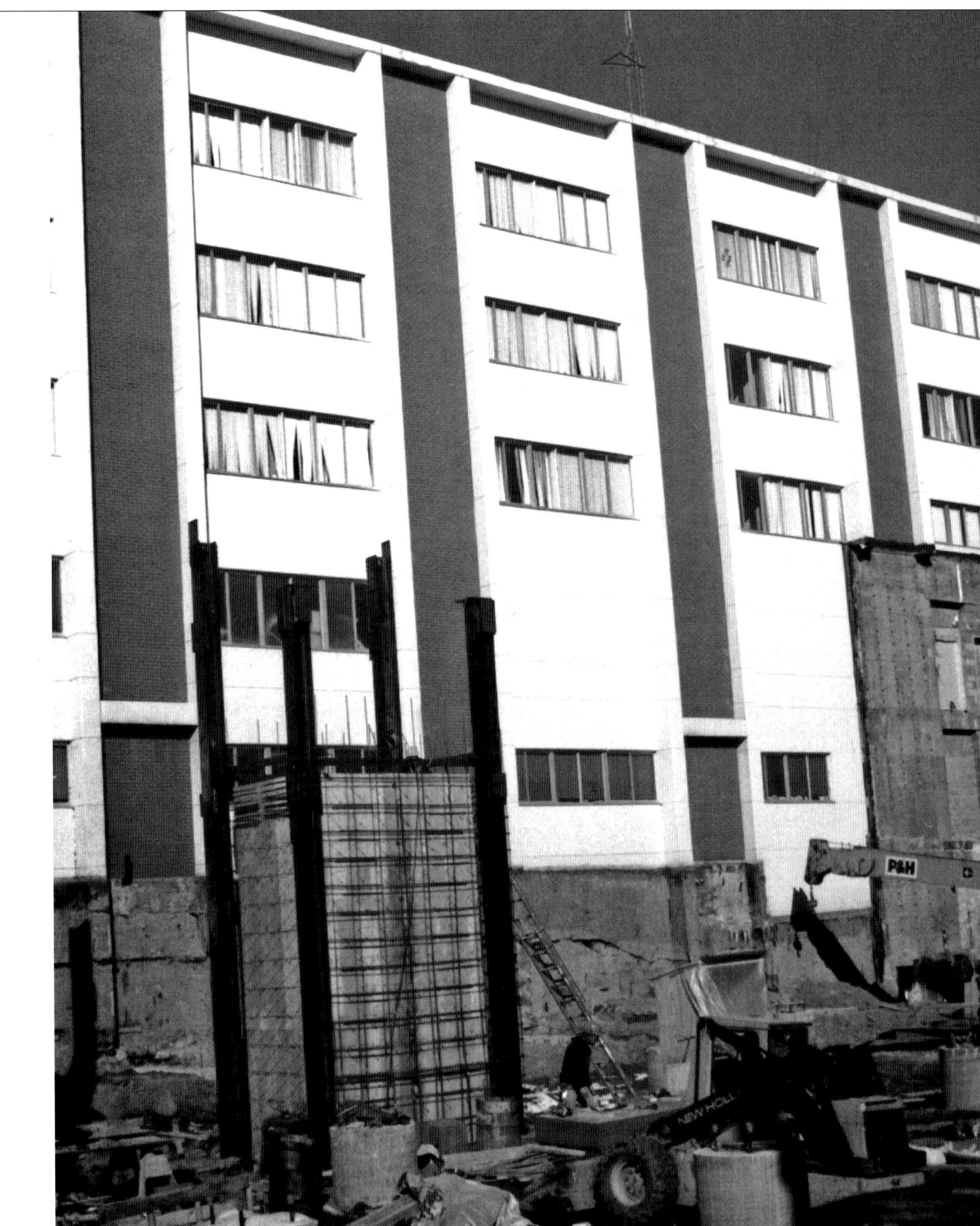

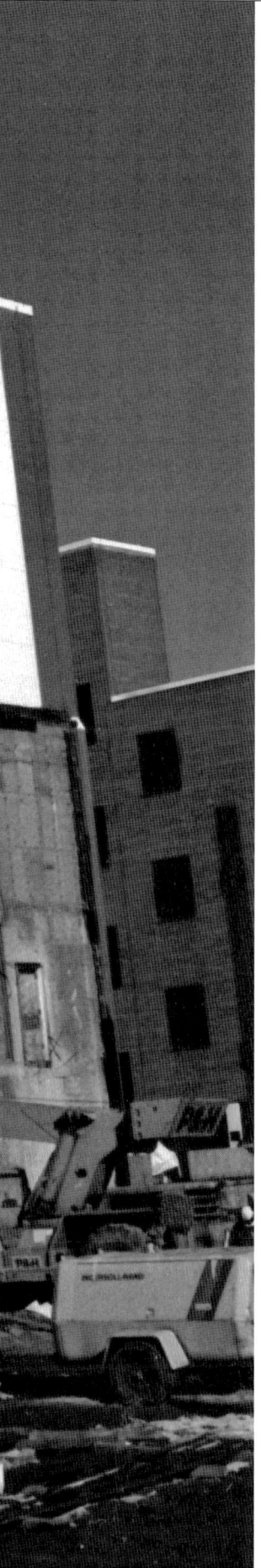

CHAPTER FIVE

From Memorial Hospital of Natrona County to Wyoming Medical Center

1960 TO 1986

In 1960, Casper, bolstered by the oil industry and new families, grew to 49,623 people, a net gain of 16,000 in a decade. Housing developments sprang up east of Country Club Road and on the west side of town centering along Poplar Street and the new Sunrise Shopping Center. The county was still primarily blue-collar with most people boasting at least a high school education. Casper College was expanding up the new "C" Hill south of town.

College and high school sports attracted large audiences both in person and through radio and television broadcasts. Each year the Natrona County Fair drew thousands with its 4-H and county extension activities, rodeo, and midway carnival. Casper was increasingly the core shopping area for a region that stretched throughout Central Wyoming.

Casper had a country club, K2 Television, and a number of radio stations, including K2 and KATI. K2 played vintage music as well as country while KATI played the new rock and roll. The radio and television stations were big supporters of local institutions including the hospital. A KATI broadcast from Sunrise Shopping Center in early May 1961 brought in $900 for Memorial Hospital.[1]

New road projects made it easier to reach Casper. The old Yellowstone Highway got new paving while all state and many county roads had blacktop as well. Natrona County Airport, on the site of the former Casper Army Air Base, had daily flights offered by Frontier Airlines.

Memorial Hospital of Natrona County continued to focus on expansion, staffing, and innovation. One highlight of the decade would be a major new wing, built in 1967, that would finally replace the 1911 central building. Management addressed

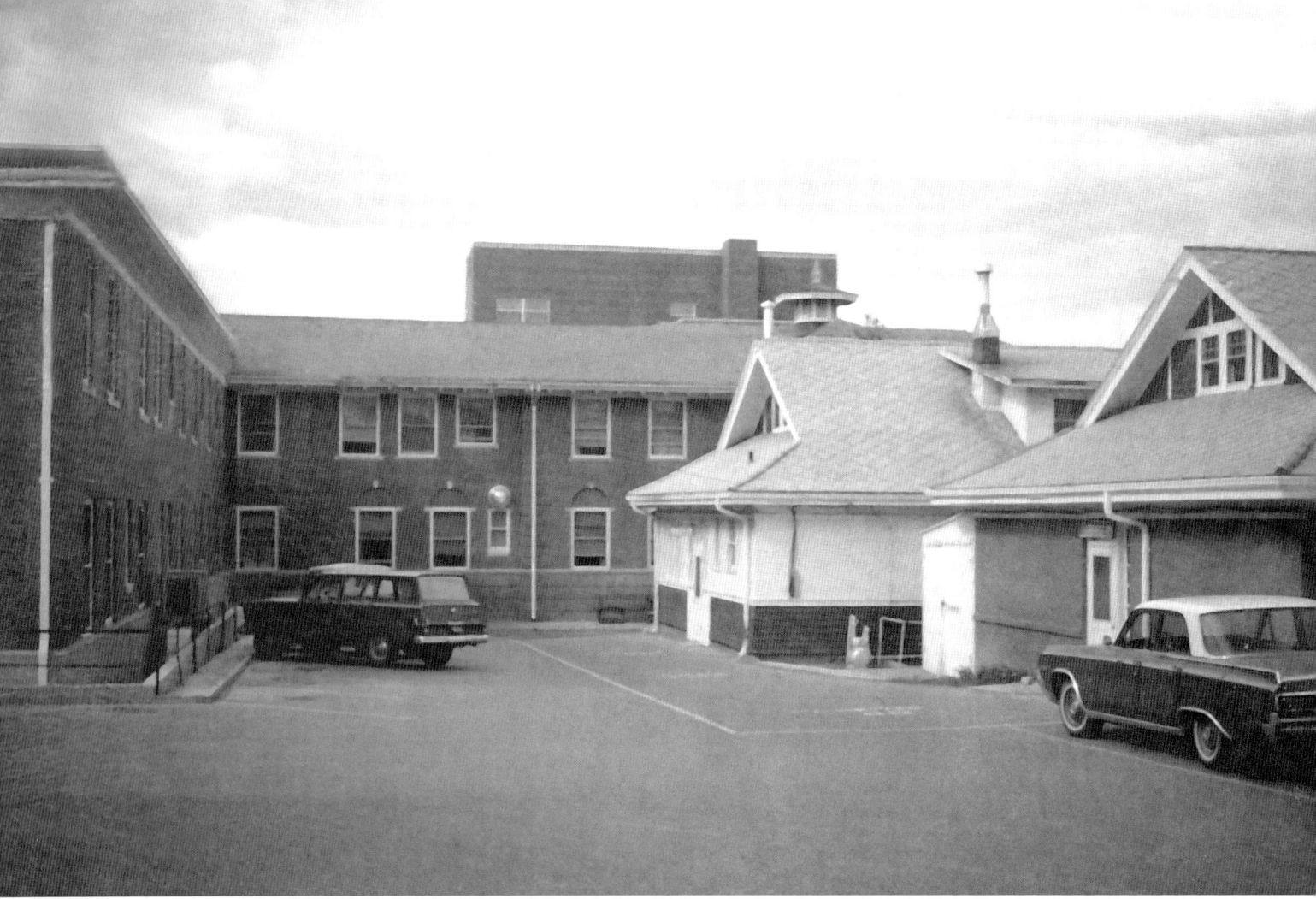

This 1960 photo shows the two nurse residence buildings that needed replacing.

staffing issues by developing creative new training programs as well as upgrading employee salaries and benefits. Collaborations with the Blue Envelope Health Fund and support of physician initiatives brought new technology and new ideas through the institution's doors.

On February 29, 1960, the Trustees met with the County Commissioners to propose a bond issue for capital expansion. While touring the Commissioners through the existing facilities, the Trustees explained the rationale for the new addition. A new building would provide more patient rooms, new laboratory space, new radiology space, and allow for the modernization of other parts of the hospital operation. Presented with convincing evidence, the Commissioners agreed to work on a bond election.[2]

In spite of the population growth, the board faced a downturn in the economy. In the late 1950s, the United States had suffered a post-war recession. Then a drop in crude oil prices occurred due to expanded production in other parts of the world. Venezuela, Iran, Iraq, Saudi Arabia, and Kuwait created the Organization of Petroleum Exporting Countries in 1960 to gain control over their production and markets.[3] This, with increasing turbulence in the world, drove oil prices down and made them more volatile.

At the same time there was a movement to reduce competition by creating ever larger petroleum companies through mergers and reorganizations. With that in mind, Standard Oil created Pan American Petroleum Corporation in 1957. Pan American's Wyoming operations became one of the area's bigger employers. When the drop in crude oil prices reduced profits, Pan American Petroleum closed its Casper operations and took its jobs elsewhere.[4] That made the idea of a major capital drive a bit daunting.

Once the board dealt with the issue of a capital funding drive, they looked at revamping the nurse training program. Mr. Carr felt that the joint Casper College and University of Wyoming four-year Bachelor of Science in Nursing program was not drawing enough students and should be replaced with a two-year Associate of Science in Nursing degree.[5] He argued that more young women would be willing to commit to a two-year program.

At the same time there were staff changes in nursing as well as in other areas of operations. Nona Pair, R.N., director of nursing services since 1957, resigned to work on a master's degree. Her assistant, Constance Nations, hoping to teach in the Casper College program, also considered leaving.[6] That left Mr. Carr looking for new nursing leadership. By the end of 1960, Anne TeKampe, R.N. joined the hospital as the new director of nursing.

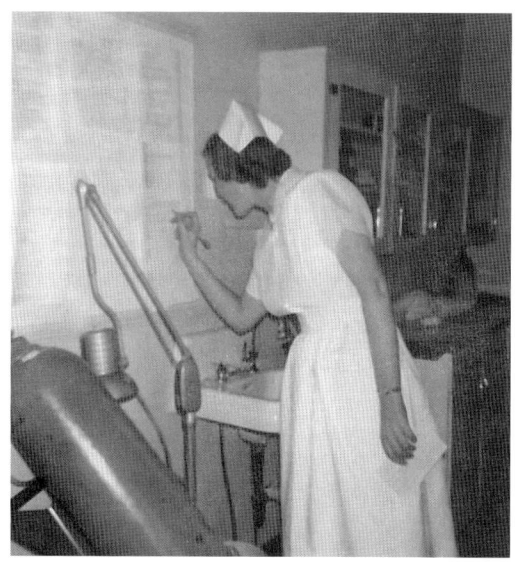

Nurses kept manual track of patients by marking on charts on the wall.

In April, Dorothy Quinlan, who had managed the Dietary Department for eight years, announced her intention to begin working part-time. She had made great improvements in food service in spite of all of the renovations during her tenure.[7] Her replacement Mrs. Gene Talbert was assisted by Rosalie St. James, Claretta Benesh, and Fern Reed.[8] Eventually, Quinlan returned to full-time work and went back to running the department until her retirement in 1991.[9]

The base rate for nurses went from $306 to $330 per month by the end of 1960. Then, in response to a salary survey of the Rocky Mountain region, the salary went up again in June 1962, this time to $350 per month for a newly hired R.N.[10]

An additional benefit change was the increase in vacation time for employees who came in the summer of 1962. The administration conducted a survey of other Wyoming hospitals, major hospitals in Denver, and vacation benefits for Casper and Natrona County employees. They concluded that Memorial Hospital, with a flat rate of two weeks per year, provided the least amount of leave. W. R. Coe Memorial Hospital in Cody had the best plan with two weeks' leave rising to four weeks after ten years of service. The recommendation that went into effect on May 1, 1962, was that vacation leave rise to three weeks after seven years of employment and then to four weeks after ten years.[11] On July 18, 1962, the nursing staff sent the board a letter thanking them for the raise and updated benefits. They believed that this would help the hospital in the long run in terms of both morale and recruitment.

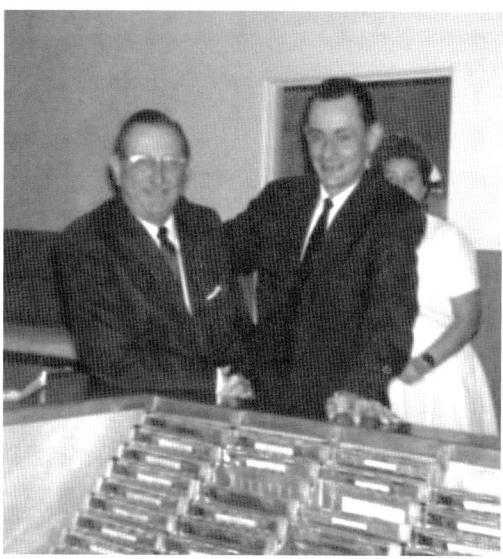

When Dr. R. P. Fitzgerald and Dr. Charles Lowe made their rounds, they consulted charts kept on clipboards at the nurses' station. In this photo, Casey Butcher, R.N. followed them on their rounds.

Hospital morale was a matter of more than pay and vacation time. Nurses worked closely with others in their specialties. Technical and support staff also formed close-knit groups. Shared holiday celebrations, birthdays, and family milestones drew co-workers closer together. At the same time, the hierarchy placed the physicians at the top. Just as patients would become partners in their own care, so too did nurses and

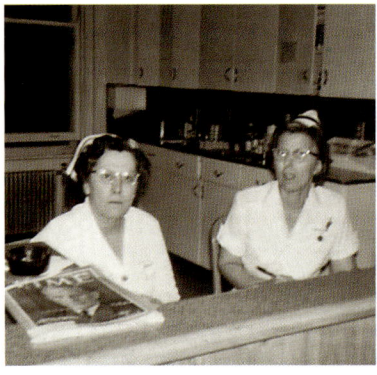
Mrs. Winship (left) and Martha Adcock (right) were staffing the nurses' station during one of their twelve-hour night shifts.

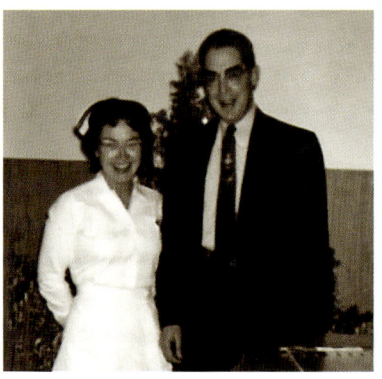
Irene Spiele and Dr. Holman posed in front of the departmental Christmas tree in 1961. Units as well as the whole hospital shared holidays.

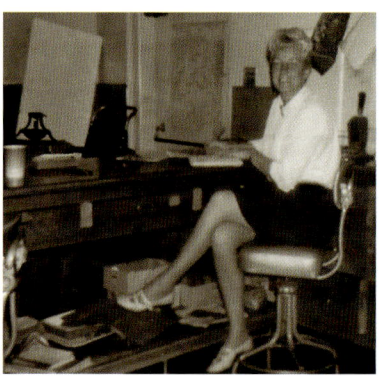
Jean Posker, ward secretary in the late 1960s, kept the medical floor running.

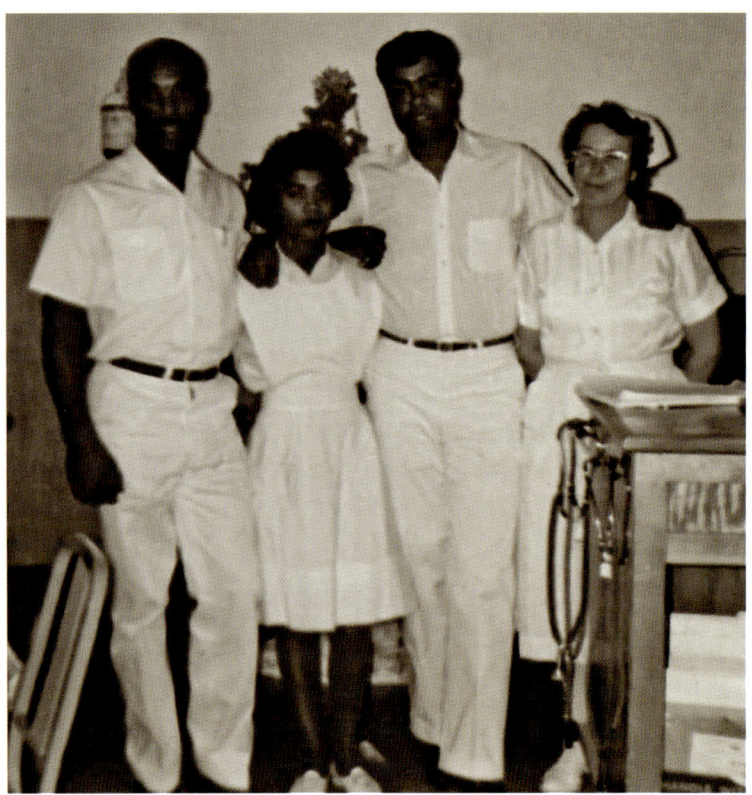
This group included Tom Johnson (left), Edna Thornton (middle left), Alb Griffin (middle right), and Leona Boyer (right).

technicians take on a larger, less subservient role in the healing process. Patients and their families saw the professional side of the hospital but they missed the internal structure that took the form of friendships that developed among co-workers, doctors, and other employees. Quality care did not just depend on training, but also on a sense of partnership and shared vision that grows in a hospital environment. People mattered.

The technological advances for the operating room in 1960 included an Ultra-Sonic unit costing $1,200 as well as a portable X-ray unit for $11,700. The nursery got an infant resuscitation unit costing $1,500.[12] The new boiler came on line and there were plans for a second one in the east building. The L. D. Liesinger Construction Company had that boiler in place and working at a cost of $18,319 in November 1961.[13]

In late March 1961, Mrs. Lewis George gave birth to her fourth child, a daughter, at Memorial Hospital. A day later during minor surgery the mother's heart stopped and the surgeon restarted it with open-heart massage. Even though she was fine, this major surgical procedure could have been prevented if the hospital had owned a heart defibrillator.[14]

By the 1960s, most cardiologists considered a defibrillator a necessary piece of medical equipment, and Memorial Hospital obtained one. After the machine arrived, it caught the attention of the *Casper Tribune-Herald*, which ran an article about training Juanita Kersting and Zora Lowe to move the machine around the hospital.[15] Approval for it had come through with the understanding that the local heart association would pay for half of the $1,200 cost.[16] Dr. Claude Beck had invented this machine in Cleveland in 1947 and first used it during surgery there.

At their January meeting in 1961, the Trustees approved a Medical Staff Research Committee to look at projects that might allow the hospital to be part of innovations that would benefit the citizens of the region. It created a process for competing for grants for research projects. The committee also provided a way to channel donations and bequests to the proper programs.[17]

The periodic Joint Commission on Accreditation of Hospitals inspection came on April 20 and 21, 1960. The reviewer found that the level of professionalism was high and recommended issuing an accreditation certificate for another three years.[18] As always happened before a JCAHO inspection, the institution spruced up and took stock of its assets and defects. Problems included the dangerous state of the oldest buildings. The building project called for demolition of the 1911 structure but did not deal with the other buildings. The big problem was how to take down the old hospital wing without disrupting vital hospital operations. In early 1961, the state fire marshal condemned the nurses' residence. Unable to decide on whether to purchase adjacent residences for housing nurses, they delayed demolition.

Acquisition of the remainder of the block began to take even greater precedence. The Trustees authorized the administrator to buy a house on the northwest corner of the block adjacent to the hospital which the County Commissioners had just purchased. Initially, after renovating it they hoped to rent it to an employee and perhaps use it for something else at a later date.[19]

As hospital physicians saw a growing number of welfare cases they asked for more space. The board offered them either the newly purchased house or space in the nurses' residence. They declined both offers, still hoping for space in the hospital basement, which still had not materialized by summer of 1961.[20]

By 1963, the Trustees delegated James Carr to run the bond election campaign. At the same time, Mr. Carr was trying to decide when and how to demolish the 1911 center section. He had a conference in early 1964 with Alan Fisher, the hospital architect since the 1950s. They were working on a plan to minimize the disruption of traffic created by new construction.

Many parts of the hospital operations, such as the kitchen, extended into the basement and first-floor sections of the old structure. One possible solution was building the new wing around the old one but at some point in the future they would still have to remove the old building. Fisher hired the engineering firm of Volk and Harrison to prepare a structural analysis. Emrick Huber, the city engineer, determined that the wood and brick construction made the building non-conforming for hospital use, meaning that it could not be salvaged and still meet new building codes. The report said, "We feel that this original center section has served its useful life expectancy."[21]

The nursery in the 1911 building was one of the most dangerous areas. During the height of the Baby Boom, hospital management realized that they needed to

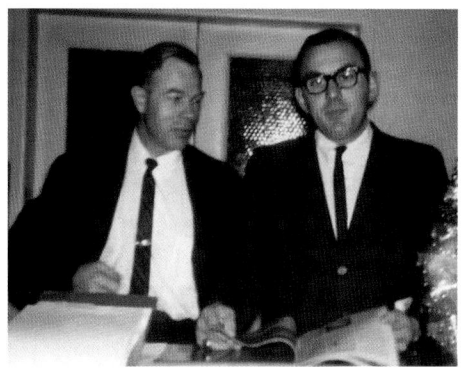

Dr. Don Mahnke and Dr. Louis Roussalis caught up on news while they checked on their patients.

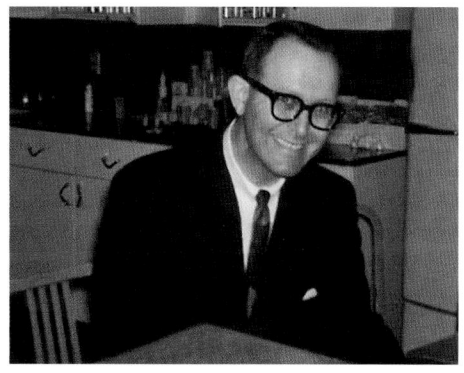

Dr. Martin Ellbogen, keeping his charts up to date.

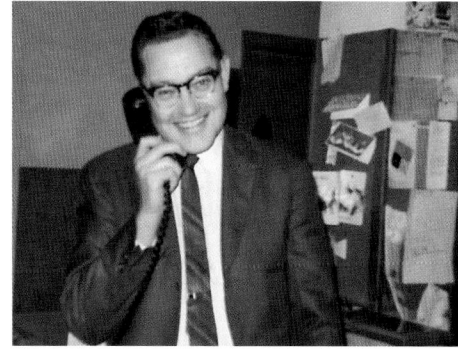

Dr. John Corbett checked his calls while visiting on the floor.

deal with these issues. Volk and Harrison consulted with Dr. Robert Fowler, head of Pediatrics, as well as obstetrician Dr. Walter Watson to determine what to do first. Code required the installation of steel beams to shore up the old construction, so as the boom tapered off in 1961, they began to look at other options.[22] Without funding, none were forthcoming.

As the hospital moved closer to holding the bond issue it looked at tapping money from the Hill-Burton Act. President Harry Truman's initiative, the Hill-Burton Act passed Congress in 1947. It granted capital improvement money to each state which then gave the money to public or private non-profit hospitals that agreed to be non-discriminatory and to provide free care for indigent patients for a period of twenty years after receiving the money.[23]

On February 12, 1964, the Wyoming State Health Department and U.S. Public Health Services toured Memorial Hospital to see if it was eligible for a grant. The evaluators agreed that the hospital was indeed a good candidate except for the old center section.[24] But since the architects were planning to replace it, the problem would solve itself.

The Hill-Burton Act free care requirement made it more important than ever to document patient demographics. In 1963, the hospital began charting where patients came from. Between 1961 and 1963, the percentage of out-of-county patients grew from 11.2 percent to 14.4 percent. Most came from towns within a hundred miles, with some towns contributing more than others. In July 1963, of 115 patients not from the county, twelve came from towns that had their own hospitals. Many of these patients came to see specialists.[25]

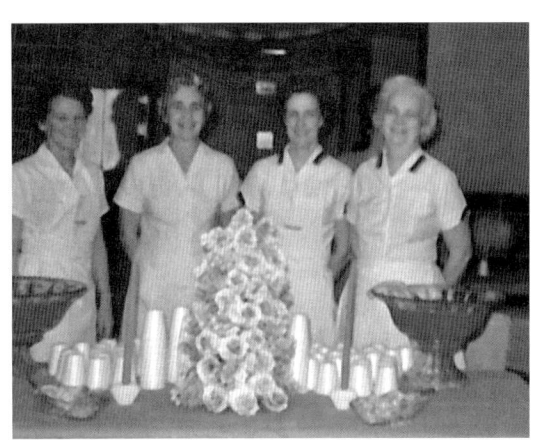

Each year, the Dietary Department held an appreciation party for the physicians at Christmas.

The increase in calls from patients and physicians outside of the county took a toll on emergency services. By 1962, the nine-year-old Pontiac ambulance had seen better days, so after considerable discussion the hospital purchased a new $8,417 Superior Pontiac ambulance. Stan Jourgensen, head of Ambulance Services, selected the vehicle's accessories.[26]

The focus shifted in the spring of 1964 from whether and when to do the bond election to how. James Carr continued to run the public relations campaign enlisting radio, television, and newspapers to get the word out. Physicians and dentists gave speeches and appeared in programs and in articles touting the building plans. The hospital developed an informational pamphlet and distributed 30,000 to community groups.[27] In response, the voters approved a $1.6-million bond fund that, combined with the Hill-Burton grant of $1 million, provided enough money to remove the 1911 center building and construct a six-story modern addition to the Memorial Hospital.

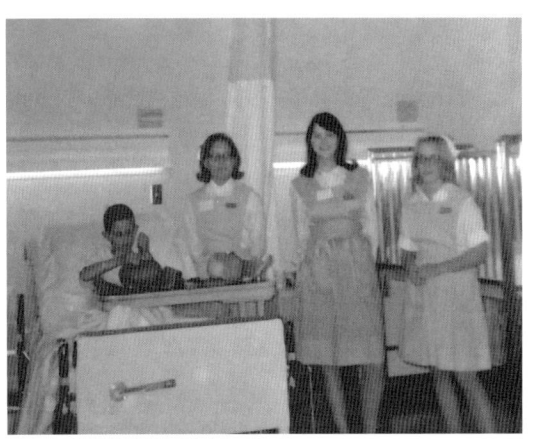

The Candy Stripers in 1968 helped the children in the pediatric ward celebrate Halloween.

Demolition of the 1911 building, coupled with new construction, made running the hospital complicated and messy, but employees and patients prevailed and on March 16, 1967, the six-story addition had its unveiling. There was considerable interest on the part of the general public in the new facility. The hospital offered well-attended tours, conducted by members of the Women's Auxiliary.

The *Casper Star-Tribune* wrote up a series of articles on opening day that detailed some of the internal changes. Nurses' stations were now in the center of a floor with patient rooms radiating off of them. Another article highlighted the new Labor and Delivery unit on the third floor. An article on the new Emergency Department noted that most patients came in between the hours of 4 and 7 p.m. and most came for treatment of injuries due to accidents. Radiology, run by Dr. Donald Jacobson with help from Dr. R. P. Mattson, Dr. Ronald Lund, and radiology technician Jerry Ressler, got its share of attention as a reporter described the Cobalt 60 Tele-Therapy unit. Construction innovations such as placing the building mechanical units in a special rooftop penthouse also intrigued the reporters. The articles documented the sheer volume of work required to run a hospital. The cafeteria served more than 600 meals per day, now on china rather than on steel plates. The snack shop served another 800 to 1,000 meals each day.[28]

All of the new technology came at a price. While Memorial Hospital budgeted for basics, they had to find outside sources for expensive or innovative items. These sources included bequests and grants and also came through the efforts of the Blue Envelope Health Fund.

The Blue Envelope Fund increasingly drew in a wide variety of people from the county's communities to raise money in door-to-door campaigns, by mail, and through large and small events. Schoolchildren saved their pennies and gave them to the program. Businessmen and housewives organized teas and lunches and bowling tournaments. The strength of the organization was that it gave virtually all it raised back to the local community, especially to Memorial Hospital and its programs.

Virtually all of the new heart monitoring equipment the hospital used came from Blue Envelope Health Fund grants. Cardiac monitors came in 1964. The Electronic Coronary Care unit in the new building received most of its funding from the Blue Envelope Fund.[29] Perhaps the biggest piece of equipment was the Magnascanner that used radioisotopes to make clear images of organs to help detect cancers.

Throughout the 1960s, Blue Envelope continued to provide support to the Strep Throat Screening Program. The hospital provided the lab analysis of all throat culture samples taken in county schools. Volunteers swabbed children's throats and then placed the samples on round covered plates that had been prepared with a mixture of agar culture and sheep's blood. JoAnn Taylor, R.N. prepared 500 to 600 blood agar culture plates per week during the school year. Area sheep men Joe Donlin, Percy Cooper, and G. G. Nicolaysen donated the sheep, which boarded at Keith Doing and James Baker's veterinary clinic. Every week the veterinarians worked with physicians to draw blood to make the agar culture medium. The Health Fund paid for all materials and even to board the sheep.[30] Matching funds came from the United States Department of Public Health. By 1968, the *Casper Star-Tribune* could report "Rheumatic Fever 'Stamped Out' in Natrona County."[31]

> *While Memorial Hospital budgeted for basics, they had to find outside sources for expensive or innovative items.*

Innovations in cancer treatments saved more lives each year. Surgery and radiation had been the mainstays of treatment, but in the early 1960s, chemotherapy became an experimental but promising approach. The Damon Runyon Foundation, in 1960, donated $5,000 to Memorial Hospital of Natrona County to create a cancer treatment room and provided experimental drugs for terminal patients. This collaboration of the Natrona County Health Fund with the Runyon Foundation, under the supervision of Dr. George Knapp, put the hospital in the forefront of cancer care in the region. The first patient to receive treatment under the program was Veronica Schuster of Edgerton and by 1963 fifty-one patients had gone through the program.[32] Over 650 patients had received treatment by 1965.

The Central Wyoming Counseling Center was the other agency to receive Blue Envelope funds. It provided psychological counseling and conducted an extensive mental health public education program.[33]

One of the agencies that collaborated with the Blue Envelope Fund and the hospital was the City of Casper-Natrona County Health Department. From its inception and through the 1960s, it had offices in the hospital or in adjoining buildings.

The same volunteerism that made the Blue Envelope Fund so successful also made the Auxiliary an important asset for the hospital. Many of the women were members of both groups. This was an era when most middle- and upper-class married women did not pursue careers. Instead they gave back to their communities

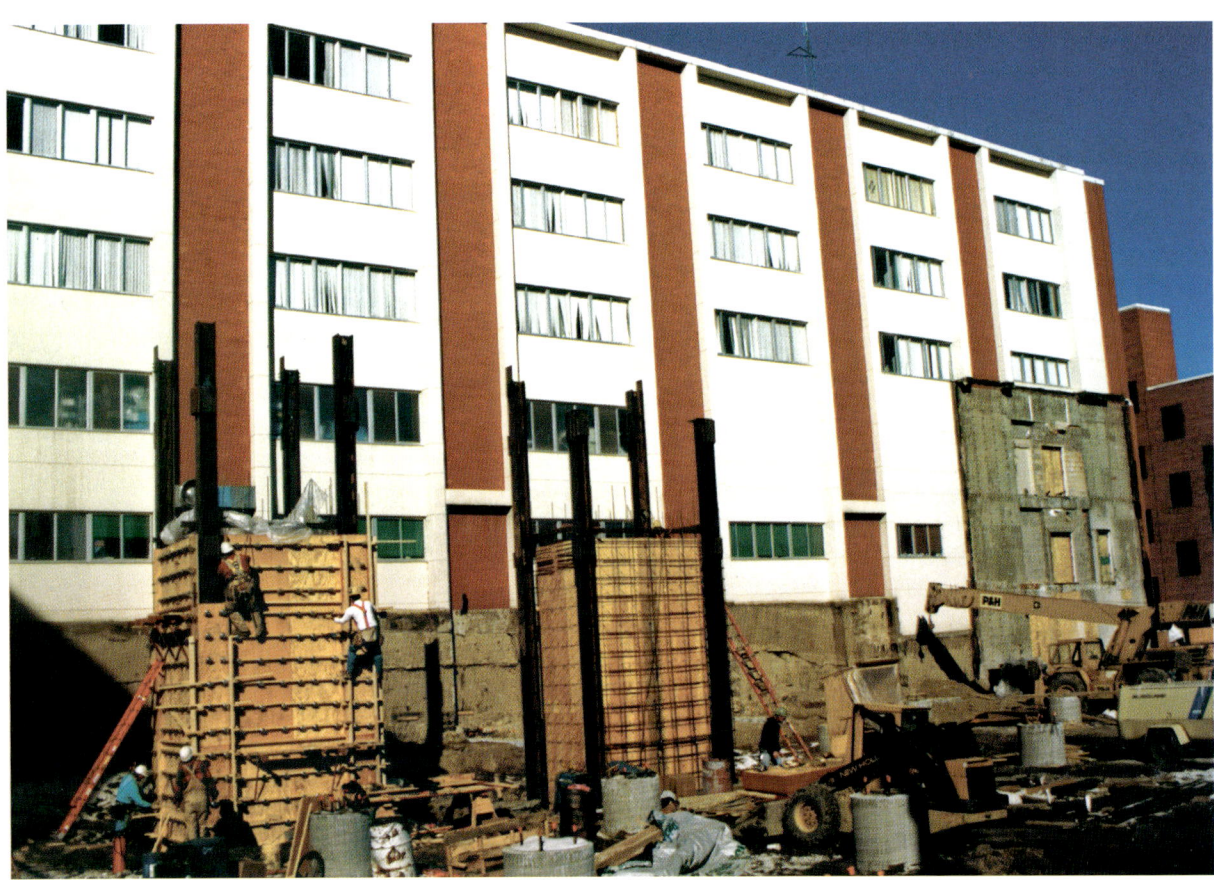

This 1997 view shows the east side of the 1967 six-story addition.

through church or community work. Each year during the 1960s, the Auxiliary members gave thousands of hours of work in the same traditional areas they had functioned in since the 1950s. They also encouraged young women to volunteer through the Candy Striper program.

Mae Reeb was an early president of the Auxiliary. She had grown up in Pennsylvania, where her mother served as a nurse. After marriage she moved to Kansas with her family and then, in 1942, to Casper. When the Women's Auxiliary formed, she joined and became one of its leaders. Her only son James became first a Presbyterian minister and later a minister in the Unitarian Universalist Church. On March 11, 1965, James Reeb died after being beaten during a civil rights march in Selma, Alabama.[34] His family dedicated a room at Memorial Hospital in the name of James and Mae Reeb to commemorate her contribution to the hospital and his to humanity. The hospital also named the chapel after James Reeb.

The Reeb family donated money to dedicate a hospital room to Mae Reeb and her son Reverend James Reeb.

As the decade of the 1960s ended, people had accomplished a great deal but there was much yet to be done. The new decade of the 1970s would not be so challenging or tumultuous.

THE 1970s: THE DECADE OF TECHNOLOGICAL ADVANCES

For years, patients experiencing kidney failure had traveled to the University of Colorado Hospital in Denver for dialysis treatment. In May 1970, Mr. Carr announced that a donor wanted to give the funds for a dialysis machine. Operating costs for a dialysis center were high, so the Trustees were not sure the program could pay for itself.[35] Matters came to a head in July when CU Hospital announced that it would no longer accept Wyoming patients since they could not continue to absorb the $23,000 cost of treating a patient for a year.[36] Memorial Hospital's management then moved to reconsider the situation.

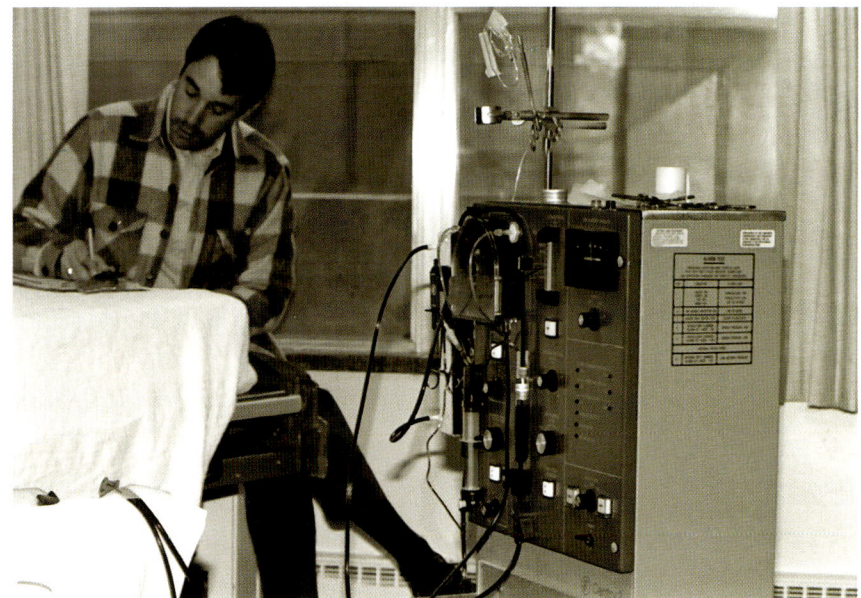

Dr. David Kahn charts a patient's progress in the dialysis unit.

The donor was Fred Goodstein, an oil and gas man who had lived in Casper since 1922. Originally from Denver, Goodstein started out in the scrap metal business but made his fortune by purchasing oilfields and making them profitable. By the end of his career, he and his wife Babe had built a fortune estimated to be $300 to $500 million. The Goodstein family began to give money back to Casper, donating a million dollars to Casper College to establish the Goodstein

CHAPTER FIVE ❖ *From Memorial Hospital of Natrona County to Wyoming Medical Center: 1960 TO 1986* 73

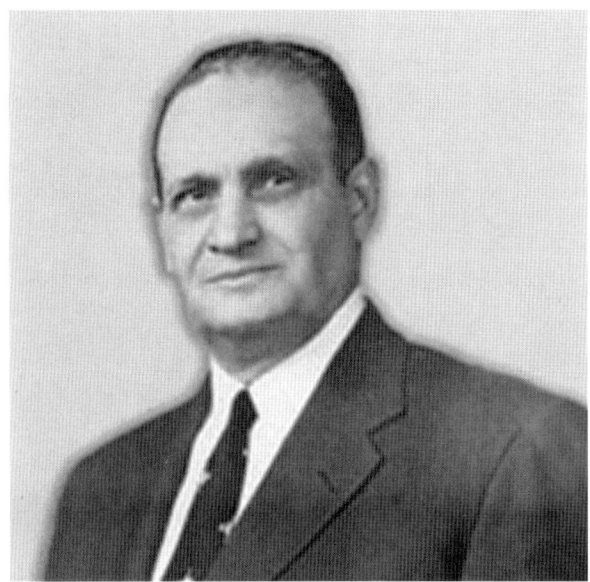

Fred Goodstein was an oil and gas developer who was one of Casper's major philanthropists. He and his wife Babe gave millions to hospitals, the arts, and education.

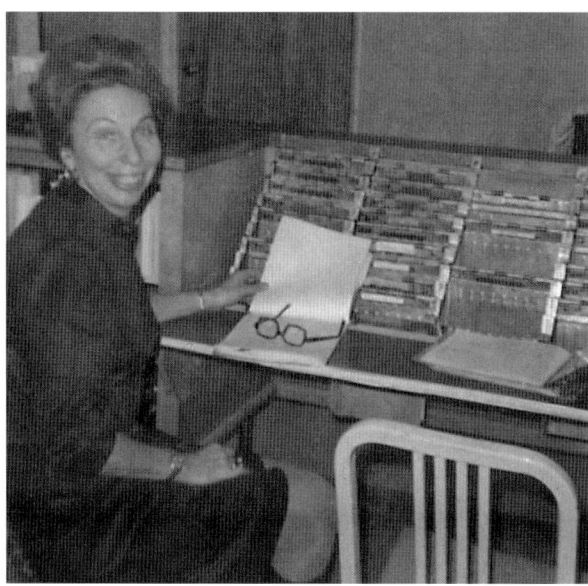

Dr. Bernice Elkin was a psychiatrist at Memorial Hospital of Natrona County for fifteen years. *Wyoming Medical Center collection*.

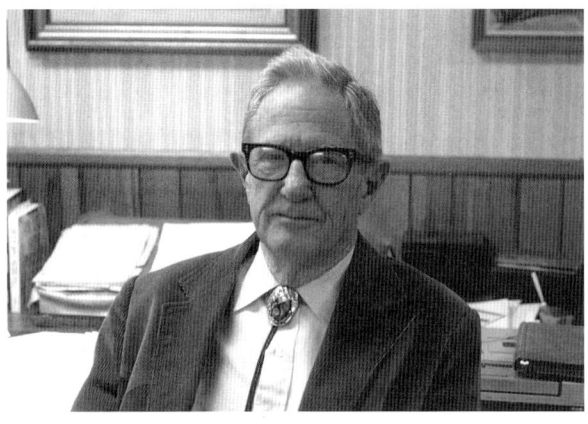

Dr. Phillip Gordy was a neurosurgeon at Memorial Hospital of Natrona County from 1973 to 1984, then established the Rehabilitation Center at the hospital.

Foundation. Grants from the Goodstein Foundation sustained numerous other community programs.[37] Goodstein later gave money for a cancer center at the hospital and to set up a hospice program. In Denver, he donated to General Rose Memorial Hospital.[38]

Memorial Hospital of Natrona County entered the computer age in the spring of 1971 when it acquired IBM computers. Most computers had about sixteen kilobytes of memory and were used for word processing and for accounting. The hospital used these first machines for keeping accounts and patient records. Personnel went to Denver to train at the IBM headquarters.[39]

The hospital's oldest X-ray therapy unit, purchased in the 1940s, was finally dying. New equipment was expensive, so in November the Trustees authorized purchase of a newer used machine from DePaul Hospital in Cheyenne at a cost of $5,000. DePaul was no longer offering X-ray therapy and so was selling the unit.[40]

When Dr. Kent Christensen requested the latest in endoscopic tools for the diagnosis and treatment of cancer, the Blue Envelope Fund purchased them. The Fund also assisted Memorial Hospital by purchasing a second lung ventilator.[41]

The strep throat program continued with the involvement of the Northern Wyoming Streptococcal Laboratory at the hospital. To honor John Tripeny, Jr., one of the Blue Envelope founders who had died earlier in the year, the hospital, in March 1971, renamed the lab the John Tripeny, Jr. Streptococcal Control Center. The center processed about 1,000 throat cultures a day from schools throughout northeastern Wyoming.[42]

One of the hospital's dentists, Dr. L. J. Williams, set up a program called Dr. Dial, where pre-recorded telephone messages gave callers advice on caring for their teeth. In March 1971, in conjunction with a program on good brushing, local pharmacies distributed toothbrushes and other dental supplies.[43]

The spring of 1971 was the end of an era. Dr. Brendan Phibbs, the cardiologist who had spearheaded the strep throat program, left for a year to teach in Arizona. The University of Arizona Medical School had appointed him as an associate professor of cardiology as well as the director of the Heart Station at University Hospital.[44] Dr. Phibbs did not return to Casper.

In 1972, a group of businessmen proposed a new competing private ambulance service. The hospital Trustees figured a private service couldn't compete financially with their publicly funded one; however, this prompted discussion of the need to update the hospital's ambulances.[45] In early 1973, Mr. Carr presented the Trustees with specifications for a van-type ambulance at an estimated cost of $11,000. They voted to replace the 1962 station wagon-style ambulance with the newer model.[46]

In 1973, the Organization of Arab Petroleum Exporting Countries embargoed oil shipments to the United States. A variety of political and economic factors led to the boycott which had a dual effect on Casper and Natrona County. While there was gas rationing, a recession, and inflation, there was also increased need for Wyoming oil. This caused a boom in the region's economy, bringing in new residents, businesses, and an improved tax base. Voters approved a 1-percent sales tax that paid for a new event center, a new museum building, an addition to the city hall, new fire stations, and a parking garage for the hospital. It also allowed the city to balance its budget.[47]

The newest boom was a mixed blessing for Memorial Hospital of Natrona County. People gave more generously to the Blue Envelope Drive or gave directly to the hospital for equipment and programs. It also meant an increased patient load and extended periods when the hospital operated at maximum capacity.

In the 1960s, the hospital had set up a blood bank in conjunction with the Cheyenne-based Blood System of Wyoming. The system was part of the larger Southwest Blood Bank of Phoenix, Arizona. On average, the hospital used thirty pints of blood per day in transfusions and during surgery. In the late 1960s, the hospital offered a hospital credit of ten dollars for each blood donation.[48]

By 1973, there was a growing concern that blood purchase programs threatened the nation's blood supplies. An increase in hepatitis cases had caused many hospitals to set up volunteer blood donor programs. Now Memorial Hospital was working on a plan of its own. Of the 1,400 pints of blood collected in 1972, only about 625 came from volunteer donors from Natrona County who had to go to the hospital laboratory to give blood. A speakers' bureau of doctors, nurses, and community leaders involved in health care issues promoted the idea of volunteer donation. By the end of 1973, the hospital hoped to only use local blood supplies for the bulk of its blood products.[49]

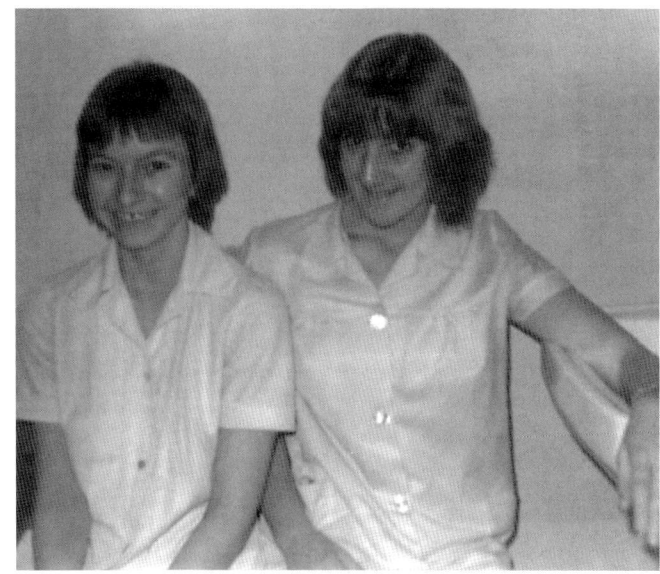

Eileen Dryer and Nancy Edelman were in nurses' training in 1974.

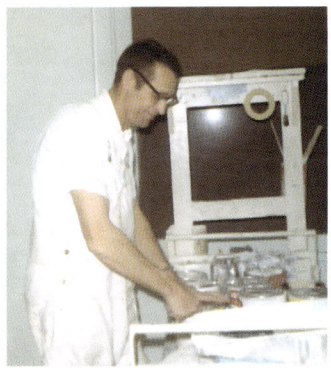
There was much behind-the-scenes work that kept the hospital running. Here the carpenter works in a patient room.

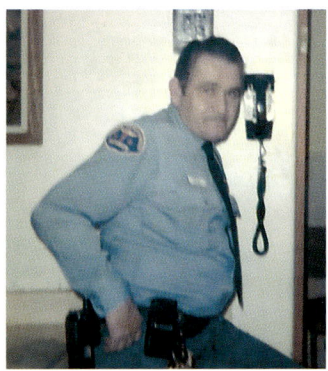
Hans Wisk was a guard assigned to deal with the rare security problem.

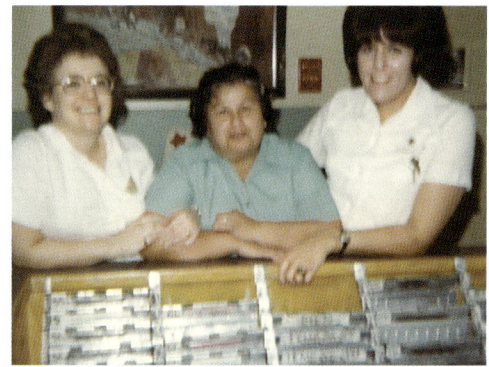
Charts stored at the nurses' station wait for further updating.

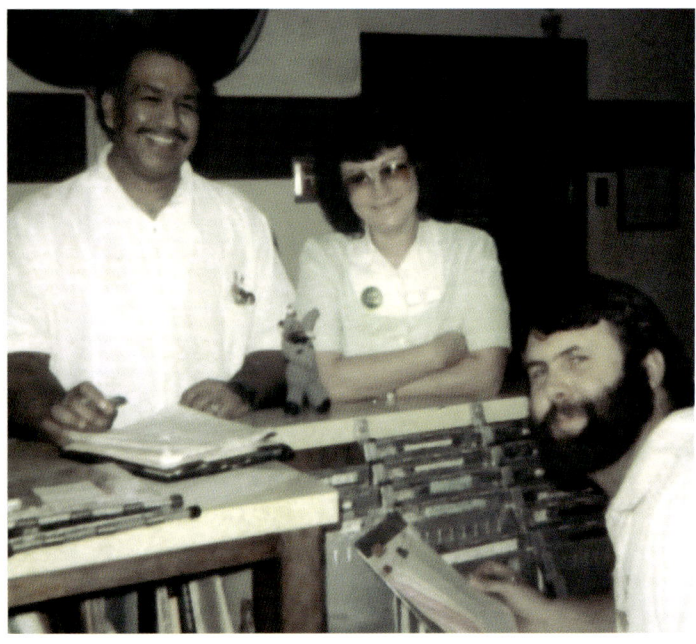
Jess Palato, Dix Edwards, and Jim Harold compare notes while waiting for further duties at the nurses' station.

The Blue Envelope Fund set up a Blood Assurance Program to assist in recruiting donors. Area clubs like Mothers of Twins asked parents to donate a pint every six months. This was a variant on the paid program since each donor family got a hospital credit against the cost of future blood needs.[50]

By 1974, Memorial Hospital had the best-equipped radiology center in the state. The *Casper Star-Tribune* documented the advances in X-ray technology including Dr. Roger Mattson's pioneering detection of joint injuries that had brought the science of athrography to the institution. This used X-rays to diagnose joint problems, many related to sports activities. Dr. Ronald Lund, who was chief of staff in 1974, used nuclear medicine to diagnose cancers.[51] Dr. Phillip Gordy was the only neurologist in Wyoming.

On February 8, 1975, the hospital and the Blue Envelope Fund collaborated on a Health Fair held at Casper College. Specialists provided health screenings, nurses immunized children and adults, and educational exhibits taught people about medical issues such as heart disease or cancer prevention. The fair focused on prevention, an area of health care that was gaining prominence in the 1970s. Prevention programs, such as the fair, encouraged patients to take more responsibility for their health rather than waiting to become ill to deal with a problem. This approach to medicine was a dramatic change from older approaches to health care where the doctor was the ultimate expert. Now patients had not just the right but the responsibility to take pre-emptive steps to stay healthy.[52]

At the end of 1975, James Carr, Jr., administrator since 1953, announced that he planned to retire after the first of the year. Carr's decision marked the end of twenty-three years of leadership. Carr had led numerous building campaigns including the

1967 six-floor addition. He had helped modernize staffing including recruiting a new generation of physicians. He encouraged use of new technology and new techniques. Mostly, he collaborated with regional governments and medical centers to increase the hospital's role in regional medicine. Finally, he gave both the public and employees a sense of stability through his leadership and his visibility.

James Carr's replacement was Lewis Spencer. He was the first administrator formally trained in hospital management. Spencer led the Memorial Hospital of Natrona County for four years, dying of cancer in 1980.[53]

In November 1975, William Barton, who had served on the Memorial Hospital of Natrona County board since 1970, died of cancer. He was a Casper native who was a veteran of World War II and a graduate of Yale Law School who had helped found the United Fund in Casper.[54] The Board of Trustees, on January 27, 1976, appointed Michael J. Sullivan to replace Barton. Sullivan, another Casper attorney, served on the board until he took up his term as Wyoming's governor in 1987. At the same meeting in January, the Trustees presented James Carr with a plaque recognizing his "outstanding leadership" for his twenty-three years as hospital administrator.[55]

The legacy of another former administrator came back to the hospital in the form of an unusual donation. Violet Dennis was the daughter of Mary Anne Eschwig Wiley, R.N., who had been the superintendent from 1926 to 1939. Dennis and her family gave an incubator to the nursery in her mother's memory.[56]

In 1976, hospital Trustees, community leaders, and members of Blue Envelope joined together to create the Memorial Hospital of Natrona County Foundation. Community leaders who led this effort were typical of the intersections of interest

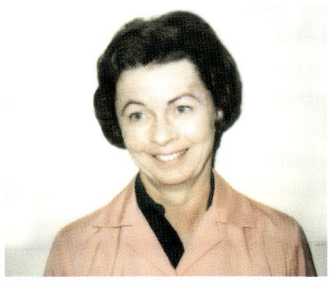

The 1976 Auxiliary president wears the trademark salmon-colored jacket.

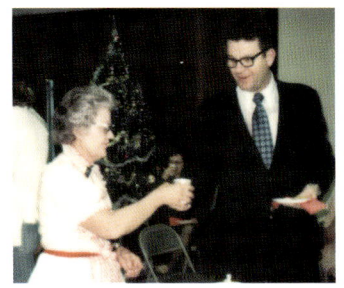

Lewis Spencer (right), Memorial Hospital of Natrona County administrator from 1976 to 1980, visits at a hospital gathering.

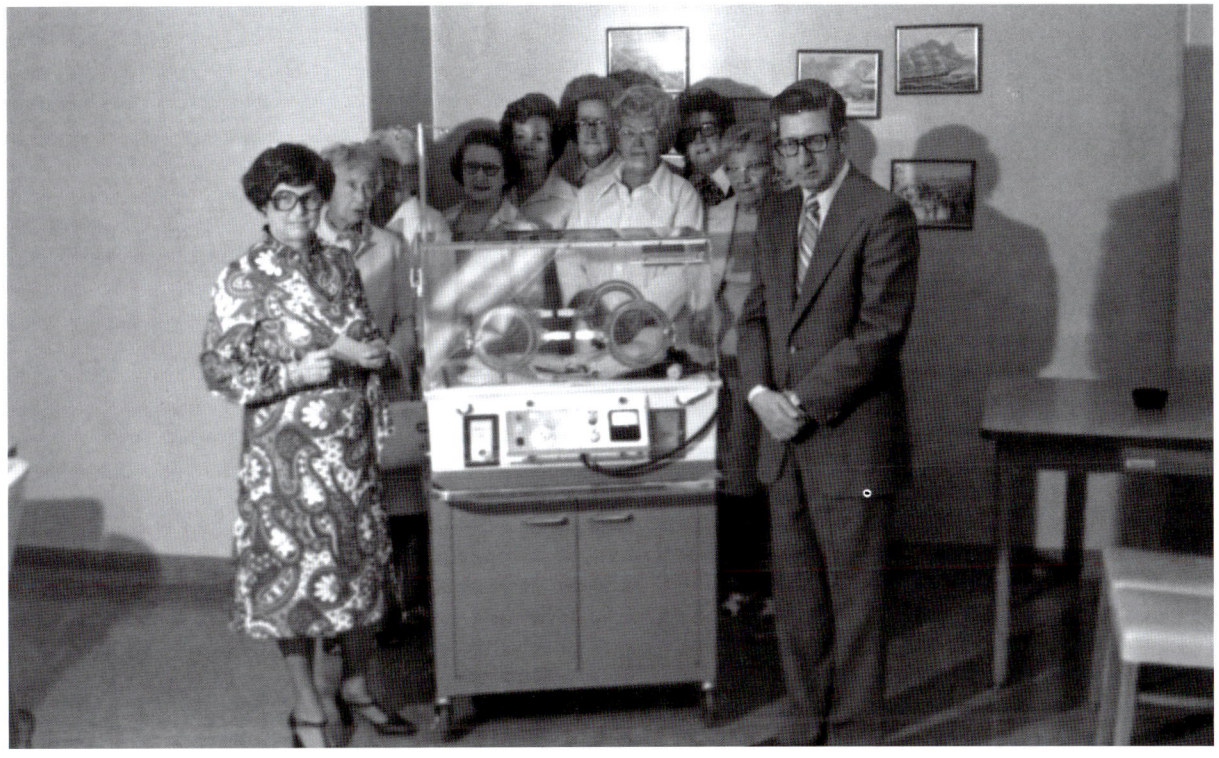

Violet Dennis (left), the daughter of Mary Anne Eschwig Wiley, R.N., and her family gave an incubator to the nursery in her mother's memory.

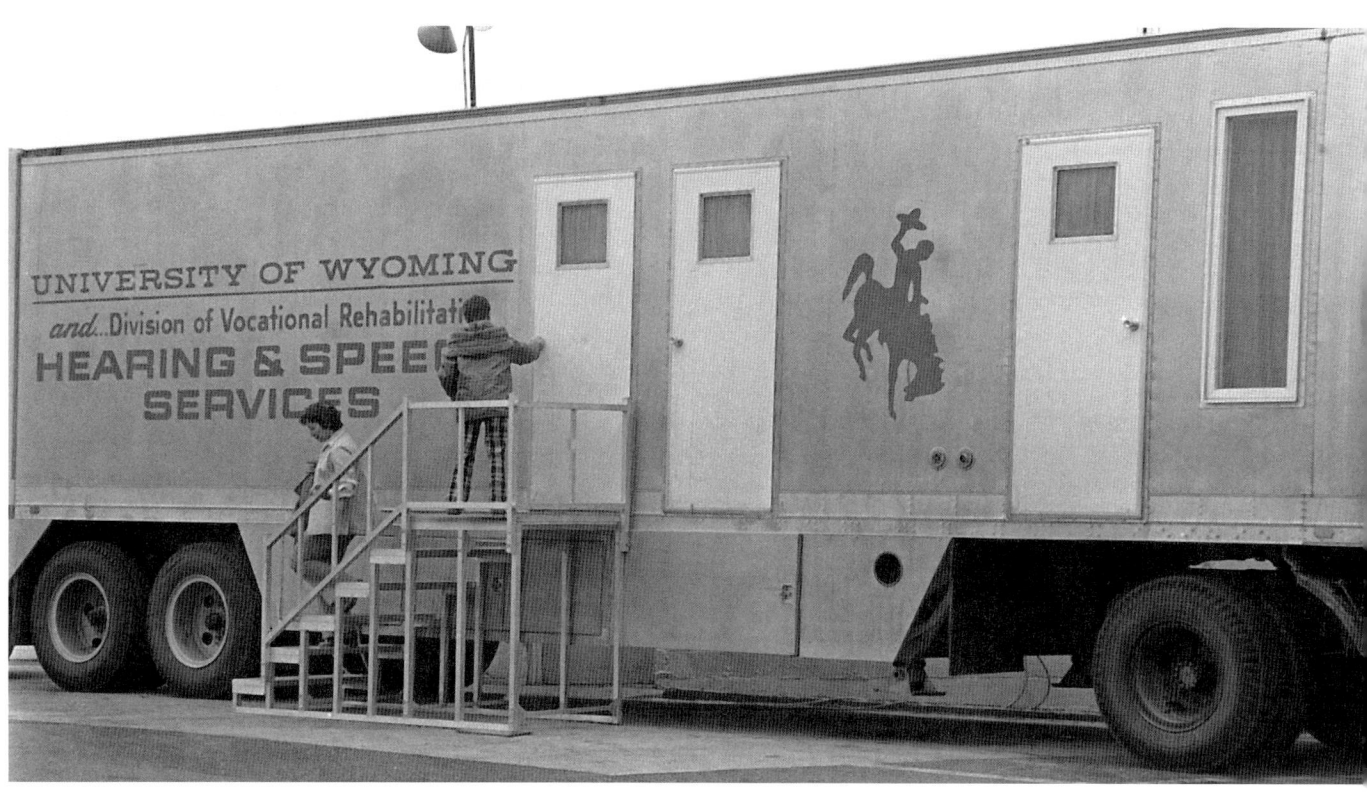

The Cleft Palate Clinic was a joint venture of Memorial Hospital of Natrona County, the Wyoming State Health Department, and the University of Wyoming.

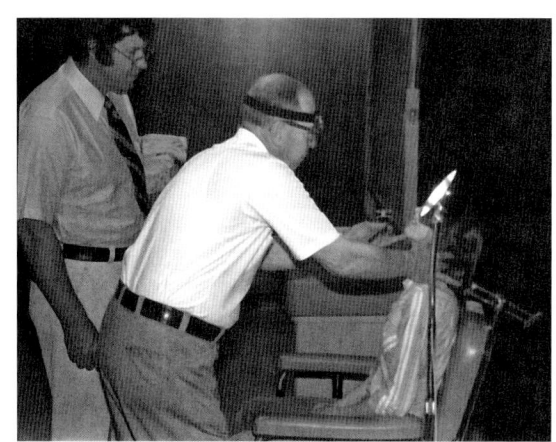

Dr. Hudgel and Dr. Slayler were visiting patients at the Cleft Palate Clinic in Casper.

in the county. The Browns, Lathrops, Hemrys, and Coopers were old-time ranching families. The Meenans represented not only the Casper Irish but were part of the intersection of law and politics. Dick Bostwick, Darrell Satterfield, and Dick Sedar came out of the business community. More women began to take on leadership roles including Virginia Lathrop, who was a member of Dr. Homer Lathrop's family. Her relative Jean Lathrop had been the first woman to serve on the Memorial Hospital board. Trula Cooper had worked with the strep throat program and she would later serve on the hospital board. Kathleen Hemry, high school teacher and historian, was a volunteer at Memorial Hospital. This organization channeled donations, held fundraising events, and supported the hospital through community contacts. It further knit Memorial Hospital to the community and the region. The Memorial Hospital Trustees president chaired the Foundation board. The chief of staff and a representative from the Blue Envelope Fund also helped govern the organization.[57]

Cardiology became a hospital specialty when in September 1976, Dr. Wesley Hiser arrived in Casper to set up his cardiology practice. Over time, cancer diagnosis and treatment became another specialty for the hospital as it attracted physicians who specialized in cancer treatment. Additionally, the Blue Envelope Fund's focus on cancer prevention meant that there was money available to purchase equipment.

In the mid-1970s, the hospital was ready to purchase a Computerized Tomographic (CT) scanner.[58] Throughout 1977, they looked at a scanner made by Philips Medical Systems of Shelton, Connecticut. Philips had begun producing its new CT scanners and had already shipped some to Europe as well as placed one in the hospital in New Haven, Connecticut, and another in Chicago. When Casper got theirs it was number twenty-one. One advantage of the machine was that it scanned in fifteen to sixteen seconds, producing good quality pictures.[59] The Philips CT scanner finally arrived in 1978, funded by $42,500 from the Blue Envelope Fund and the remaining $352,500 from the Foundation.

On April 27, 1978, the hospital dedicated the William Barton Memorial Computerized Tomographic Center. Dr. Ronald Lund, chief of Radiology, explained the benefits of the CT scanner to a gathering of local dignitaries and the interested public. According to Dr. Lund, the machine looked into the body's tissues and gave a three-dimensional picture of normally hidden features. This gave physicians a non-invasive way to diagnose a patient's problems.[60] By the summer of 1978, the laboratory performed an average of five scans as day. Eighty-five percent were brain scans.[61]

At the same time that the hospital was dedicating the scanner, it received a gift to purchase a Siemens Medical Laboratories Mevatron XII linear accelerator for the cancer center. The donation came from Fred Goodstein and his brother J. M. Goodstein through the Goodstein Foundation.[62] The linear accelerator used Cobalt radiation to kill cancerous tissue. Its most innovative quality was that the patient stayed stationary while the machine moved around, hitting the tumor from all sides in very concentrated doses. The images supplied by the CT scanner allowed the radiologist to know precisely where to aim the radiation. Dr. Lund noted that there was a new cancer specialist, Dr. Carol Fellows, who had come to the hospital in 1977 to direct treatments. Memorial Hospital now had a perfect combination of expertise and equipment for treating cancer. Before the cancer center could open a number of federal and local agencies needed to approve the donation. The hospital also had to renovate the Radiology Department to make room for the accelerator.[63]

> *On April 27, 1978, the hospital dedicated the William Barton Memorial Computerized Tomographic Center.*

In 1977, to explain these innovations to the public, the hospital hired journalist Elaine Hough to run the Marketing Department. One of her first initiatives was to produce the institution's first hospital newsletter. *Outreach*, later called *Hi-Lites* and then *High Lights*, documented the daily life as well as the major accomplishments of Memorial Hospital. Hough was a native of Buffalo, Wyoming, who had received her journalism degree from the University of Colorado in Boulder. Before coming to the hospital she was a reporter and editor at the *Casper Star-Tribune*.[64]

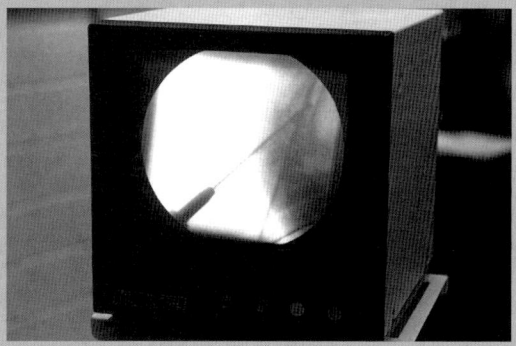
The fluoroscopy machine generated the image seen on this screen.

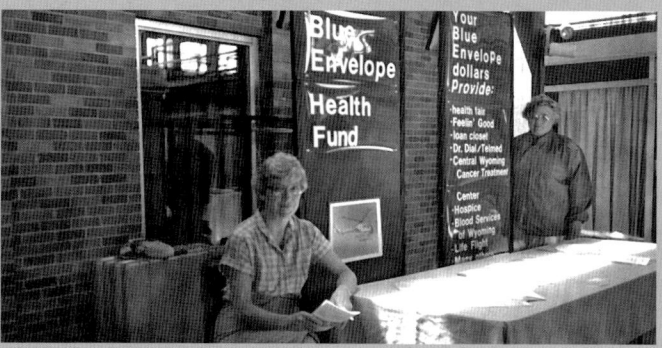
This Blue Envelope volunteer was soliciting contributions during the 1977 campaign.

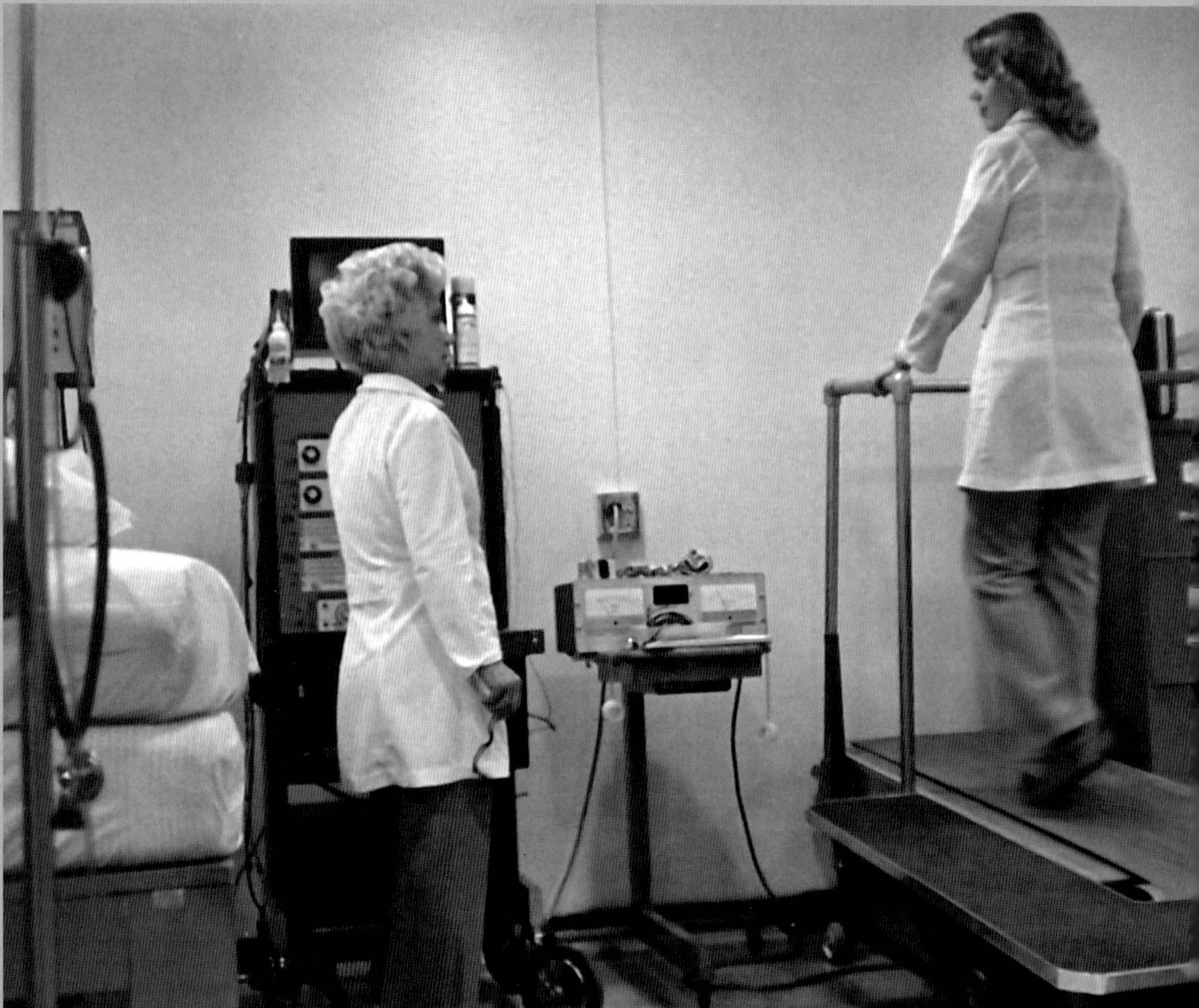

Hospital staff demonstrate the heart station treadmill.

80 *Wyoming Medical Center:* A CENTENNIAL HISTORY

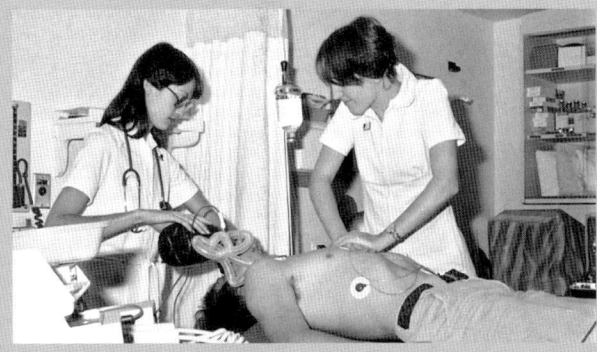
Nursing students practice cardiopulmonary resuscitation.

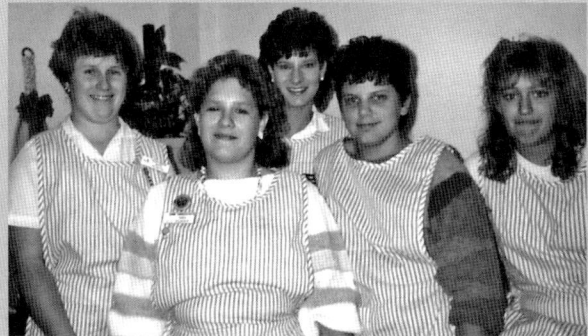
These are some of the 1970s Candy Striper volunteers.

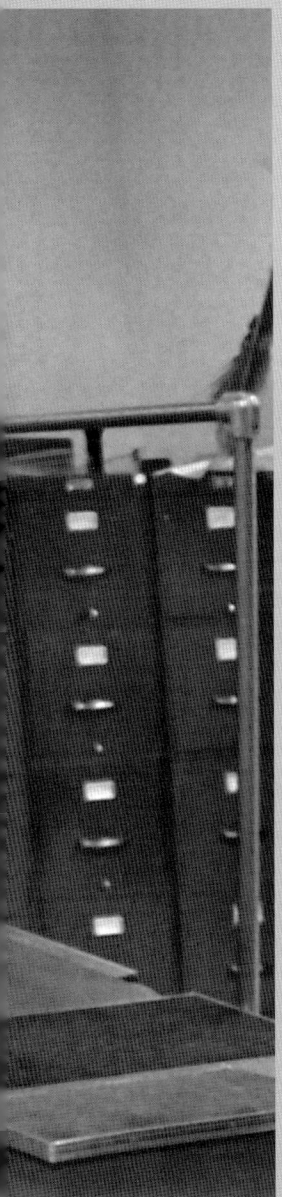
The C Arm fluoroscopy amplifier, an X-ray technology, provided clear images of soft body tissue.

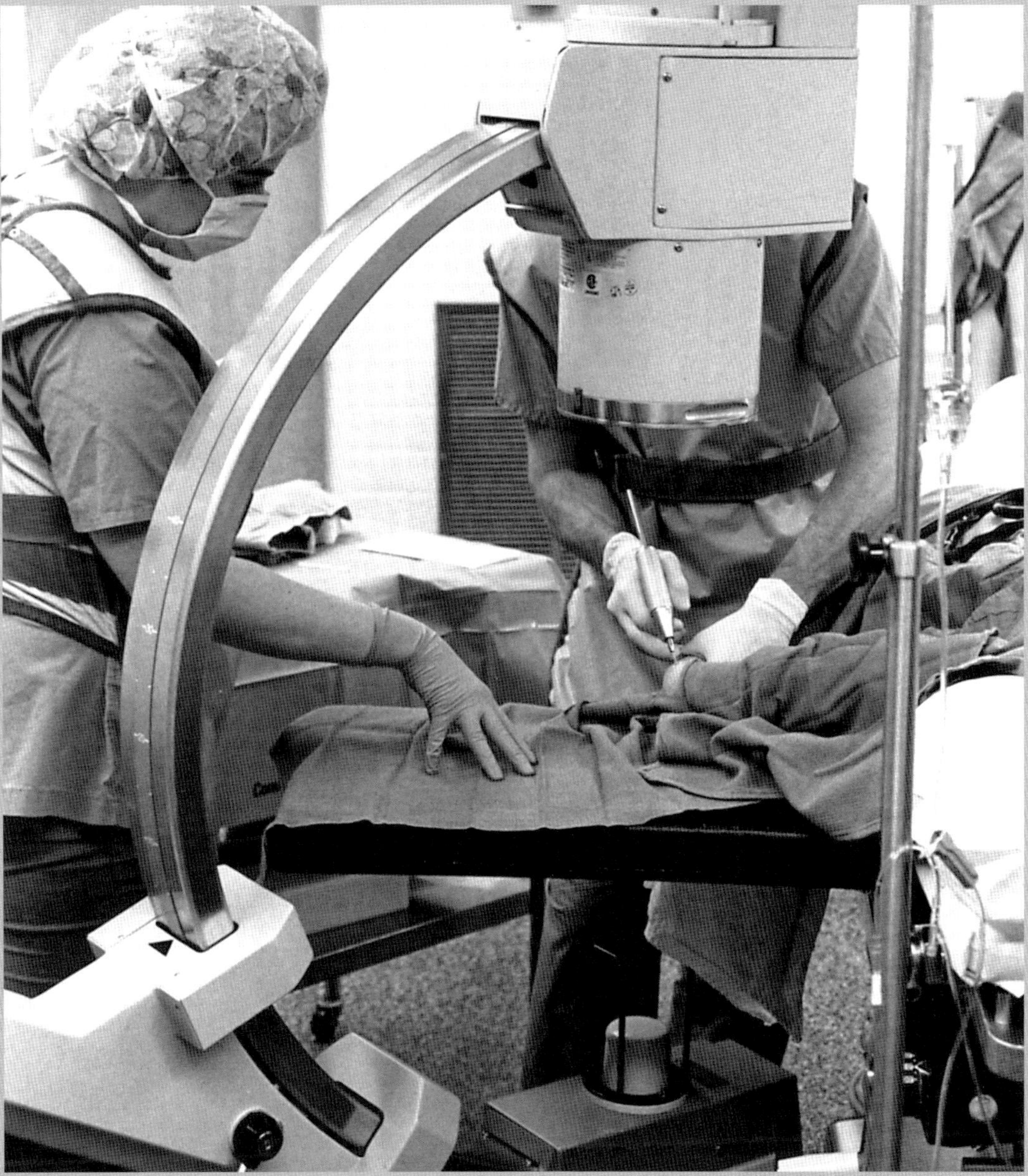

CHAPTER FIVE ❖ *From Memorial Hospital of Natrona County to Wyoming Medical Center:* 1960 TO 1986 81

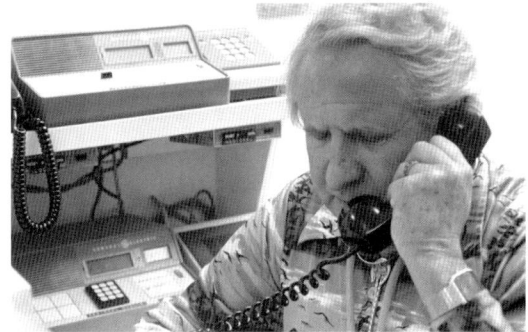

Dr. Cleve Beller, head of Emergency Services at the hospital, receives an emergency call.

The hospital continued to focus on training the next generation of hospital professionals. This time, in July 1977, they developed a collaborative program to train physical therapists. The University of Puget Sound had a physical therapy training program that wanted to work with the hospital to provide oversight of clinicals.[65]

Medical research in the 1970s proved that smoking was implicated in many diseases including cardio-vascular problems, lung cancer, and oral cancer. Researchers found that nicotine was dangerous to a fetus so urged expectant mothers give up smoking, at least while pregnant. Later research began to link second-hand smoke to childhood illnesses and allergies.

Based on this research, the administration, in November 1977, decided to stop selling cigarettes and other tobacco materials in the hospital. By January 1978, they had also banned smoking in most areas of the building, setting up designated smoking zones. They felt they were serving as role models to the community as well as looking out for the health of patients and employees.[66]

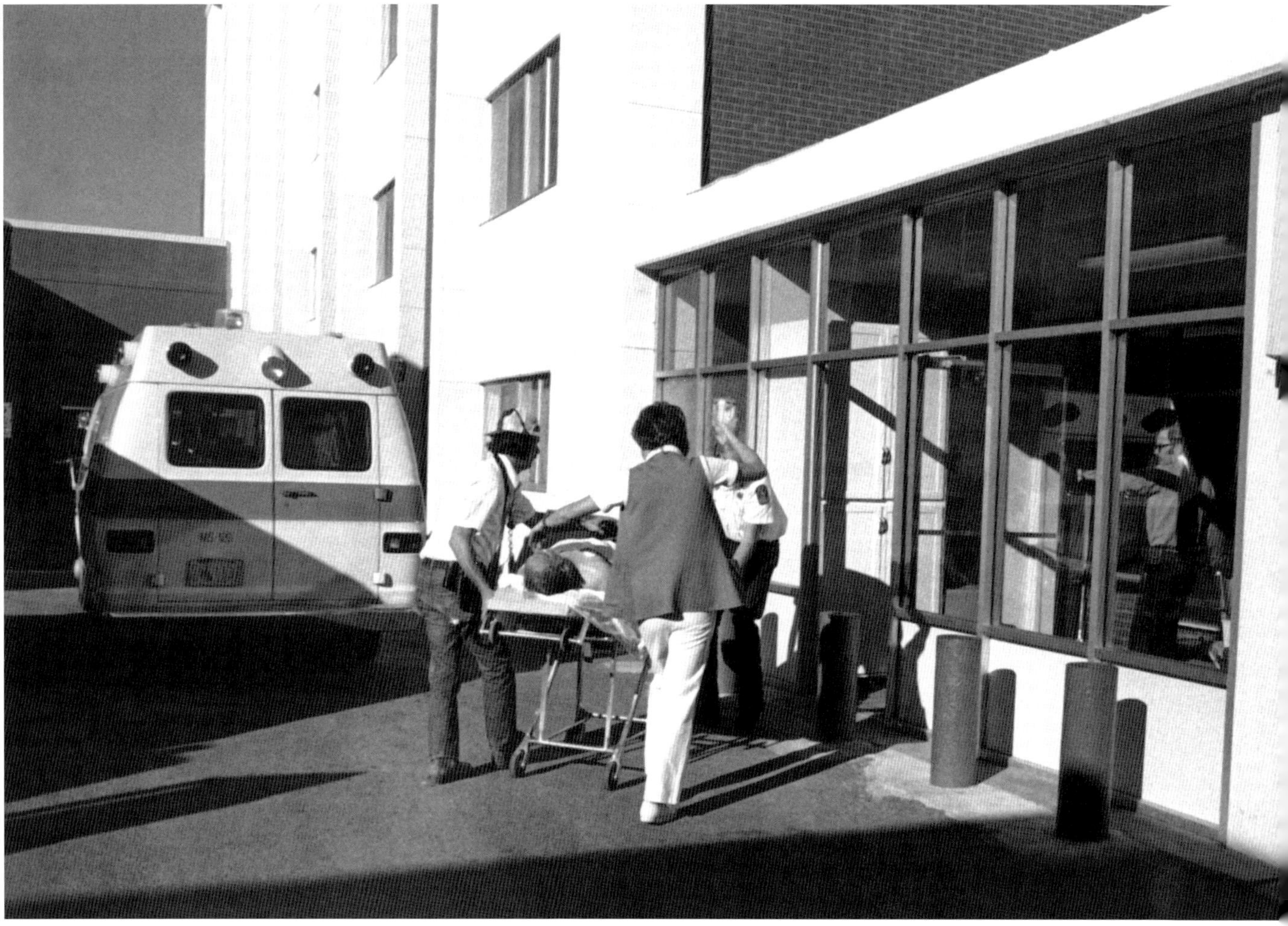

A patient arrives at the emergency entrance at Memorial Hospital of Natrona County in 1977.

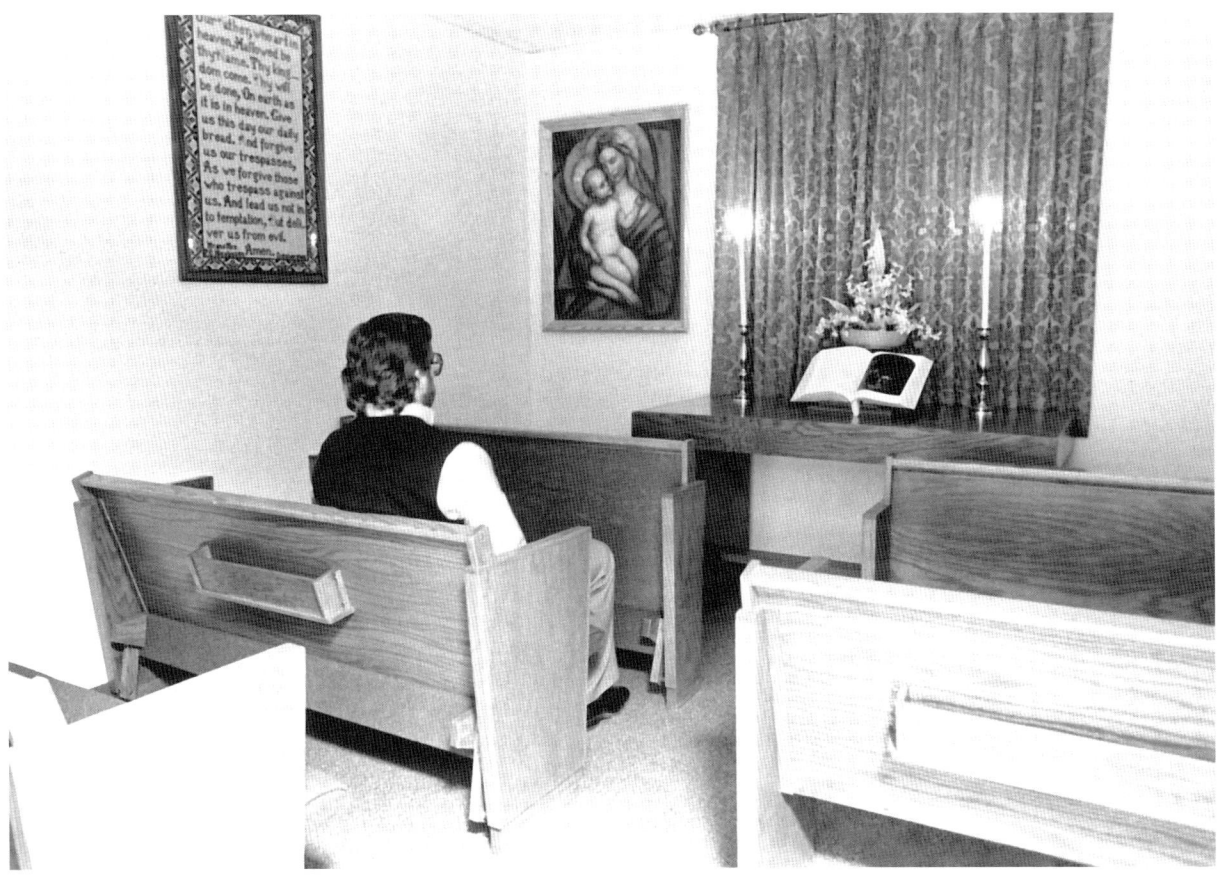

The hospital chapel bore the name of slain minister James Reeb. Hospital chapels gave visitors a space for prayer and meditation.

The Auxiliary marked its twenty-fifth anniversary in 1978. Now referred to as the "Pink Ladies," they continued to provide thousands of hours of service each year to the hospital. The anniversary provided an opportunity to reflect back on the origins of the program in 1953 and to look at the progress both the Auxiliary and Memorial Hospital of Natrona County had made in the quarter-decade that had just passed. Events included a blood drive among Auxiliary members, the revival of the Candy Striper program that had been so popular in the 1960s, and a new volunteer information station near the Intensive Care Unit (ICU)/Critical Care Unit (CCU).[67]

The broader interpretation of its mission that the hospital developed in the 1970s taxed the physical plant in many ways. The administration now had to face one issue that had been unresolved for many years: the hospital needed more parking. In late 1978, the board moved to start planning for a parking structure based on the One Cent Sales Tax program and revenues that would be available upon completion of the Natrona County Health building.[68] The new parking building would stand on the southeast corner of Third and Conwell streets and would have 487 parking spaces. It would have reserved spots for physician parking as well as parking for visitors and patients. In February 1979, the process began that would produce the parking garage by June 1980.[69]

The City of Casper-Natrona County Health Department building opened in May 1979 in a new building near the hospital. The structure allowed for consolidation of a number of programs that had been housed at Memorial Hospital:

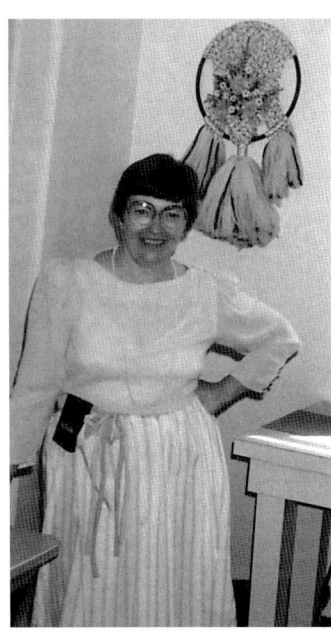

Elaine Hough became the head of Marketing and Public Relations at the hospital in 1977.

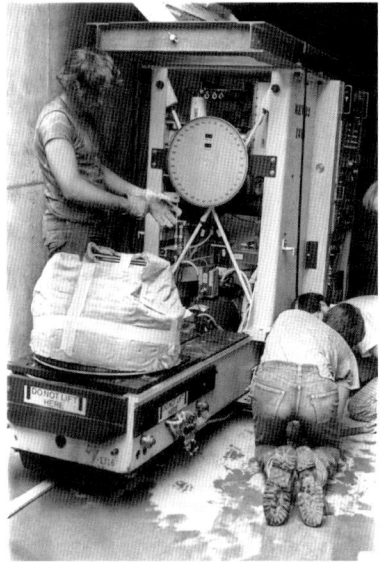
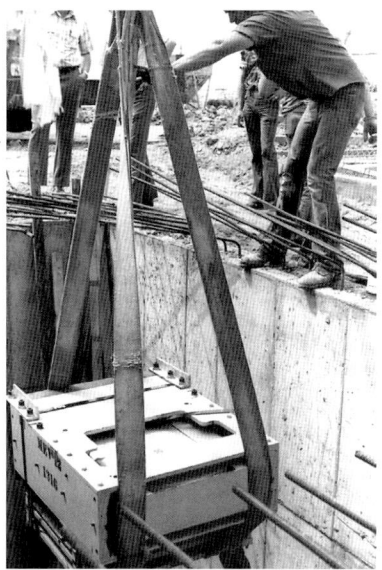

The cancer center got a linear accelerator in 1978. These photos show workers installing the accelerator radioactive core.

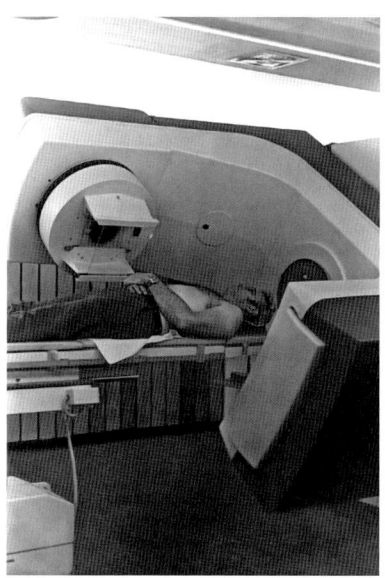

This is the linear accelerator as it looked set up in the hospital cancer center.

some that were public health programs, and others that were hospital programs. These included the Central Wyoming Counseling Center, Memorial Hospital data processing, the Pharmacy Clerkship Program, and United Blood Services of Wyoming. The Blue Envelope Fund also had offices in the new building. When the Health Department moved, the strep throat laboratory moved as well.[70] This freed space and personnel within the hospital building to address the issues of the 1980s.

1980 TO 1986: THE HOSPITAL TAKES WING

Since the United States Supreme Court had upheld a woman's right to choose whether or not to continue a pregnancy, there had been a growing split on religious and ethical grounds on whether women should have access to abortions at Memorial Hospital. In early 1980, the anti-abortion group Right to Life asked the hospital to end all abortions except to save the life of the mother. The board president responded that the board would consider the request but did not guarantee action.[71]

This led Memorial Hospital to spend more time dealing with ethical issues that arose as health care innovations allowed physicians and other personnel to diagnose and treat illnesses in ways unimagined by earlier generations. Also in October, the board had to consider how having accepted the Hill-Burton grant for the 1967 addition might have new implications in light of a recent Congressional ruling. In 1979, the United States Congress had revised the free care provisions of the Hill-Burton Act. It now required hospitals to document that they were providing roughly 10 percent of their original federal grant in free care each year. This came to about $100,000 for the hospital. The

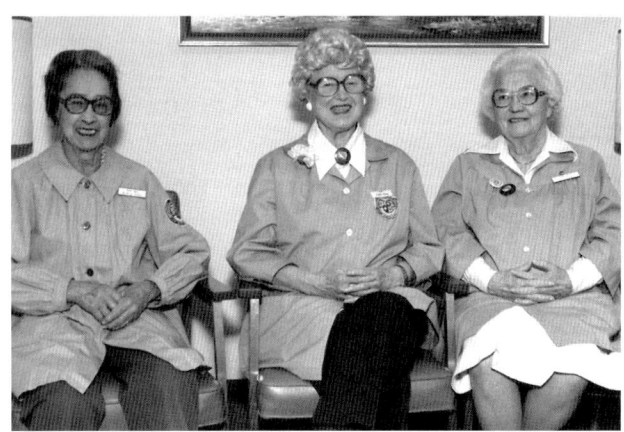

These Memorial Hospital of Natrona County volunteers wait for their next assignment. Kathleen Hemry is in the center.

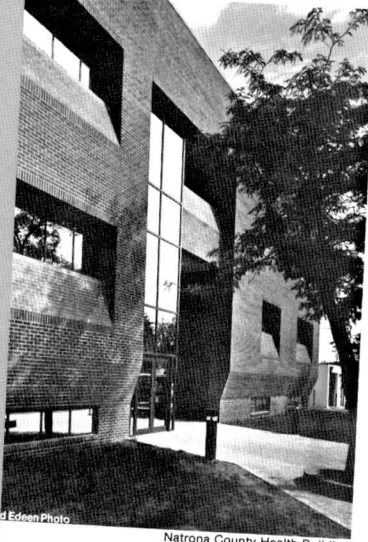
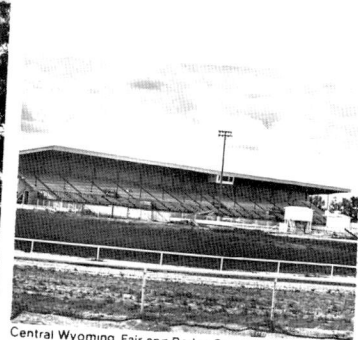
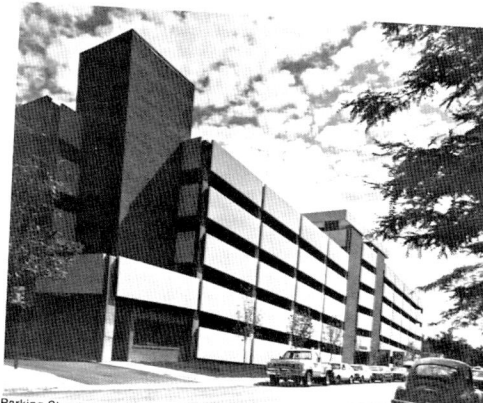
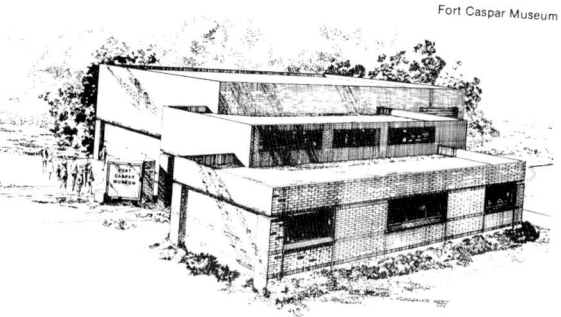
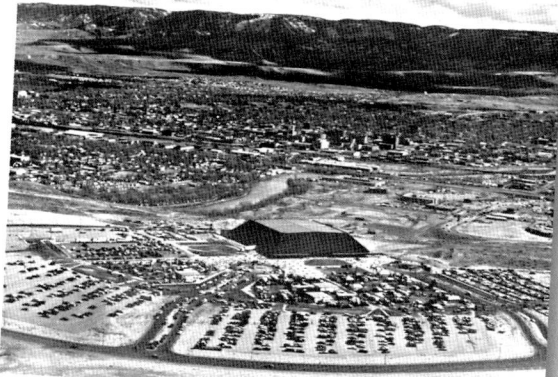

This advertisement highlighted buildings built in the early 1980s using One Cent Sales Tax money including the parking garage at the hospital.

original provision attached to the 1967 construction grant required them to provide free care for twenty years and to provide an "open door" policy, which they'd been doing. The new regulations set specific targets, and the hospital theoretically had to advertise for more indigent patients to meet its marker. In March 1980, Wyoming's attorney general ruled that the federal government couldn't retroactively change the rules. The federal government disagreed and there was a court case pending. The Wyoming Hospital Association was building a war chest to fight the case in court, and asked Memorial Hospital to give $4,112 as its share.[72]

At the end of 1980, the hospital dedicated the linear accelerator. Dr. Carol Fellows explained the benefits of the photon and electron treatments the machine provided which could cure patients with cancer, especially when combined with surgery and chemotherapy. When the patient could not be cured, the radiation still provided pain relief. Dr. Fellows noted that the machine aided her philosophy: "To cure sometimes, to relieve often, to comfort always."[73]

After Lewis Spencer died of cancer on August 16, 1980, Robert Manville reluctantly agreed to serve as acting hospital administrator. In March 1981, the Executive Committee of the Trustees recommended that they appoint Manville as the new administrator.

The board began long-range planning for a new wing in February 1981. They selected TriBrook Group, Inc. of Oakbrook, Illinois, to guide the planning. TriBrook worked with a core group of organizational leaders including Robert Macy of the Trustees, Jerry Wetherbee, Dr. Charles Wood, Dr. Lyford, Dr. Robert Patrick, Steve Ott and Tom Meyers from the community, and Robert Manville.[74]

TriBrook submitted their report on the next building project in March 1982.[75] In 1983, staff members began working with TriBrook to "present a functional program and space plan." The working group estimated that the project would cost $14 million without a fourth floor or $19.5 million for the whole project.[76] After consideration the committee revised the plans to reduce the cost to $17.6 million. The new building would be in the west parking lot and construction would be done in December 1986.[77] The firm selected for the project was the Gorder/S Group of Denver which included the architects John Reece, G. Fred Peterson, and Hillary M. Johnson (Fisher, Reece and Johnson, Architects).[78] They had built the parking garage. By early 1984, the Trustees had decided to defer the bond issue due to a recession that severely hurt the local as well as national economy. Additionally reduced patient load had cut back the need for new space.[79]

In the mid-1980s, the hospital continued its ongoing commitment to training. On a formal basis they began to look at training respiratory therapists. Western Wyoming Community College wanted to work with Memorial Hospital to provide clinicals for a respiratory therapy technician (RTT) program. Casper College was

> *In the mid-1980s, the hospital continued its ongoing commitment to training. On a formal basis they began to look at training respiratory therapists.*

COMMENDATION

WHEREAS, the immediate family of our late departed mother feels an endearment to all the personnel of Fifth Floor Central Nursing of Memorial Hospital of an intensity far surpassing the norm; and,

WHEREAS, it is perceptibly clear that the discharge of duty was to a degree of devotion far exceeding any type of tender loving care known to any of us; and,

WHEREAS, in partial recognition of your exemplary performance we have created a perpetual scholarship fund for students involved in the nursing arts as a token appreciation of our heartfelt gratitude; and,

WHEREAS, we feel that such effort merits the attention of the entire hospital administration for it well could serve as a model to be emulated,

NOW THEREFORE BE IT RESOLVED: That the family of our mother, Mrs. Eleanor Broadhurst, proffers our most sincere appreciation for the efforts of all.

We request this citation be posted in a conspicuous place so all will know the extreme regard in which you are held.

Eleanor Broadhurst Family

Katharine Zavell
Michal Sommer
John Stewart

cc: Natrona County Hospital Administration
Attention: Robert Manville

In 1982, Eleanor Broadhurst's family wrote this commendation for the nurses of Fifth Floor Central in honor of the great care given to their mother.

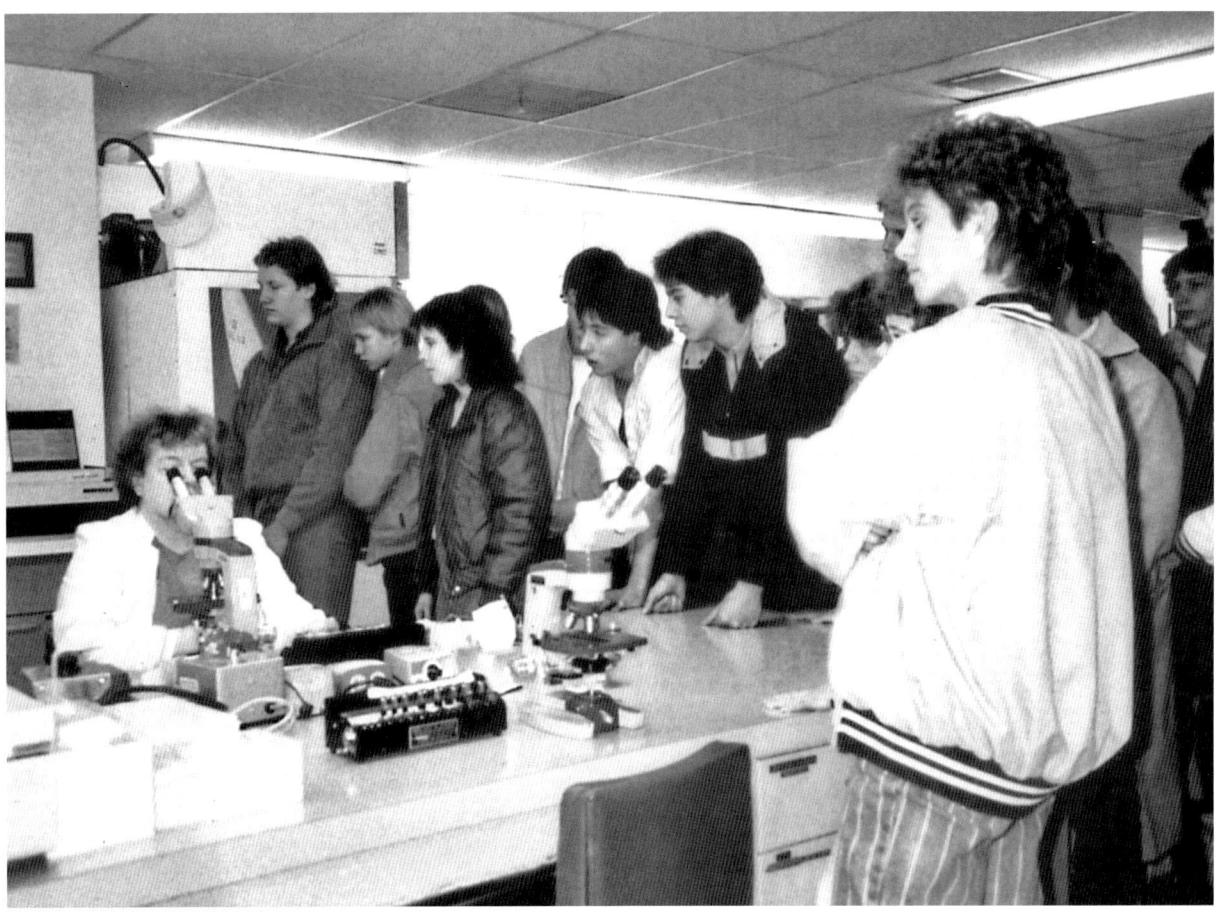

Volunteers conduct tours for students interested in health care careers.

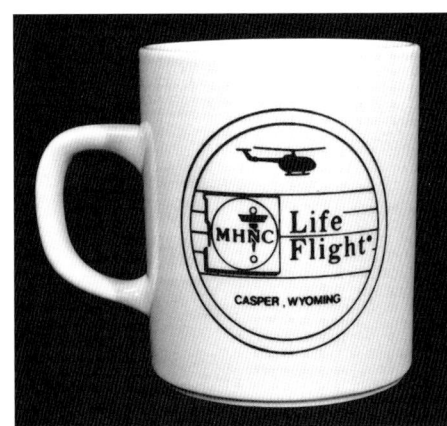

This coffee mug commemorated the start of Life Flight.

also setting up an RTT program. Neither college could proceed until the state legislature voted to authorize such a program.[80]

Whenever possible, the hospital tried to encourage young people to go into health care work. The local Boy Scout Council had Explorer posts that enrolled older teens including Medical Explorer Post 99. Sponsored by Memorial Hospital, it gave the young people opportunities to help out. In 1983, the Scouts helped raise $500 for Blue Envelope. At the annual Scoutarama, they gave tours of a hospital ambulance, took the blood pressure of other attendees, and helped out with a blood drive.[81]

The biggest event of 1983 and one of the most important innovations in the history of Memorial Hospital was the beginning of Life Flight, the helicopter and airplane patient transport service. As the hospital continued to draw patients from a broad region of the state, it needed a faster way to reach critically ill or injured people. Road transportation took time to get to outlying areas and those in the back country, whether hikers, snow mobilers, or hunters, often could not be reached for hours or days. Many people lived on ranches far from main roads. The hospital and other emergency personnel looked at ways to better collaborate in reaching patients in remote areas.

In March 1983, the hospital ambulance service did a market analysis to determine if a helicopter program would be economically feasible. Ninety-five flights a year would allow the program to break even. Based on the number of calls that came in each year from remote areas, planners anticipated that they would make 200 runs in the first year, jumping to 250 and then to 300 by 1985.[82]

The next step was to decide if purchase or lease was the best option. Evergreen Helicopters of Oregon provided a contract service and would lease a helicopter to the hospital.[83] Initially, that was the approach they took with money coming from the Blue Envelope Fund.

Life Flight was scheduled to begin service on June 1, 1983, but its first run was at 2 a.m. on May 15, 1983. Soon the pilots were so busy that ambulance service managers realized that purchasing a helicopter would save money in the long run. The best model for high altitude work was a Messerschmidt-Boelkow-Blohm Model BO 105CB, a German-made helicopter that had proven very reliable in service in Switzerland. In September 1983, Betty Holmer of the Blue Envelope Fund presented the Memorial Hospital of Natrona County with a check for $100,000 to help buy the new helicopter. That ensured that the program would have the right equipment to do the job.[84]

It became increasingly important to provide for better communication among first responders. The hospital paid $10,000 for a radio base station to allow common communications with the Wyoming Highway Patrol, the sheriff's office, and the fire department. The sheriff's department paid $2,500, the county another $2,500, and the hospital picked up the rest of the cost.[85]

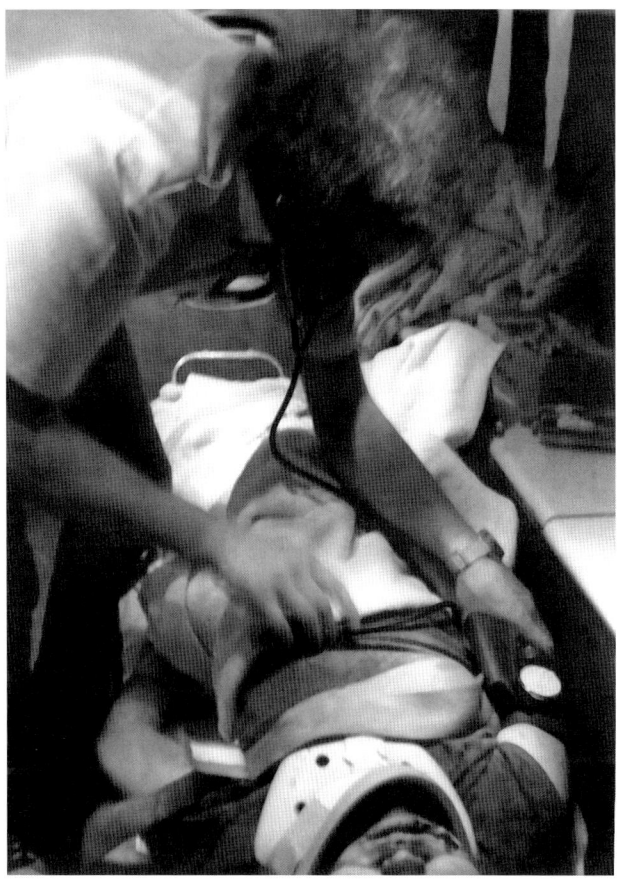

Hospital Emergency Medical Technician Rob Hendy tending an accident victim.

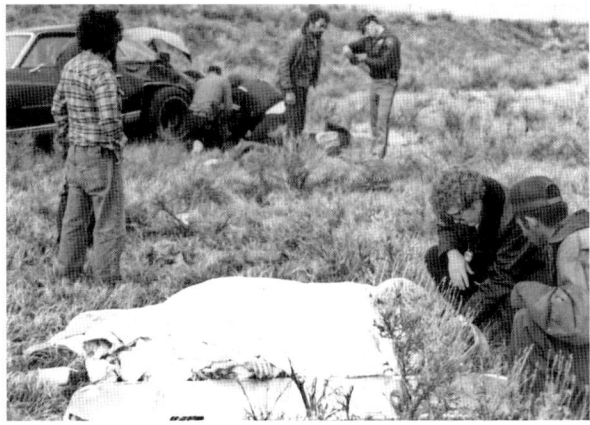

Emergency Department personnel responding to an automobile accident north of Casper.

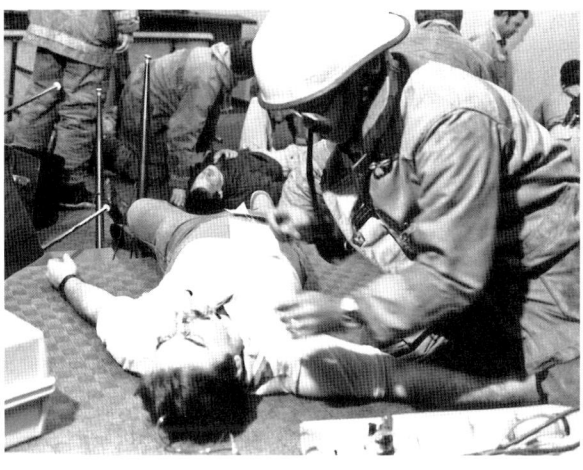

Disaster drills prepared hospital personnel for the real thing.

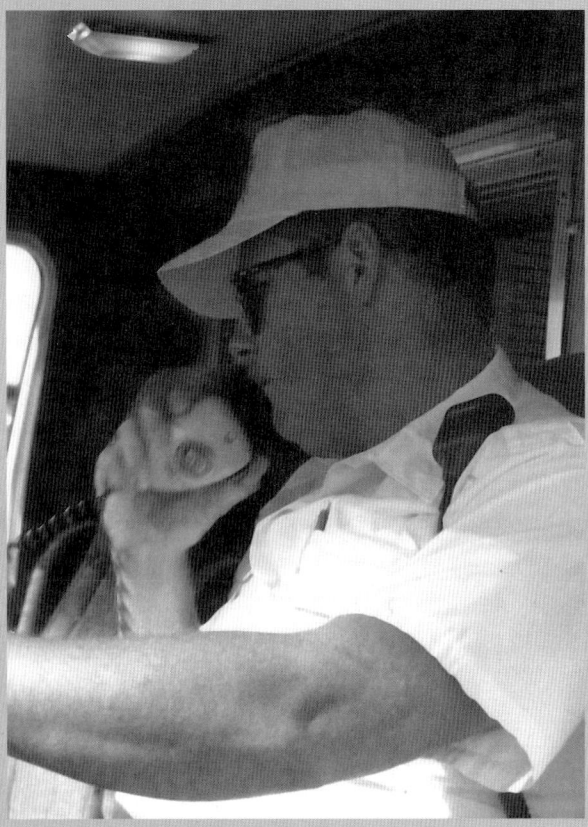 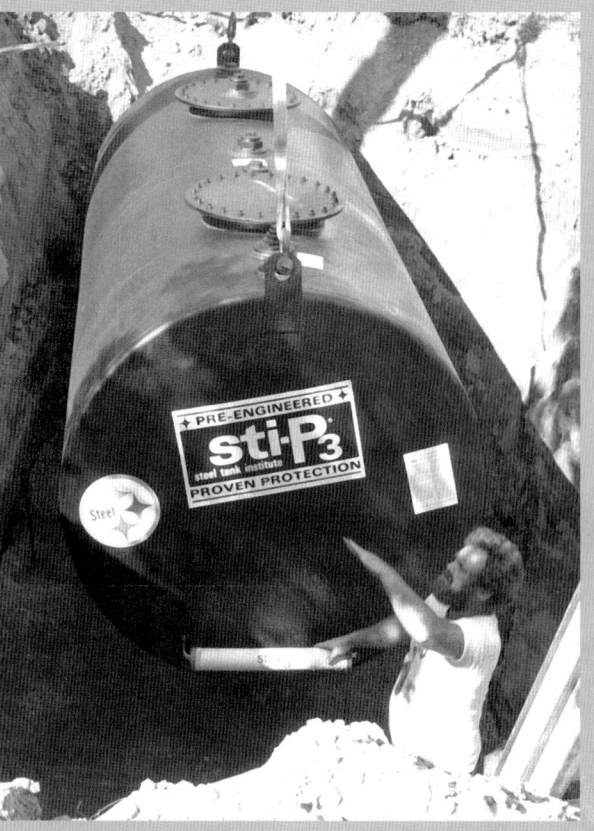

Emergency Medical Technician Tim Weaver using the radio system on the new four-wheel-drive ambulance.

Workers installed a flight fuel tank at the hospital to refuel the Life Flight aircraft.

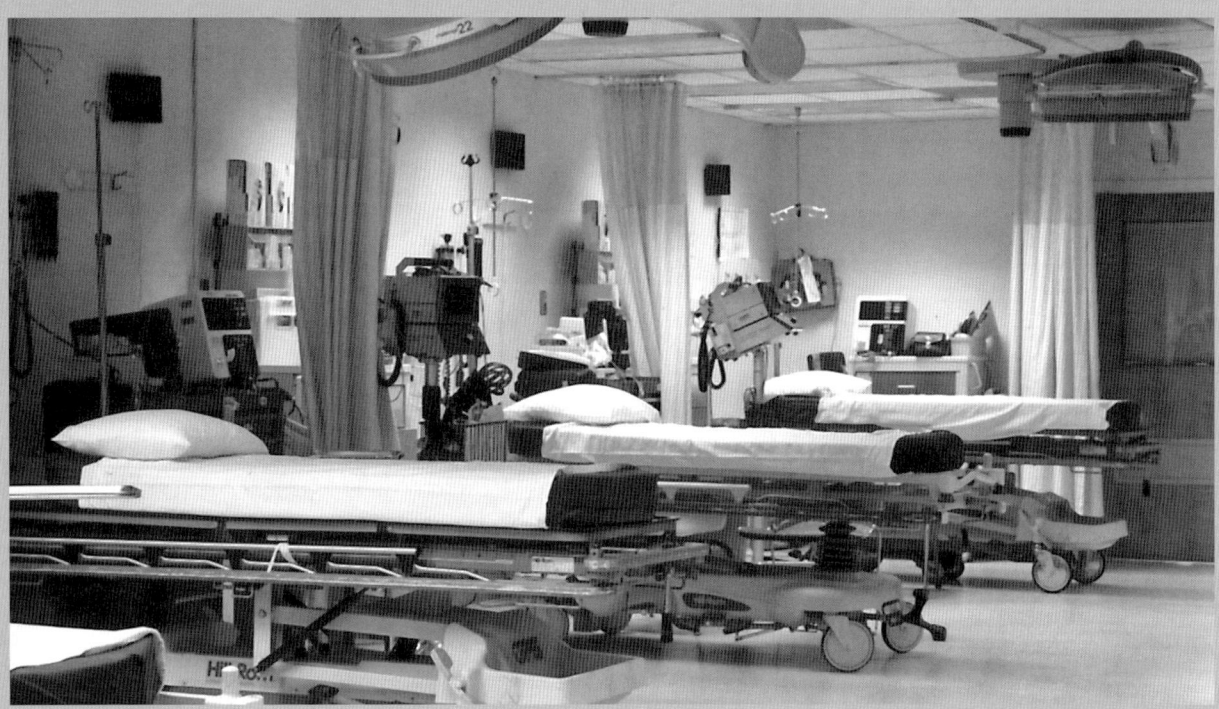

The Emergency Department was a ward where curtains separated patients and privacy was minimal.

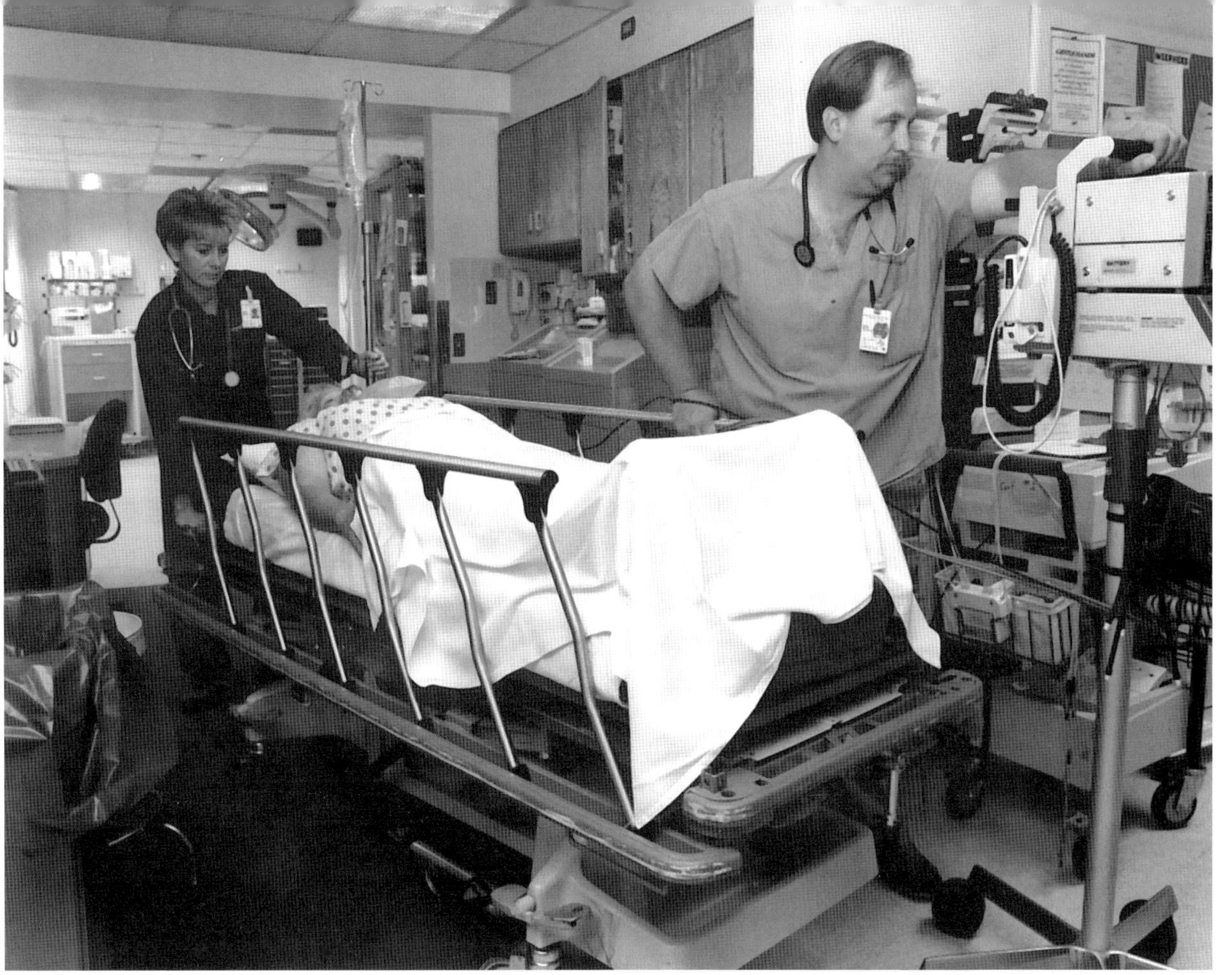

Transporting a patient out of the emergency room.

In 1983, a rancher had a heart attack during a big snowstorm. There was not access by road and emergency crews did not know exactly where the ranch was located. The helicopter pilot flew to where the sheriff had his lights flashing then counted the ranches until he got to the right one. The man lived, but this led to plans to create a file card system for each ranch in Wyoming. Global positioning systems (GPS) and computers were not yet in common use in emergency services so a card system was the only option. When the system was complete the cards provided location accuracy to within fifty feet. In early 1984, the Trustees approved purchase of TI-9100 Loran C Navigator gear for Life Flight. The hospital Foundation donated $5,720 towards the navigation equipment. Finally, to provide increased regional ambulance service, the hospital purchased its first four-wheel-drive ambulance. A Foundation donation covered the $40,000 price of the ambulance.[86]

Now that the hospital had better equipment, it was time to get better-trained emergency personnel. Emergency medical technicians (EMTs) received special training to be able to take physicians' orders and carry them out in the field. The next step up was paramedic training. Few institutions offered this so Tim Weaver and some of the other EMTs went back to school. The best program at the time was at Swedish Medical Center in Denver so Weaver and others moved to Denver for the four-month course, returning to the hospital when their training was complete.[87]

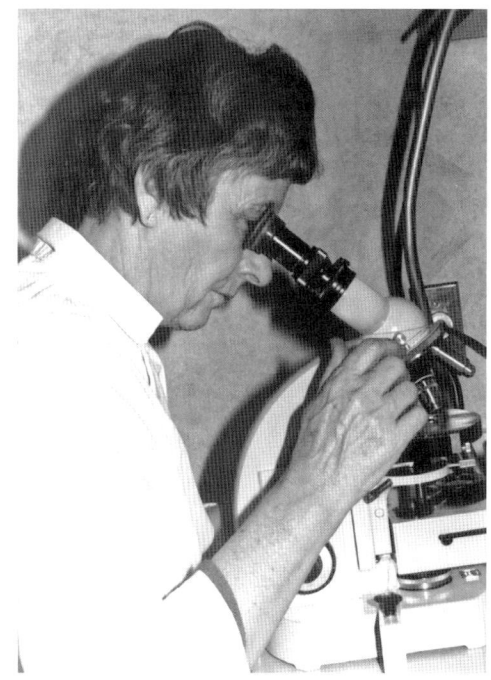

Memorial Hospital of Natrona County pathologists and technicians analyzed samples brought from surgery.

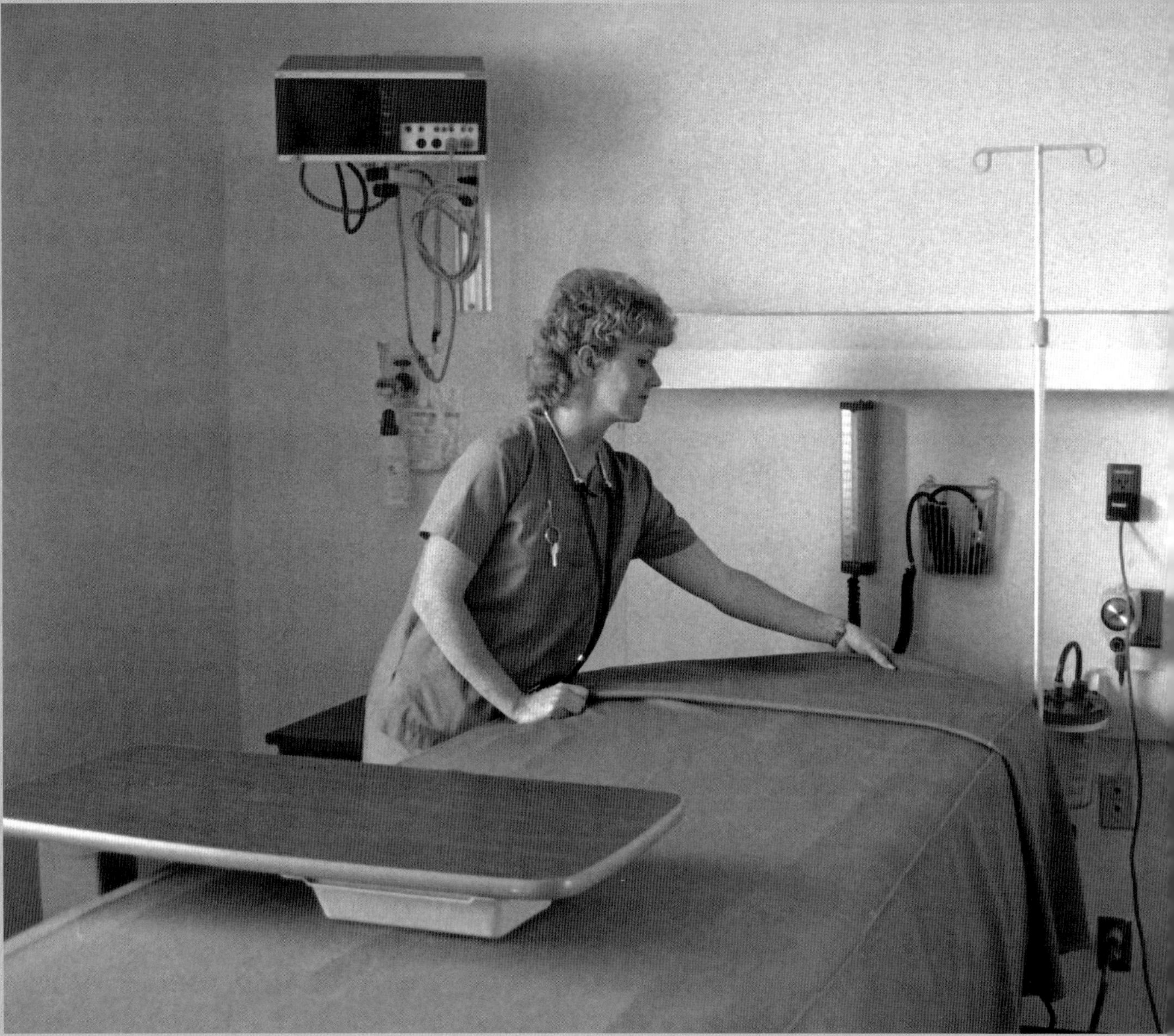

Diane Hubbard, R.N., working in a private room in Memorial Hospital of Natrona County.

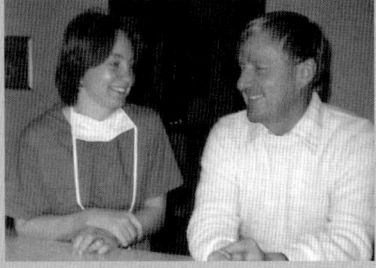

Young physicians like Dr. Abigail Rayner and Dr. Edward Reasoner came to the hospital in the 1980s.

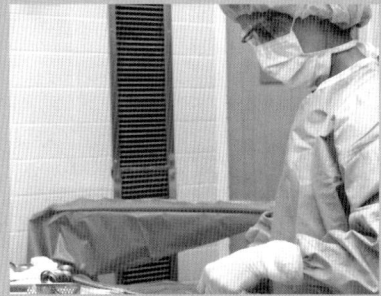

Dana Miller sets up for surgery in one of the old operating rooms.

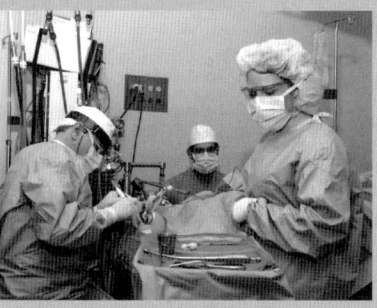

Surgeons and a scrub nurse operate on a patient in one of the old operating rooms.

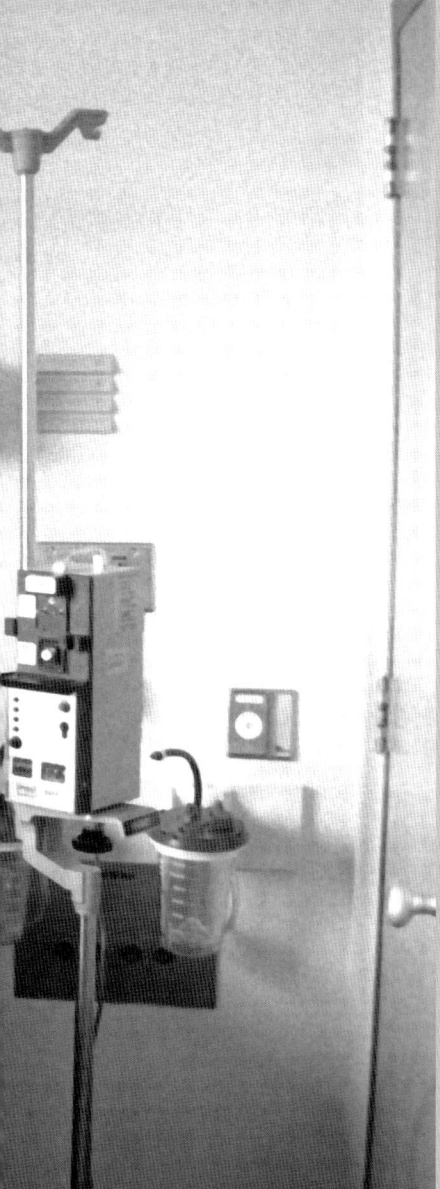

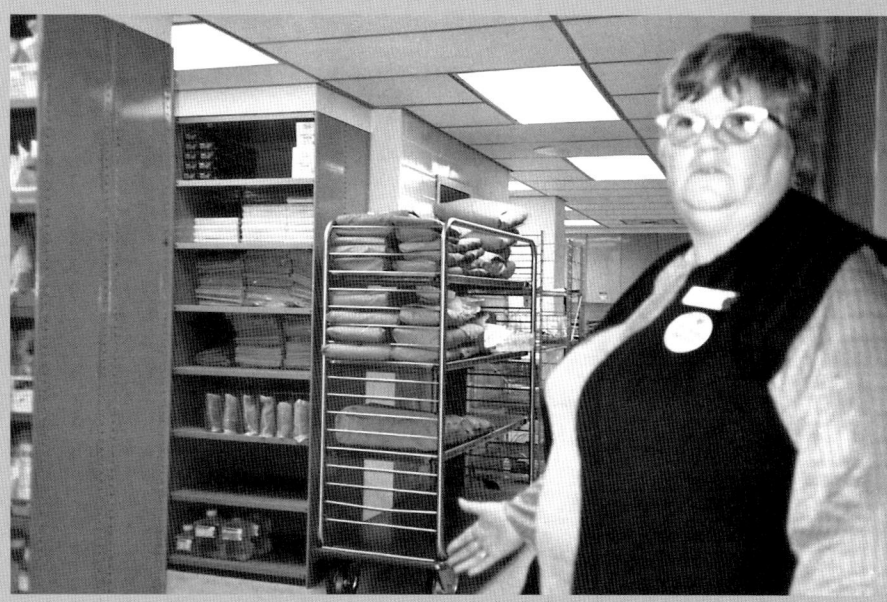

Central Services provided one place for all needed hospital supplies. Organization mattered.

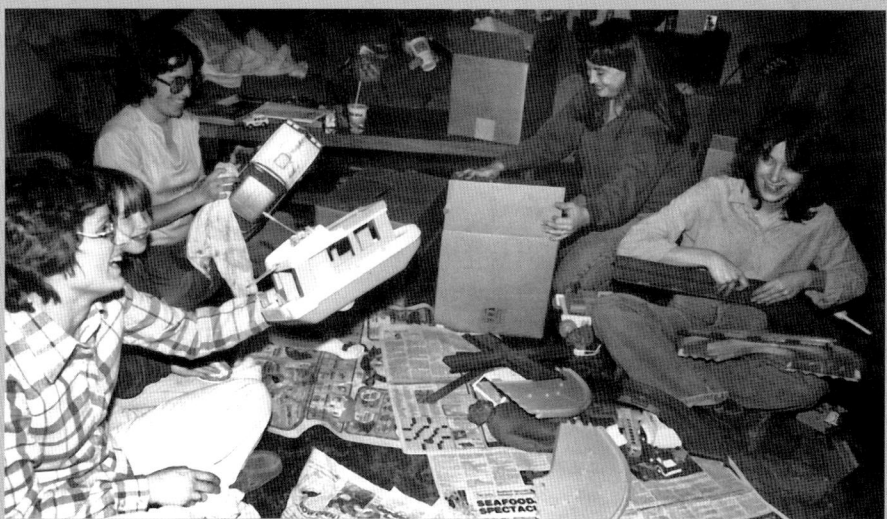

Hospital staffers in 1985 wrap presents for children who would not otherwise get presents.

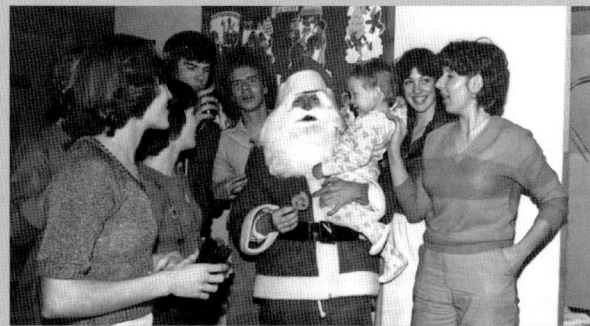

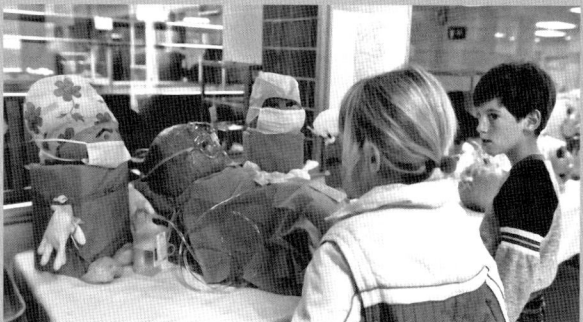

Holidays were very important at the hospital as these photos of Santa and Halloween jack-o-lanterns attest.

CHAPTER FIVE ❖ *From Memorial Hospital of Natrona County to Wyoming Medical Center:* 1960 TO 1986   93

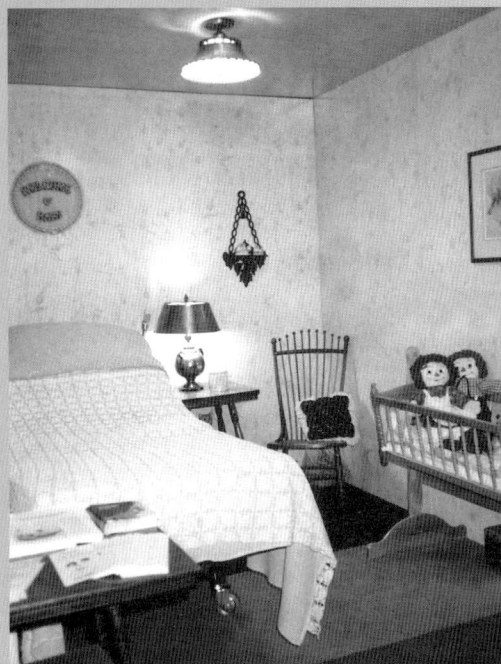
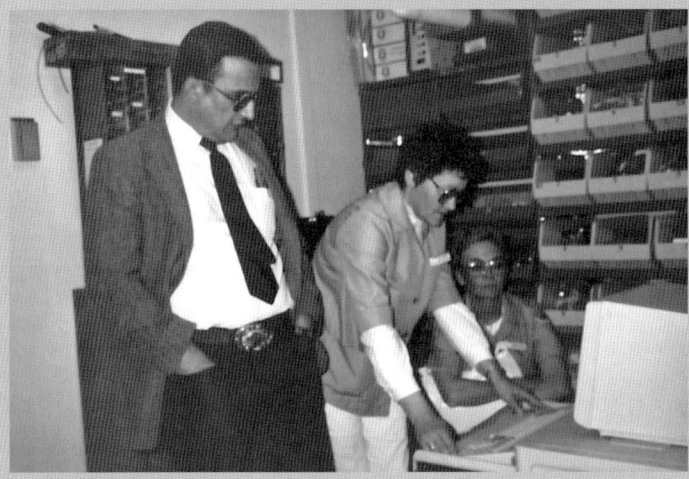

The hospital set up the Lifeline program directed by Ned Byers and staffed with volunteers.

Left: Birthing rooms gave an expectant family a home-like atmosphere for the delivery.

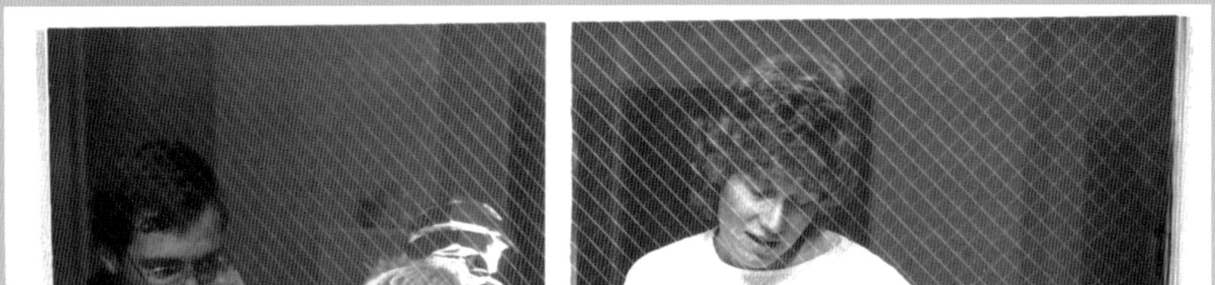

Relaxed rules in Labor and Delivery allowed older siblings to view the new baby through the nursery window.

For a decade, parents and childbirth advocates had been promoting a greater role for parents, especially fathers, in the birthing process. Lamaze classes prepared fathers to coach the mother in the labor room. Many mothers opted for limited or no pain killers during delivery. Birthing rooms allowed for a more homelike setting for the event. Increasingly, older siblings shared the childbirth experience with their parents. In September 1983, the Trustee Executive Committee agreed to allow fathers into the operating room to observe Cesarean-sections.[88]

The Cottage Gift Shop opened in 1984, generating income that returned as grants for programs and equipment. This provided an additional volunteer opportunity for the Auxiliary. Volunteers helped with purchasing, sales, and decorating the shop.

Beginning in 1985, the Blue Envelope Fund leadership and community physicians began to debate whether to continue the Strep Throat Screening Program. With rheumatic fever virtually eliminated, only those with an active sore throat needed to be screened. Many parents simply took their children to family doctors when they or their child had a severe sore

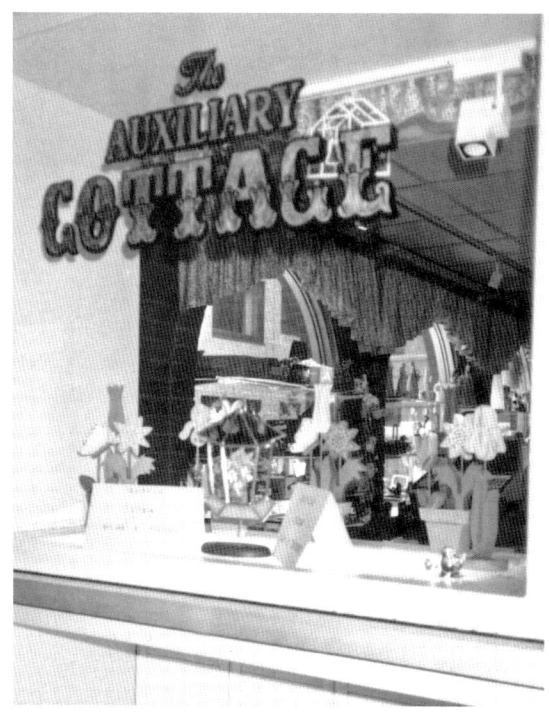

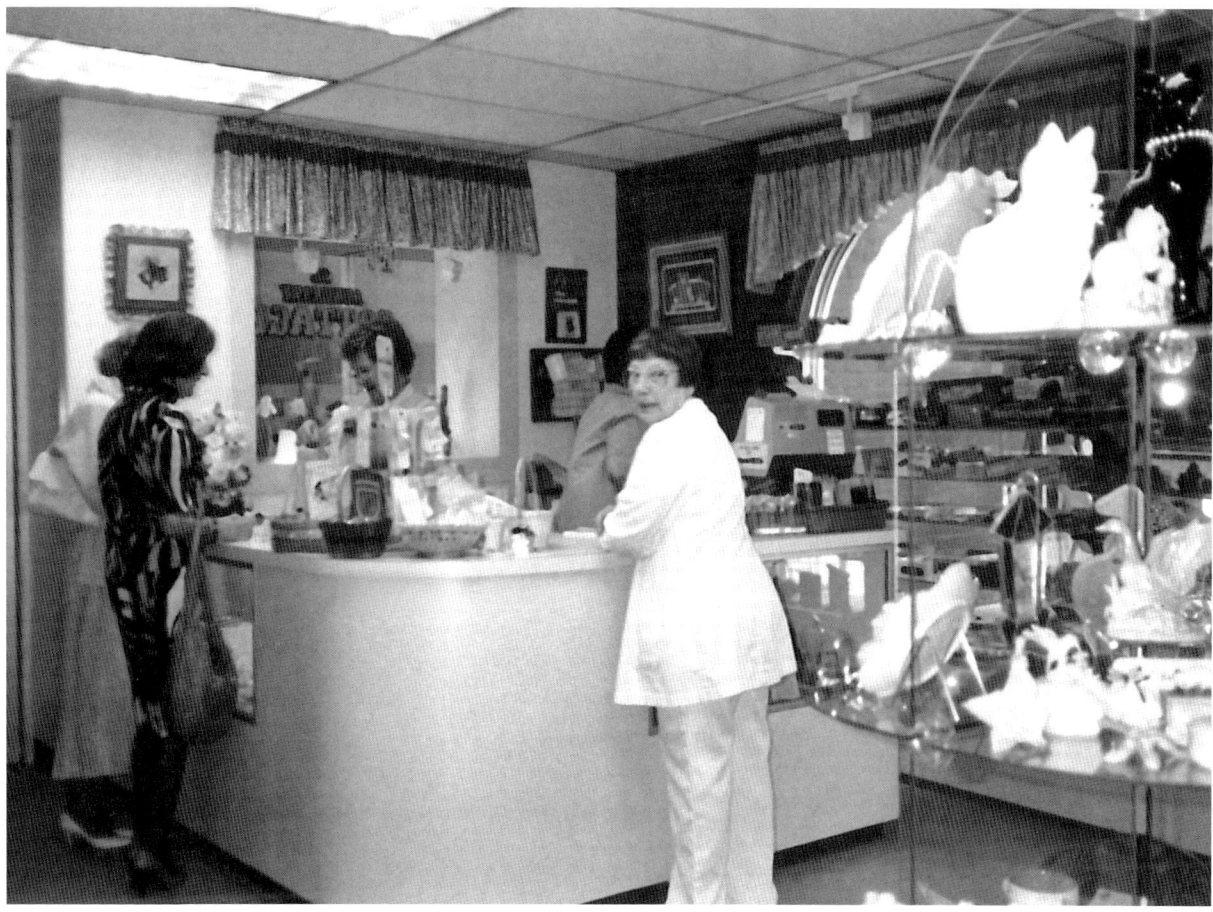

The Auxiliary opened the Cottage Gift Shop in 1984.

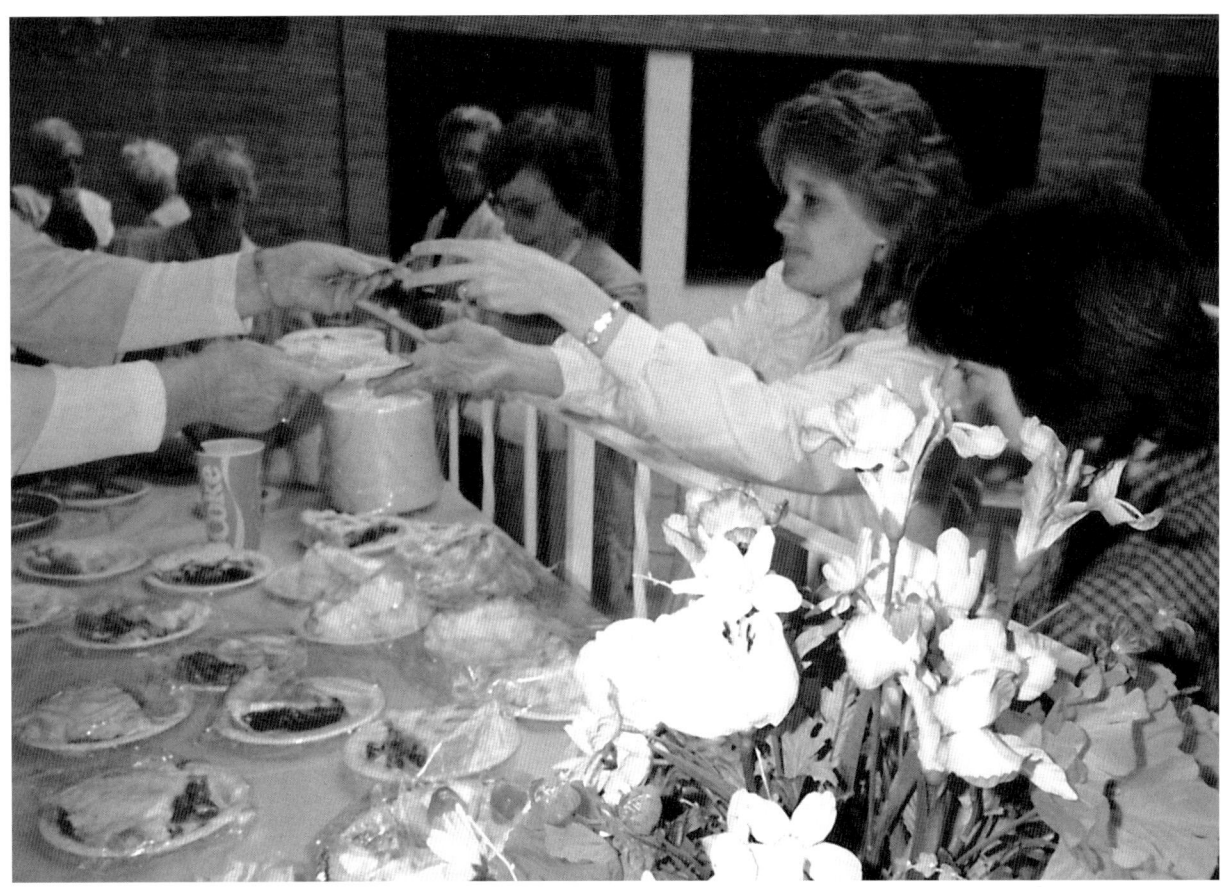

Volunteers enjoy pie while they are honored for their hard work.

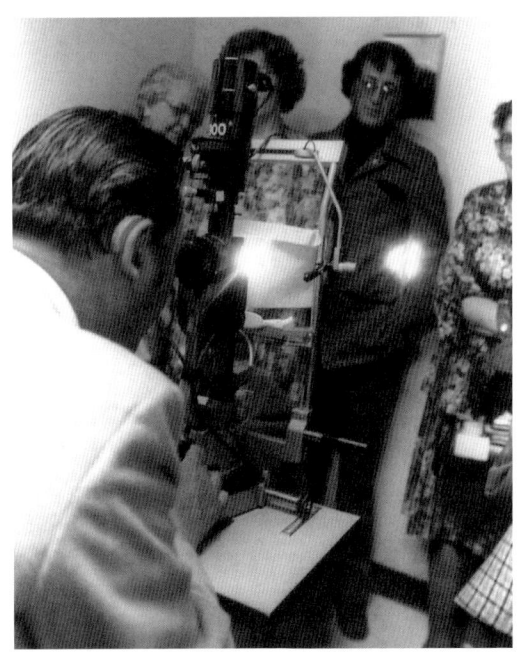

Nat Fowler, M.D. demonstrates a slit laser lamp to hospital volunteers.

throat. After a year of debate, the Fund decided to eliminate donations to the program.[89] In anticipation, the strep throat program moved back to Memorial Hospital, which now offered free throat swabs through the emergency room.[90]

This was just one of many changes ongoing in the community. The new building plans, the evolving community, and new leadership on the Board of Trustees led to reconsideration of the corporate structure of the Memorial Hospital of Natrona County and its relationship to Natrona County. The end result would be a new organization, Wyoming Medical Center.

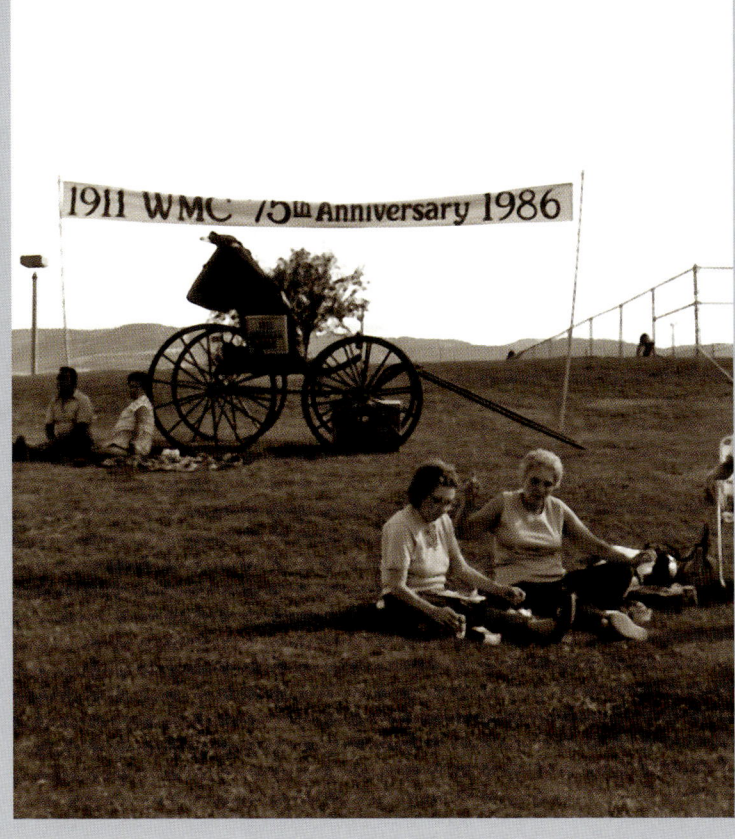

The 1986 summer picnic was a celebration of the seventy-fifth anniversary of the hospital's founding in 1911.

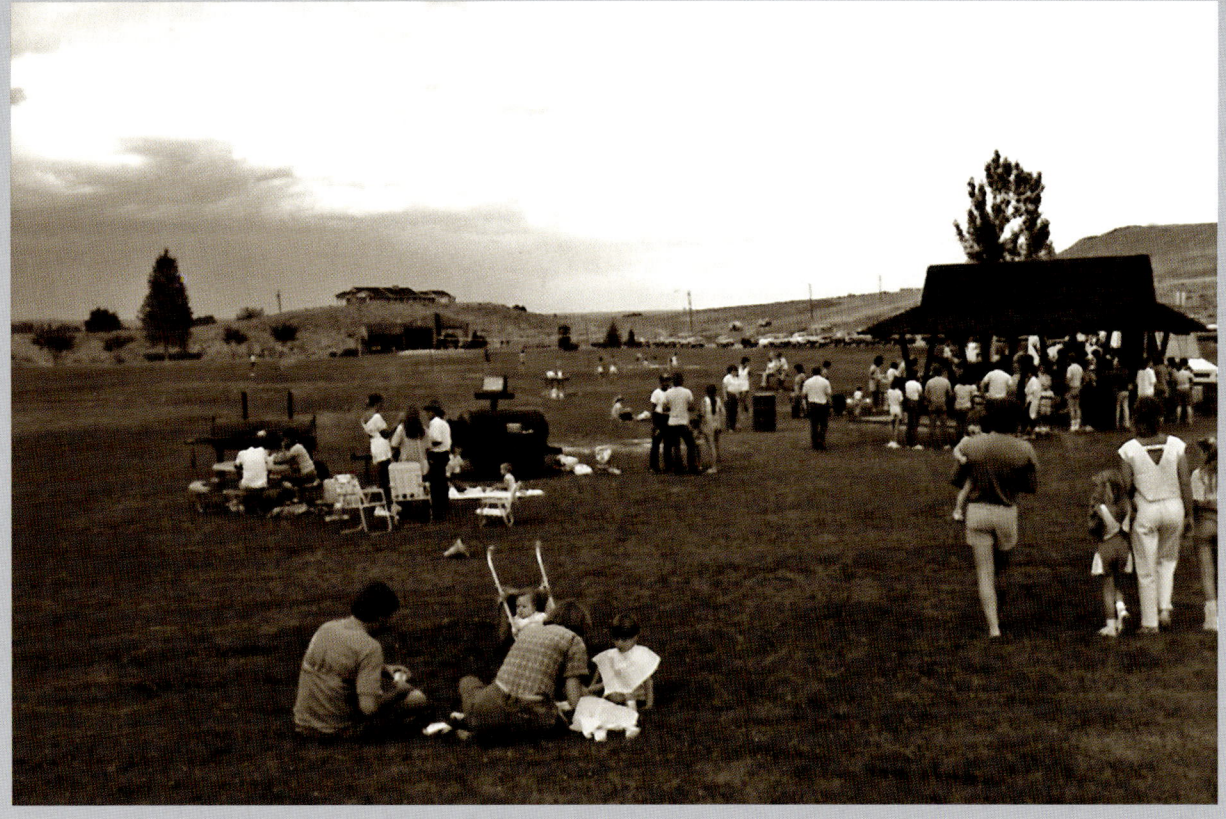

CHAPTER FIVE ❖ *From Memorial Hospital of Natrona County to Wyoming Medical Center:* 1960 TO 1986

NOTES

1 "KATI Radio Fundraiser nets $900 for Hospital," *Casper Star-Tribune*, May 5, 1961.

2 Board of Trustees Minutes, February 29, 1960, p. 1.

3 OPEC, "A Brief History," 2010, http://www.opec.org/opec_web/en/about_us/24.htm.

4 Amoco Corporation, Corporate History, 2010, http://www.fundinguniverse.com/company-histories/Amoco-Corporation-Company-History.html.

5 Board of Trustees Minutes, May 26, 1960, p. 1.

6 Board of Trustees Minutes, February 29, 1960, p. 1.

7 Board of Trustees Minutes, April 18, 1960, p. 1.

8 "Memorial Hospital of Natrona County Operations," *Casper Star-Tribune*, 1962.

9 Ann Burns. "Quinlan leads Nutrition Services through four decades," *Hospital Hi-Lites*, Wyoming Medical Center, September 1991, p. 1.

10 Board of Trustees Minutes, October 31, 1960, p. 1; Board of Trustees Minutes, June 27, 1962, p. 3.

11 Natrona County Memorial Hospital vacation benefit survey and recommendations, May 1962.

12 Board of Trustees Minutes, April 18, 1960, p. 2.

13 Board of Trustees Minutes, August 21, 1961, p. 1; Board of Trustees Minutes, November 27, 1961, p. 1.

14 *Casper Tribune-Herald*, December 16, 1961.

15 Irving Garbutt. "Surgery Restores Life to Mother," *Casper Tribune-Herald*, December 16, 1961.

16 Board of Trustees Minutes, June 30, 1961.

17 Board of Trustees Minutes, January 16, 1961, p. 1.

18 Kenneth Babcock, M.D. Recertification report, JACHO, June 15, 1960.

19 Board of Trustees Minutes, August 21, 1961, p. 1.

20 Board of Trustees Minutes, June 30, 1961, p. 2.

21 Volk and Harrison. Engineering report, Memorial Hospital of Natrona County, February 28, 1964.

22 Board of Trustees Minutes, December 22, 1961, p. 1.

23 The Hill-Burton Act, 2010, http://en.wikipedia.org/wiki/Hill%E2%80%93Burton_Act.

24 Board of Trustees Minutes, February 12, 1964, p. 1.

25 Board of Trustees Minutes, July 1963, p. 1.

26 Board of Trustees Minutes, March 19, 1962, pp. 1–2.

27 Board of Trustees Minutes, July 13, 1964, p. 1.

28 "New Wing Opened," *Casper Star-Tribune*, March 16, 1967.

29 "New Coronary Care Hospital Unit Like Science Fiction Lab," *Casper Star-Tribune*, April 1, 1967.

30 "Health fund Aids Local Diagnosis," *Casper Star-Tribune*, March 27, 1964.

31 "Rheumatic Fever 'Stamped Out' in Natrona County," *Casper Star-Tribune*, March 6, 1968.

32 "Cancer Cause and Cure Being Researched Here," *Casper Star-Tribune*, March 20, 1963.

33 Blue Envelope Health Fund, "A Report to the People of Natrona County," 1967.

34 Duncan Howlett. *No Greater Love: The James Reeb Story*. Boston: Skinner House Books, 1993.

35 Board of Trustees Minutes, May 26, 1970.

36 Board of Trustees Minutes, July 28, 1970.

37 Robin Beaver. "He turned lemons into lemonade: Fred Goodstein used his largesse to benefit those who had little," *Made in Wyoming*, http://www.madeinwyoming.net/profiles/goodstein.php.

38 Irving Garbutt. *History of Casper and Natrona County, Wyoming, 1889–1989*, Vol. 1. Dallas: Irving Media, 1990, p. 53.

39 Board of Trustees Minutes, April 27, 1971.

40 "Blue Envelope Buying Equipment for Hospital," *Casper Star-Tribune*, April 1971.

41 "New Lung Respirator Breathes for Patient," *Casper Star-Tribune*, 1971.

42 "Lab Named for Tripeny," *Casper Star-Tribune*, March 21, 1971.

43 "'Dr. Dial' Draws 6000 in Week," *Casper Star-Tribune*, March 1971.

44 "Noted Casper Doctor Takes 'Sabbatical,'" *Casper Star-Tribune*, March 5, 1971.

45 Board of Trustees Minutes, August 30, 1972.

46 Board of Trustees Minutes, March 29, 1973.

47 Garbutt, *History of Casper and Natrona County*, p. 68.

48 "Donors give blood for $10 credit for donee," *Casper Star-Tribune*, November 14, 1968.

49 "All-volunteer donation blood program outlined," *Casper Star-Tribune*, January 1973.

50 "Mothers of Twins members will participate in blood drive," *Casper Star-Tribune*, April 1973.

51 "Special X-ray procedures make hospital state referral center," *Casper Star-Tribune*, March 1974.

52 "Health Fair set Feb. 8," *Casper Star-Tribune*, February 1975.

53 Rebecca Hunt. Interview with Elaine Hough regarding Wyoming Medical Center, December 18, 2009.

54 Elaine Hough, *MHNC Outreach*, Vol. 1, No. 2 (Spring/Summer 1978), p. 4.

55 Board of Trustees Minutes, January 27, 1976.

56 "Special interest gift," *Casper Star-Tribune*, c. 1977.

57 Wyoming Medical Center Foundation, 2010, http://www.wyomingmedicalcenterfoundation.org/index.php.

58 Hough, p. 7.

59 Board of Trustees Minutes, April 27, 1976.

60 Board of Trustees Minutes, February 22, 1977.

61 Hough, pp. 1–3.

62 Board of Trustees Minutes, August 15, 1978.

63 Hough, p. 4.

64 Hunt, interview with Elaine Hough.

65 Board of Trustees Minutes, July 19, 1977.

66 Board of Trustees Minutes, January 17, 1978.

67 Hough, p. 5.

68 Board of Trustees Minutes, November 21, 1978.

69 Board of Trustees Minutes, February 20, 1979.

70 Robert Johnson. *A Look Backward, A Step Forward: The Quiet Impact of Fifty Years, City of Casper-Natrona County Health Department, 1954–2004*, Casper, Mountain States Lithography, 2004, p. 43.

71 Board of Trustees Minutes, February 19, 1980.

72 Board of Trustees Minutes, October 21, 1980.

73 "Accelerator Dedication is Tomorrow," *Casper Star-Tribune*, 1980.

74 Board of Trustees Minutes, February 17, 1981.

75 Board of Trustees Minutes, March 24, 1982.

76 Board of Trustees Minutes, October 30, 1983.

77 Board of Trustees Minutes, December 20, 1983.

78 Board of Trustees Minutes, January 18, 1983.

79 Board of Trustees Minutes, January 30, 1984.

80 Board of Trustees Minutes, February 28, 1983.

81 "Medical Explorers to Help at Scoutarama," *Casper Star-Tribune*, April 1980.

82 Board of Trustees Minutes, March 15, 1983.

83 Board of Trustees Minutes, April 19, 1983.

84 Board of Trustees Minutes, September 20, 1983.

85 Board of Trustees Minutes, September 20, 1983.

86 Board of Trustees Minutes, January 17, 1984.

87 Rebecca Hunt. Interview with Tim Weaver, September 6, 2009.

88 Board of Trustees Minutes, September 13, 1983.

89 "Choice to end swabbing hard for Blue Envelope," *Casper Star-Tribune*, March 23, 1986.

90 *Casper Star-Tribune*, July 1985.

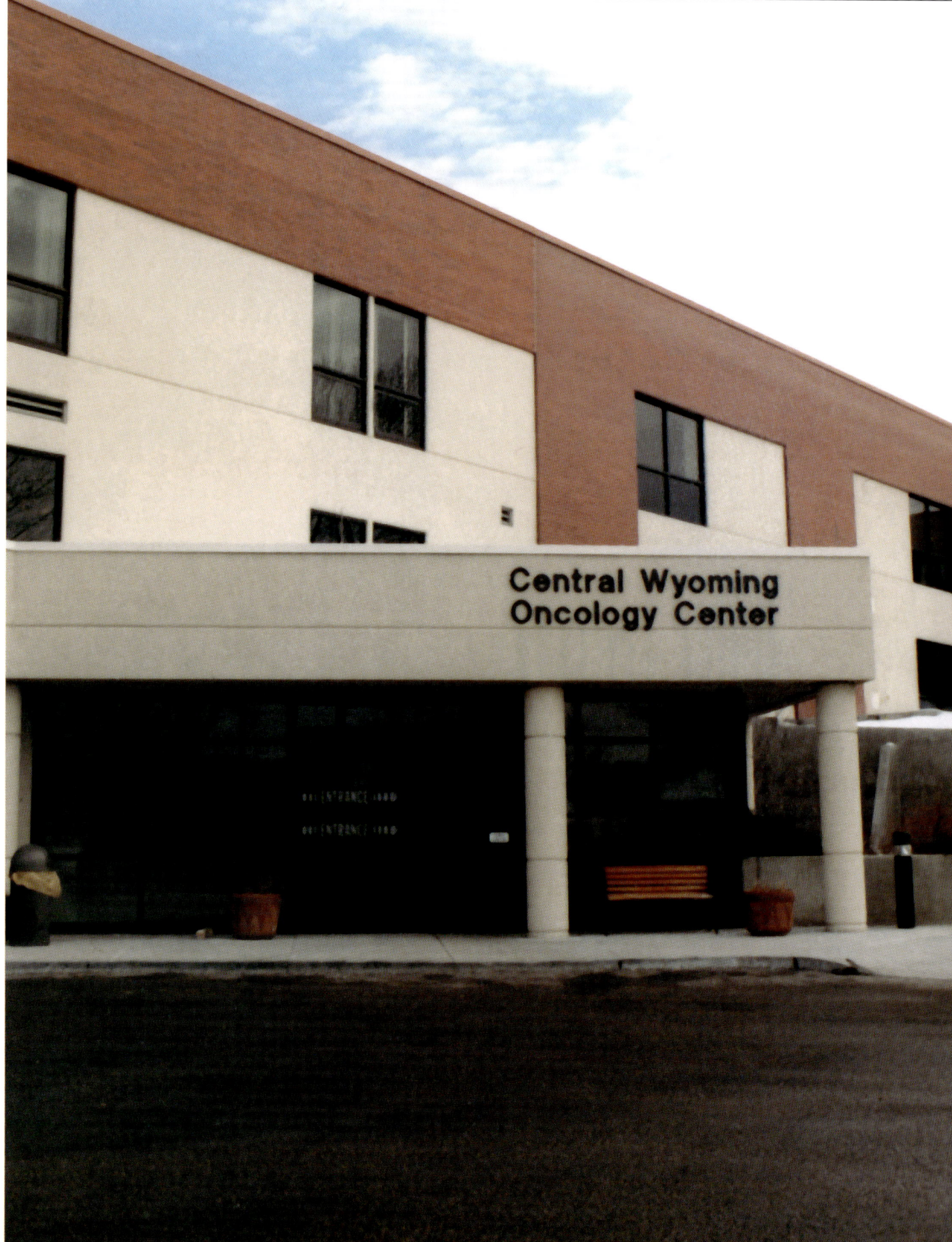

CHAPTER SIX

Wyoming Medical Center

1986 TO 2010

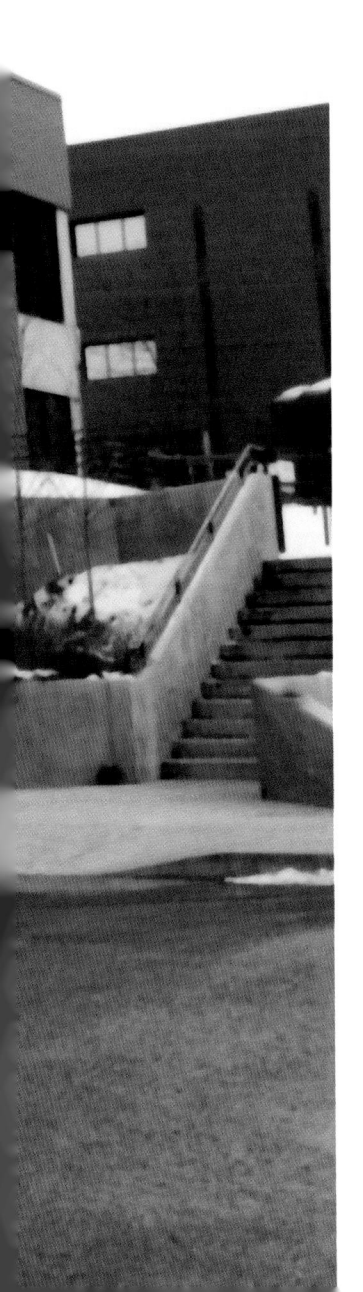

The old relationship between the hospital and the county was complex. Natrona County owned the buildings, and the Memorial Hospital of Natrona County Board of Trustees and the hospital administration made sure money was there to operate and that there was a vision to keep the institution current in staffing and facilities. At the same time, Wyoming's laws limited what hospitals could do to modernize because they limited possible partnerships.

Mike Sullivan, Trustee and Wyoming's governor-to-be, helped manage the reorganization process. The end result was Wyoming Medical Center, a non-profit corporation that had responsibility to the Trustees, to the county, and to its people. This corporate structure brought in new business principles and a new era of accountability, as well as a flexibility that allowed it to meet the challenges of the future.

Wyoming Medical Center's board operated in tandem with the Memorial Hospital of Natrona County board that reported to the county. The Medical Center board had seven appointed members. The Commissioners appointed two, another two were physicians working at Wyoming Medical Center, and the business community selected the last three members. Since it was an independent entity, the board could build partnerships with and get input from physicians in ways not previously possible.[1]

The county had the Medical Center pay rent on the buildings by absorbing the cost of providing indigent care. Free care amounted to $700,000 in 1987, with Wyoming Medical Center also absorbing about $2 million in bad debts. The Medical Center board then raised money for new facilities and remodeling.[2]

In 1986, J. Douglas Bird, who had been the hospital's chief financial officer, took over as president. He replaced John Bohler, who replaced Robert Manville in 1985. Bird brought in some new upper management, including Len Gross, who

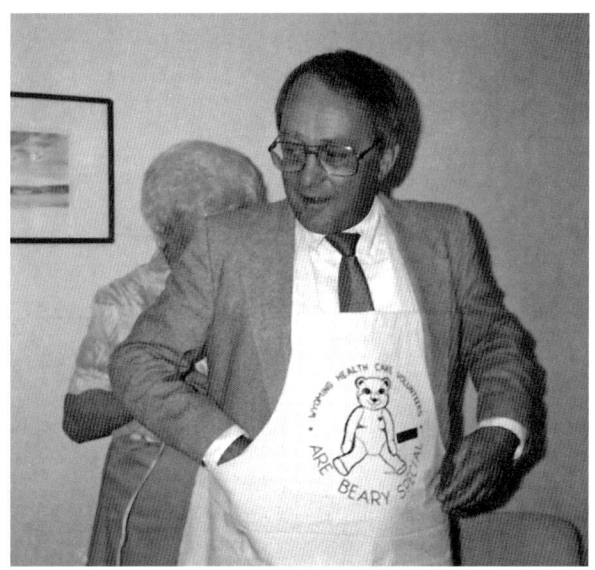

Doug Bird took over as president of Memorial Hospital of Natrona County in 1983.

became Human Resources director in early 1987.³ Gross was hiring nurses at a time when there was a nationwide nursing shortage, so Human Resources offered a $1,000 bonus to any employee who recruited a registered nurse to the Medical Center.⁴ Gross also developed a new maternity leave plan that gave women six weeks of paid leave plus the right to take three months total.⁵

Recruiting and keeping nurses led the hospital to provide continuing education that developed local talent. Wyoming Medical Center's Perioperative Nursing Residency Program was a six-month course of study that included classes and clinical experience for registered nurses who wanted to learn surgical nursing. The free program required the nurses to commit to one year of service at Wyoming Medical Center at the end of their training. A similar program trained nurses for work in critical care. The first classes graduated in April 1989 and included Jill Deane, R.N., Elizabeth Jones, R.N., Judith Kraen, R.N., Patrick Parmenter, R.N., Sandra Puder, R.N., and Michel Vance, R.N.⁶

Elaine Hough became director of Volunteer Services in 1987, coordinating volunteer activities and editing their newsletter.⁷ In 1987, the Auxiliary changed their name to the Auxilians. They continued to contribute to the Medical Center through volunteer hours, fundraising, greeting visitors, and assisting in the departments in myriad ways. They also helped out with the Blue Envelope Drive Health Fair.⁸

Volunteers working at Wyoming Medical Center formed strong bonds of friendship with each other, with hospital nurses, and with other employees. Some had been active for years. They combined community, support, and service in their interactions with the hospital and with each other.

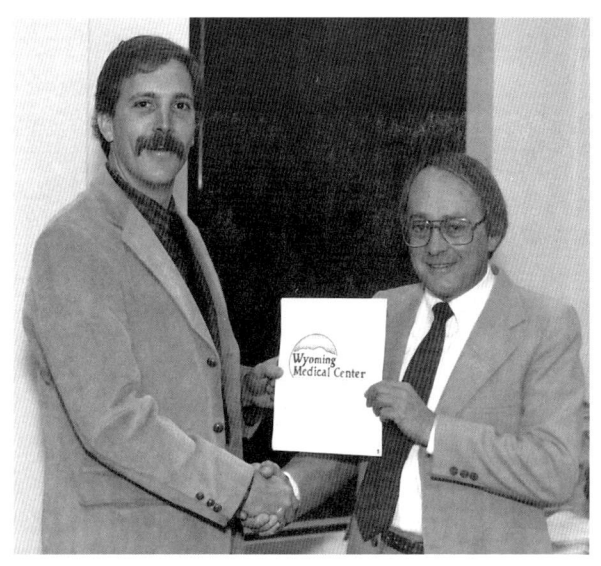

Wyoming Medical Center needed a logo. Here, Doug Bird gives the award for the best design.

Employees gave back to the community in many ways. They helped out with the United Way and the Blue Envelope Health Fair. They taught in Sunday schools, volunteered for Boy and Girl Scouts and in their children's schools, and they took meals to shut-ins.⁹ An annual program called "Paint Your Heart Out," in conjunction with Casper Neighborhood Housing Services, encouraged employees to paint a house for someone who needed assistance. In August 1987, the Medical Center fielded a team for the Seventh Annual Great River Raft Race on the North Platte River. The race raised money for a number of Casper organizations including the Girls' Club and the Natrona County Firefighters' Burn Fund.¹⁰

The Medical Center programs received support from many sources. Blue Envelope made donations directly as well as to Wyoming Medical Center Foundation which in January 1987 distributed $10,000 to the Life Flight program. Money from the 1987 campaign went to Dr. Dial, to the Central Wyoming Cancer Center, to the hospice, and to blood services.¹¹

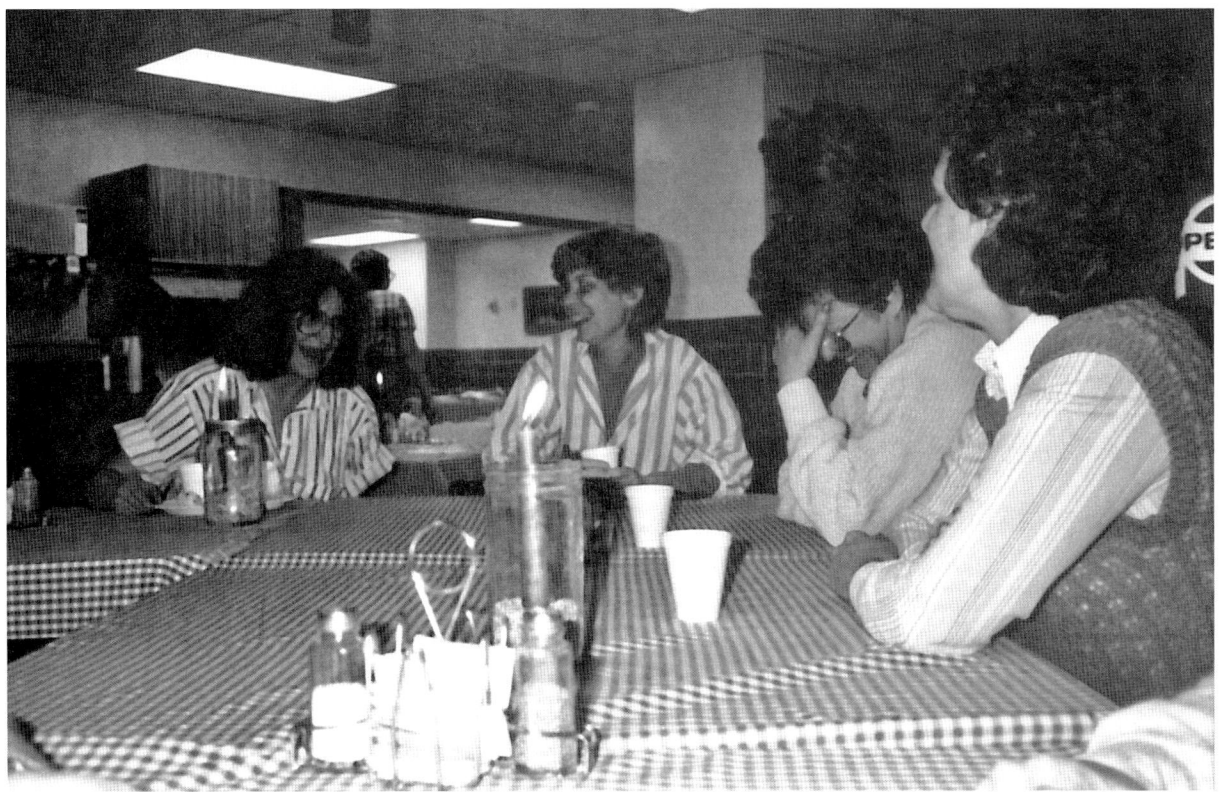

Nurses at the Medical Center take a break in the cafeteria.

Donations in early 1987 allowed the Medical Center to purchase a mammography machine for the early detection of breast tumors. Equipment that attached to the CT scanner screened for osteoporosis. This new technology allowed the hospital to become a center for women's health.[12] Since women's health was a new concept, an extensive public education program acquainted patients with both screening techniques.

Actual or planned construction projects dominated the remainder of the decade. A new Central Services building was going up on the east side of Conwell Street that would house boilers, a chiller, the laundry, and the Materials Management Department.

Wyoming Imaging Center was nearing completion and installation began on the Magnetic Resonance Imager (MRI). The Imaging Center leased the building and the MRI machine in the first joint venture allowed by Wyoming Medical Center's new corporate structure. A number of regional hospitals, physicians, the Medical Center Foundation, and Wymedco bought shares. The center expected to scan around 1,500 patients in the first year of operation at $550 per scan.

In addition to the Central Services building and the Imaging Center, construction began on a south bank of elevators connecting the parking garage to the hospital. A tunnel connected the Central Services building with the area near the new elevators. Construction slated for the future included new east and west wings. A groundbreaking ceremony was tentatively scheduled for July 1988.[13]

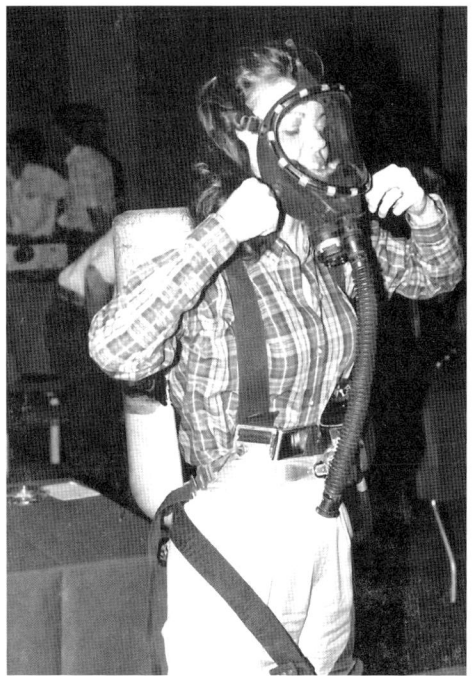

Kathy Simons, R.N. demonstrates the emergency air pack as part of a training exercise.

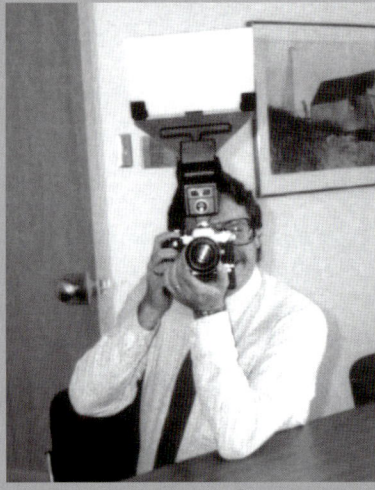
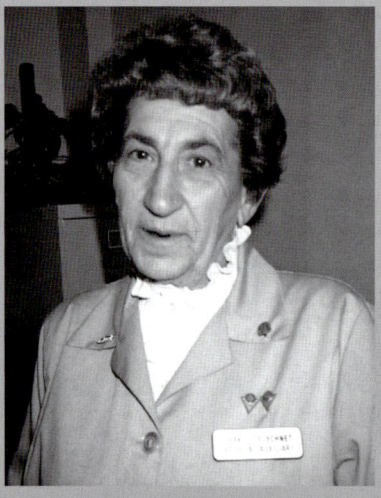
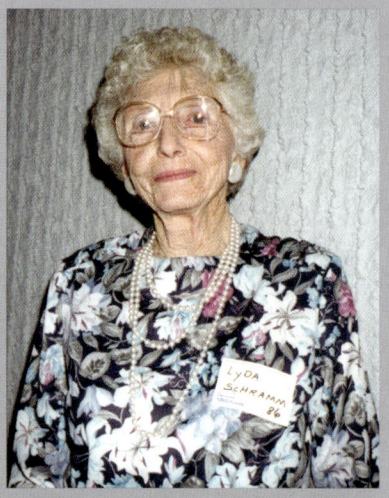

Mike Moore was the hospital photographer through the 1980s.

Volunteers like Charlotte Bohnet were essential to Wyoming Medical Center operations.

Lyda Schrann was another volunteer who gave thousands of hours of work.

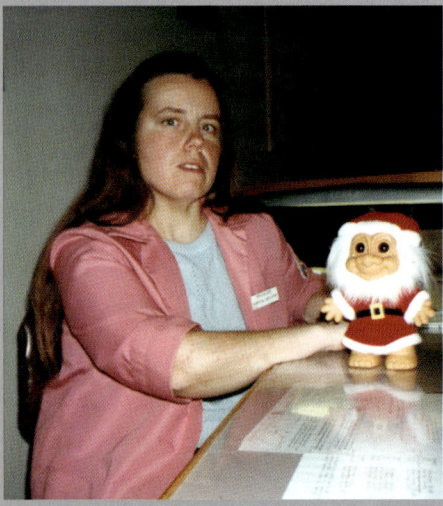

Nita Balser represented the new generation of volunteers.

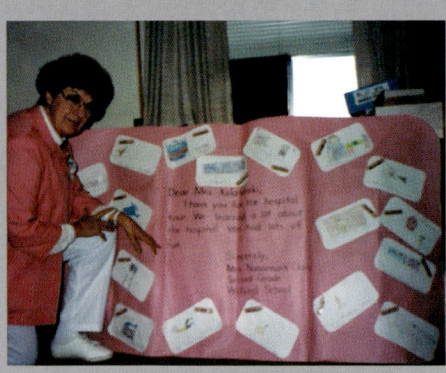

Joanne Kolasinski shows off her letters received from students she had toured through the hospital.

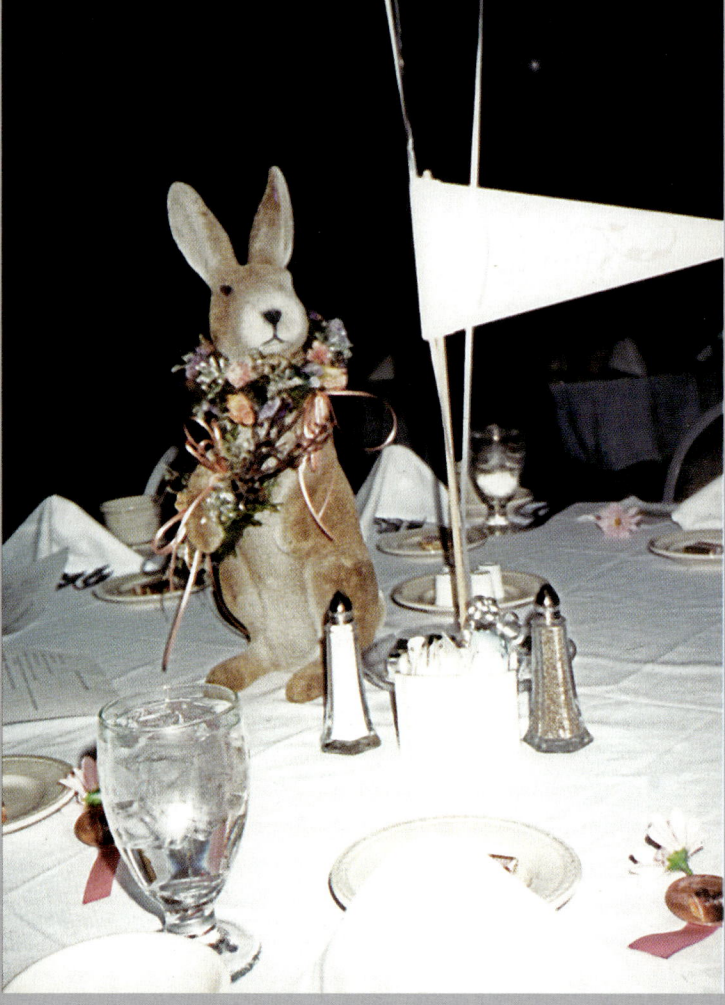

Volunteer appreciation lunches represented the fun side of the Auxiliary.

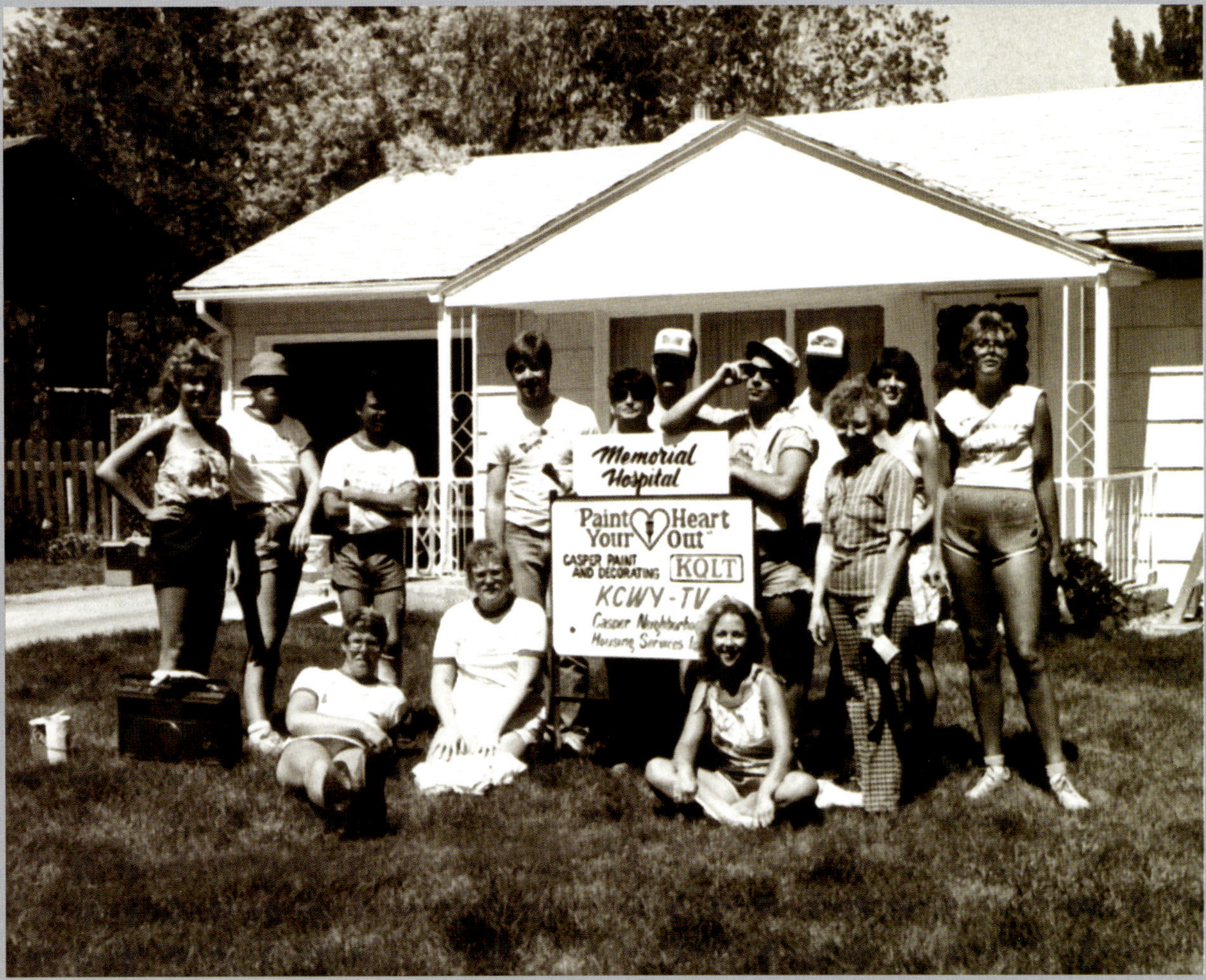

Hospital staff each year painted a house for a senior citizen. This picture is from the 1987 event.

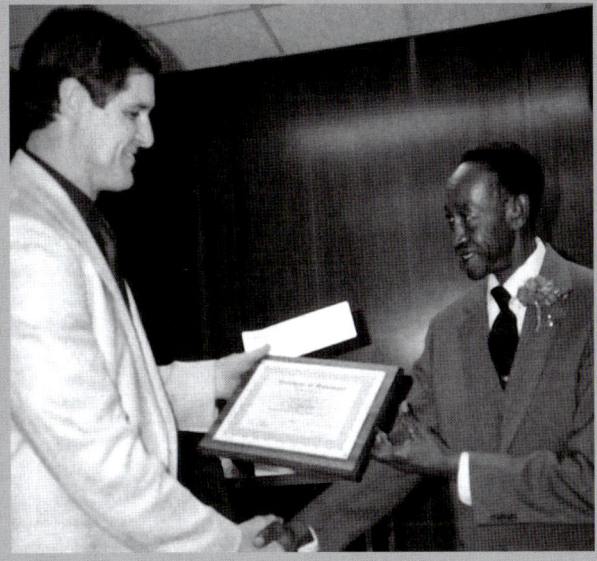
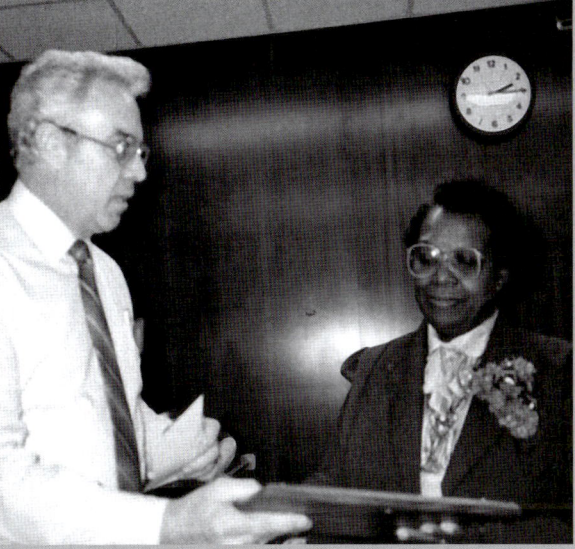

Marion and Myrtle Rucker had worked in the hospital for many years. They retired in 1986.

CHAPTER SIX ❋ *Wyoming Medical Center:* 1986 TO 2010

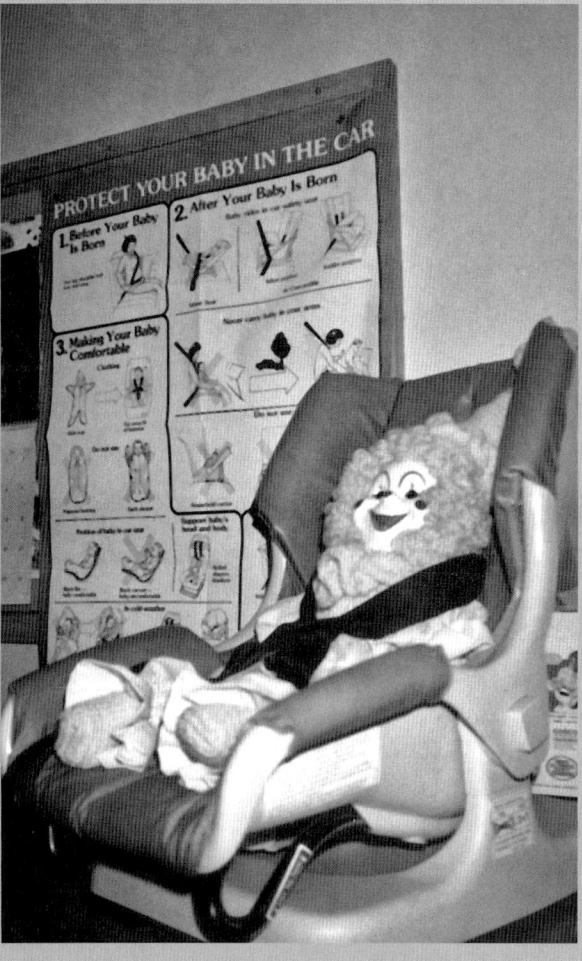

Every family with a newborn infant leaving Wyoming Medical Center needed to have an infant car seat. The hospital donated them to families who could not afford the expense.

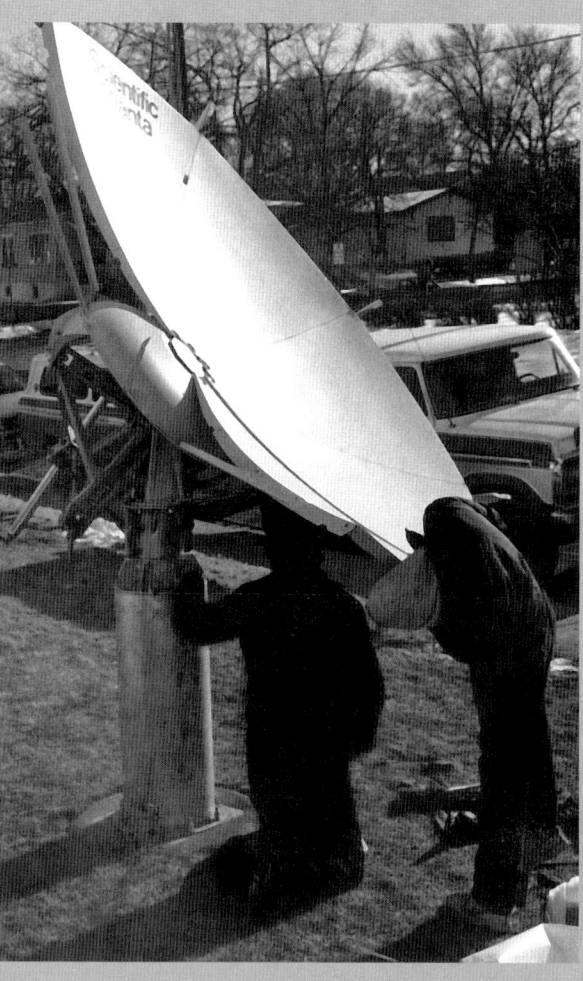

Communication in the late 1980s depended on satellite connections. Here, workers are installing a satellite dish at the Medical Center.

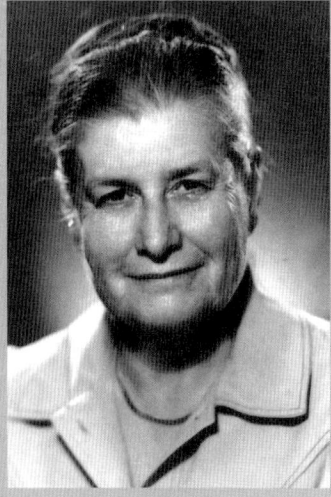

Trula Cooper joined the Trustees in 1986.

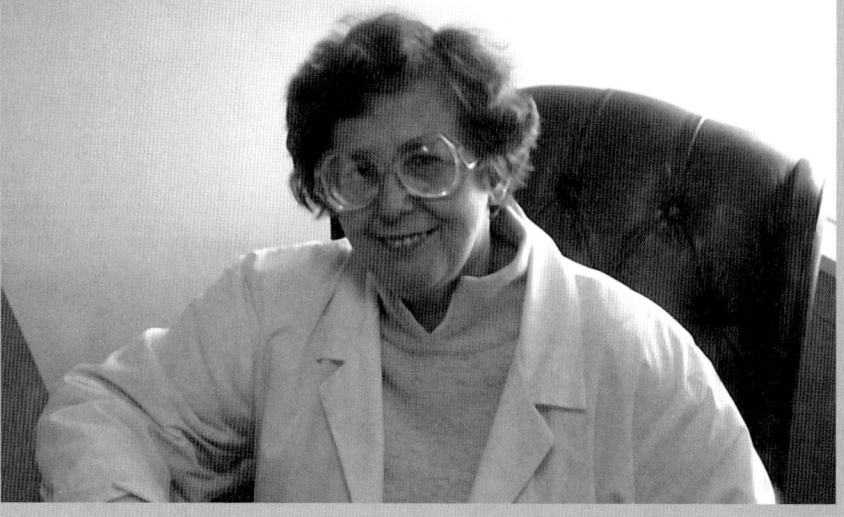

Dr. Raisa Gringauz was a rehabilitation psychiatrist at Wyoming Medical Center.

The Wyoming Farm Loan Board and $1.6 million left from the 1982 One Cent Sales Tax fund were the primary funding for the Central Services building and the elevators. However, these did not provide funding for the east and west additions.[14]

National Cash Register began installing the Mednet computer system at Wyoming Medical Center in August 1988. Training followed for emergency, nursing, and financial personnel as soon as the system arrived at the Information Services offices in the Natrona County Health building.[15] The system's computerized patient charting appealed to most nurses since it allowed them to spend less time on paperwork and more time with patients.

Wyoming Medical Center board members who oversaw all of these changes combined new with familiar faces. Dr. Charles Lyford, William Kidd, Charles Chapin, and Trula Cooper, the second woman to serve, were ongoing members. Hardy Ratcliff and Dr. Paul Johnson were the newest members.[16]

THE 1990s: PINCHING PENNIES AND CHANGING LEADERS

The 1990s was a pivotal decade for Wyoming Medical Center. The 1986 Nichols Plan called for replacing or updating all of the old buildings including the 1967 addition, to accommodate changes in health care including the hospital's new high-technology equipment. Finding financial resources was complicated. The capital bond election scheduled for November 1991 would hopefully get voter approval for an additional one-cent sales tax. That funding proved elusive.

In the meantime, cost-cutting measures became a way of life at the hospital. All departments found ways to pinch pennies. The hospital incinerator burned medical waste and paper trash from hospital departments. That powered the boiler to provide steam to run the laundry or heat the hospital during mild weather. The hospital offered to incinerate medical waste for county residents, serving the double purpose of building public regard and providing more fuel for the boiler.[17]

The newly restructured Marketing and Public Relations Department, under Ann Burns, published *Wyoming Medical Center Hi-Lites*, which conveyed a sense of mission and community building while telling the stories of the hospital's many accomplishments.[18] During this era, management used business terminology to urge employees to think of themselves as members of unit teams as well as of the broader Medical Center team. Articles encouraged employees to achieve their personal best in working with the people who came through the doors.

Douglas Bird's resignation as Wyoming Medical Center president, following a vote of no confidence, was the most dramatic event of 1991. Although employees supported Bird with a mass rally in Conwell Park, he submitted his resignation and moved back to Utah.[19] The board then began a search for a CEO and found Lin

> *In the meantime, cost-cutting measures became a way of life at the hospital. All departments found ways to pinch pennies.*

Carriger, an experienced administrator with a strong business focus. Carriger served as CEO until June 1995, when on a team-building trip with senior staff his raft overturned and he drowned.[20]

Carriger's tenure was challenging on a number of levels. He helped the Medical Center accomplish longstanding goals such as the Central Wyoming Oncology Center, High Plains Psychiatric Center, and the Home Health Department. He employed the Deming Method of continuous quality improvement to restructure the staff and provide leadership opportunities to a new generation of employees. At the same time, his use of terms like "customer" for patient and "product line" for program bothered more traditional hospital workers.[21]

Carriger's "reengineering" tried to place the right people in the right places, doing the right jobs. As Laurie Sanftner, a former Medical Center respiratory therapist, said in an interview, "the ability to learn and grow was high."[22] To accomplish this, Carriger brought in managers such as Barbara Ringhouse, who questioned the way everything had been done in the hospital, looking for savings and better practice. Carriger's leadership moved the hospital forward and helped rebuild its reputation in the community.

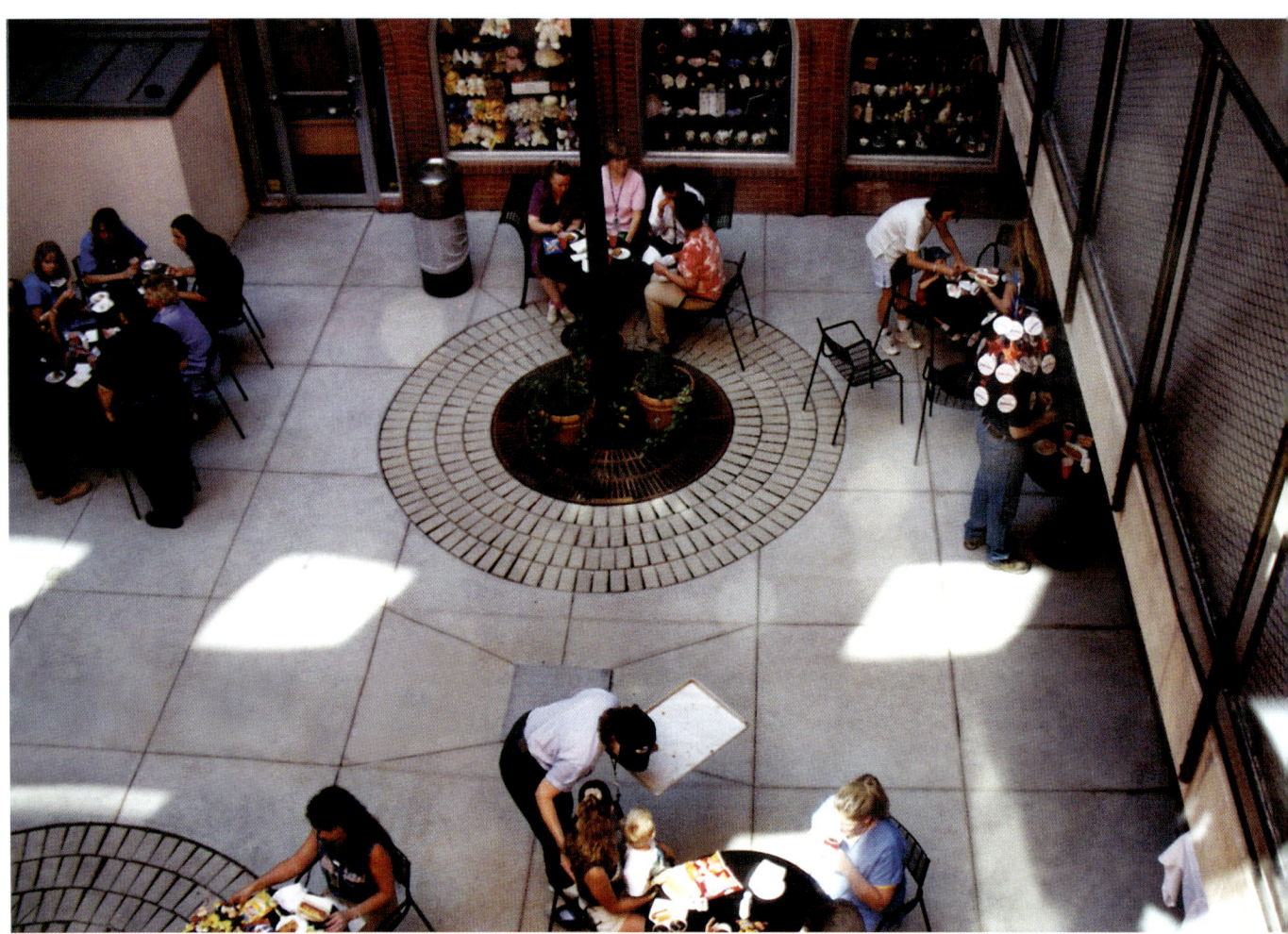

The first-floor interior courtyard was a gathering place surrounded by the old and new hospital wings.

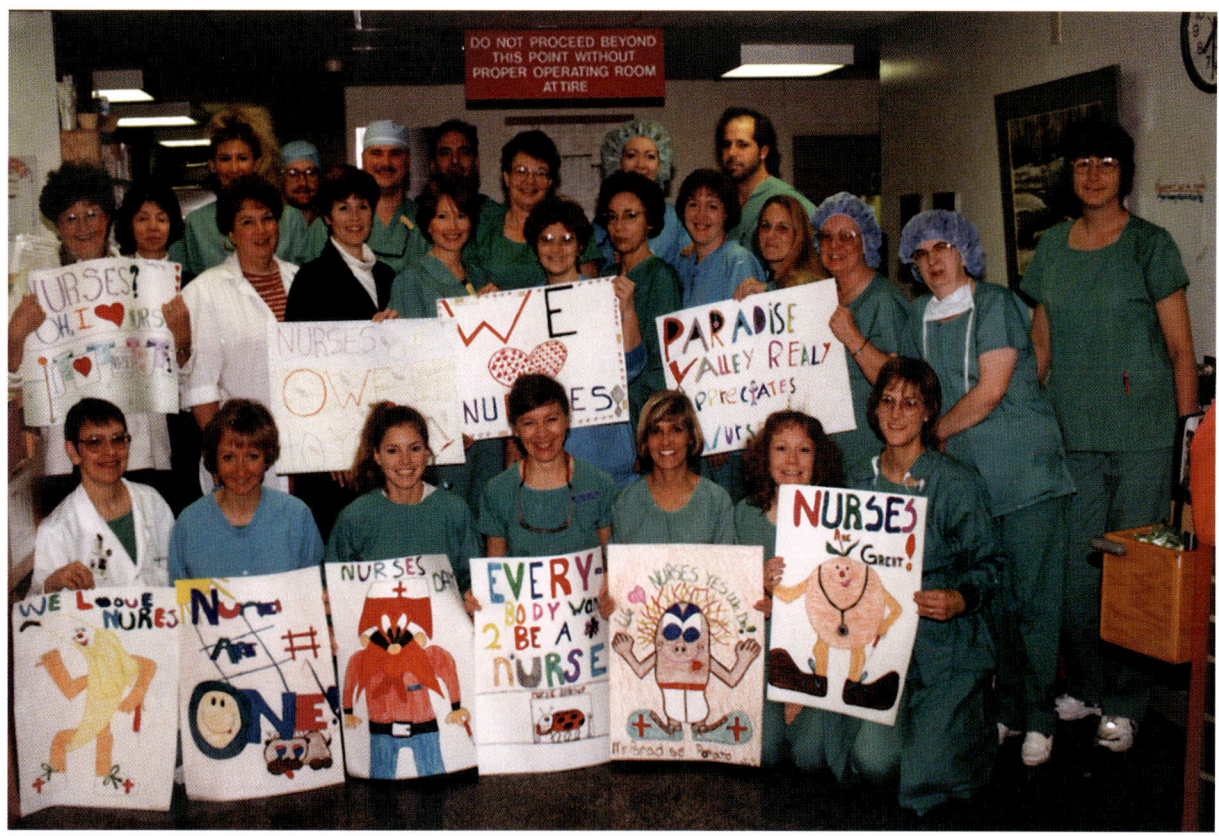

Operating room nurses display the signs schoolchildren made for them during Nurses' Week festivities.

The 1990s was an era of physician shortages. Older doctors, many of whom had arrived in the 1950s, were retiring. To attract new physicians, Casper needed something extra. That "extra" was the higher quality of life in Natrona County. Many doctors appreciated the slower pace of life in a small city as well as the scenery and outdoor activities that were possible in Wyoming. Casper offered reasonable housing and office prices, decent schools, and a low crime rate. The corporate structure of Wyoming Medical Center also allowed for innovative collaborations among physicians and between public and private entities. Finally, since many small towns in Wyoming lacked doctors, especially specialists, there was the possibility of branch offices around the state. The hospital recruited physicians from around the world.[23]

Some of the new physicians were Casper natives who were coming home. Mary MacGuire, M.D., a general surgeon, arrived in 1991, bringing expertise in endoscopic and laparoscopic surgical techniques.[24] Robert Tobin, M.D. returned to run the Central Wyoming Oncology Center, which opened in September 1992.[25] The cancer center provided a balanced program of high technology and personalized care. In June 1998, when Dr. Diane Turner arrived, she was the first woman oncologist on staff. She joined Robert Tobin, M.D., Dr. Paul Johnson, and Dr. Vaughn Cipperly at the Oncology Center.[26]

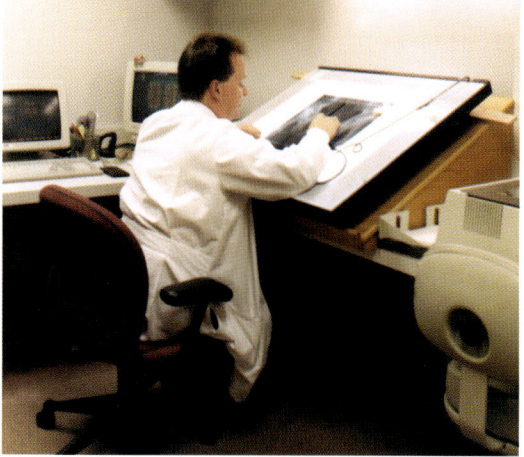

The Central Wyoming Oncology Center blended personal care and new technology.

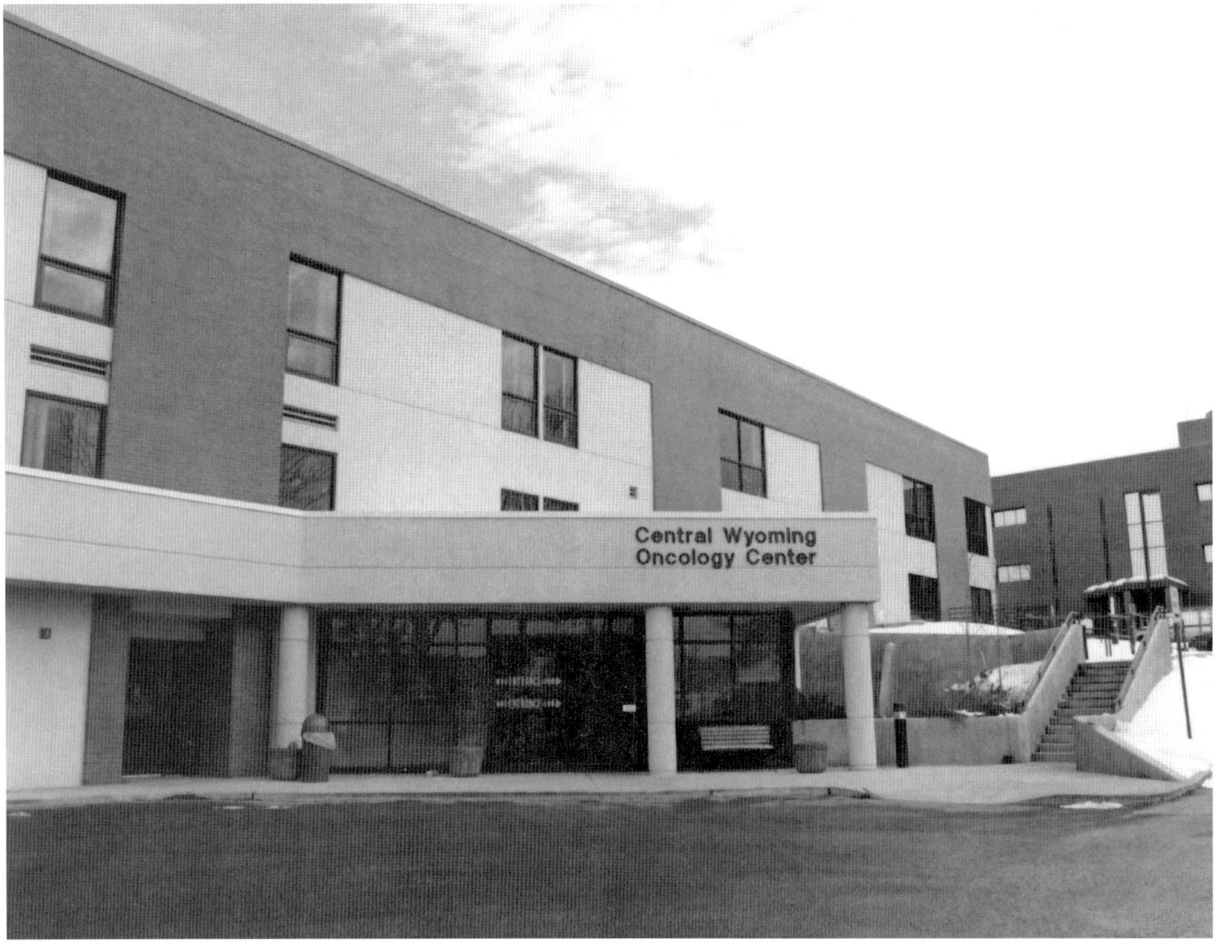

The Central Wyoming Oncology Center provided the best in cancer treatment for Wyoming residents.

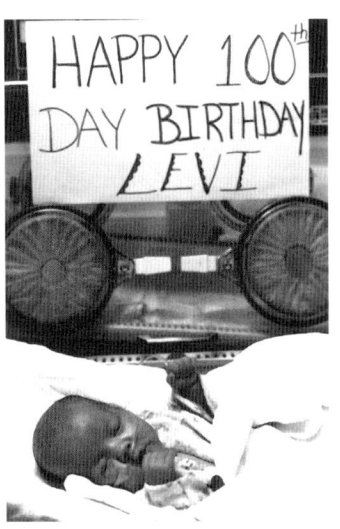

Levi Harmon was one of Wyoming Medical Center's successes. He later returned to celebrate his first birthday with the nurses.

Some of the Medical Center's personnel were in the Wyoming National Guard. When the United States entered the First Gulf War in 1991, the Guard called up Bill Shugart and Debbie Gronning, two Wyoming Medical Center employees. *Hi-Lites* articles chronicled the adventures of Shugart, a Life Flight nurse, and Gronning, a surgical nurse, both of whom were stationed in Saudi Arabia.[27] As the war dragged on, other employees had sons, daughters, and other family members serving in the military and the newsletter kept track of those people as well.

To make it easier to balance the needs of work and family, in 1991 the Medical Center decided to build and staff a child care center. The four-person staff offered full- and part-time care twenty-four hours a day, 365 days a year. The Next Generation Child Care Center opened in June 1992 with seventy-five to one hundred children per day, under the direction of Lorrie Larson.[28]

Patients continued to flood into the Medical Center in the 1990s, reflecting expanded use by people from around Wyoming. In 1991 alone, the Medical Center staff saw more than 45,000 patients in all of its programs.[29] Human Relations Director John Ysebaert organized a Guest Relations Program in May 1991. As part of the program, *Hi-Lites* printed notes from patients and their families that detailed their good experiences. Employees who excelled also received recognition in the newsletter.[30]

Each month, *Hi-Lites* focused on an employee. Some were retiring. Dorothy Quinlan had worked at the hospital since 1952. Medical Technologist Shirley Hunter, described as "a laboratory legend," retired in 1992 after thirty years.[31] Other articles focused on current employees such as Roy Hayford, who helped keep the facilities running through his carpentry and committee work.

New technology brought new skills to the Medical Center. Once a pharmacist's greatest skill was mixing powders and herbs to make medicines by hand. In 1992, new chief pharmacist Carmel Tice worked in a computerized pharmacy where pre-made medicines were barcoded and then matched with barcoded patient bracelets, ensuring that the right medicine in the correct dosage got to the right patient.[32]

Nurses and other technical personnel continued to take more coursework and receive certifications in their areas of expertise. An evolving area of medical care was respiratory therapy. Many patients came in with lung problems, but at some point, all surgical patients need help with their breathing. Respiratory therapy training was another Medical Center joint venture with Casper College.[33]

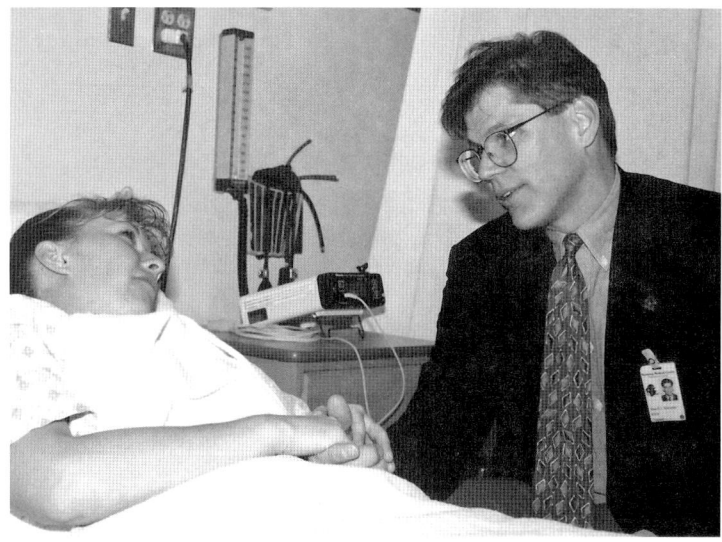

Hospital Chaplain Dana Schroeder led the chaplaincy program from 1994 to 2000.

In 1992, construction began on a new Emergency Department, operating rooms, and Intensive Care Unit. At the same time, the hospital began moving other departments from the east wing in preparation for demolition followed by the construction of the five-story addition, theoretically scheduled for November 1993. While there was money for the relocation and demolition, there was not yet money for building the new building.[34] Fundraising for the new east wing was going slowly, so it would be the summer of 1997 before demolition started.[35]

On April 6, 1993, the Life Flight plane crashed in a snowstorm, killing the pilot Tom Rickert, paramedic Dennis Patrick, and emergency room nurse Tom Wolfe, as well as the patient, Hank Williamson. This was the first fatal crash in Life Flight's ten-year history. The community responded in May with a series of events to raise funds for the staffers' families. Donations from forty-four area restaurants, as well as a community car wash, raised $4,300.[36]

In August 1995, Wyoming Medical Center leased a new fixed-wing plane, a Beechcraft C-90 King Air, to replace the MU2 that had crashed. The plane, leased from Corporate Jets of Pittsburgh, could fly in conditions that the helicopter could not and carry more equipment and patients. It could also transport physicians to branch clinics.[37]

Physicians had an additional way to reach outlying areas. Telemedicine connected Wyoming Medical Center specialists with physicians in other parts of the state. The system used computers, cameras, and speakers to connect, allowing exchange of X-rays

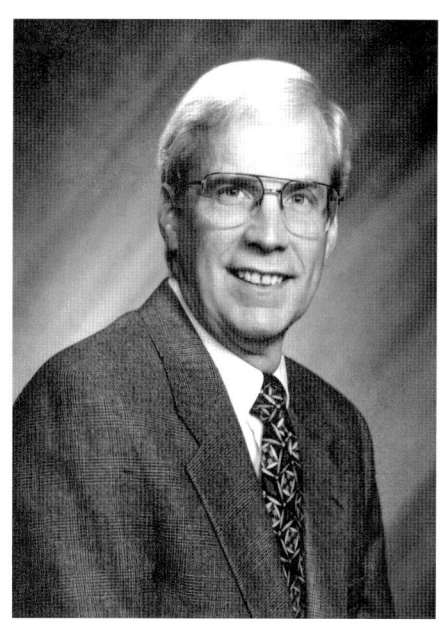

Michael Schrader was the Wyoming Medical Center CEO from 1995 to 2000.

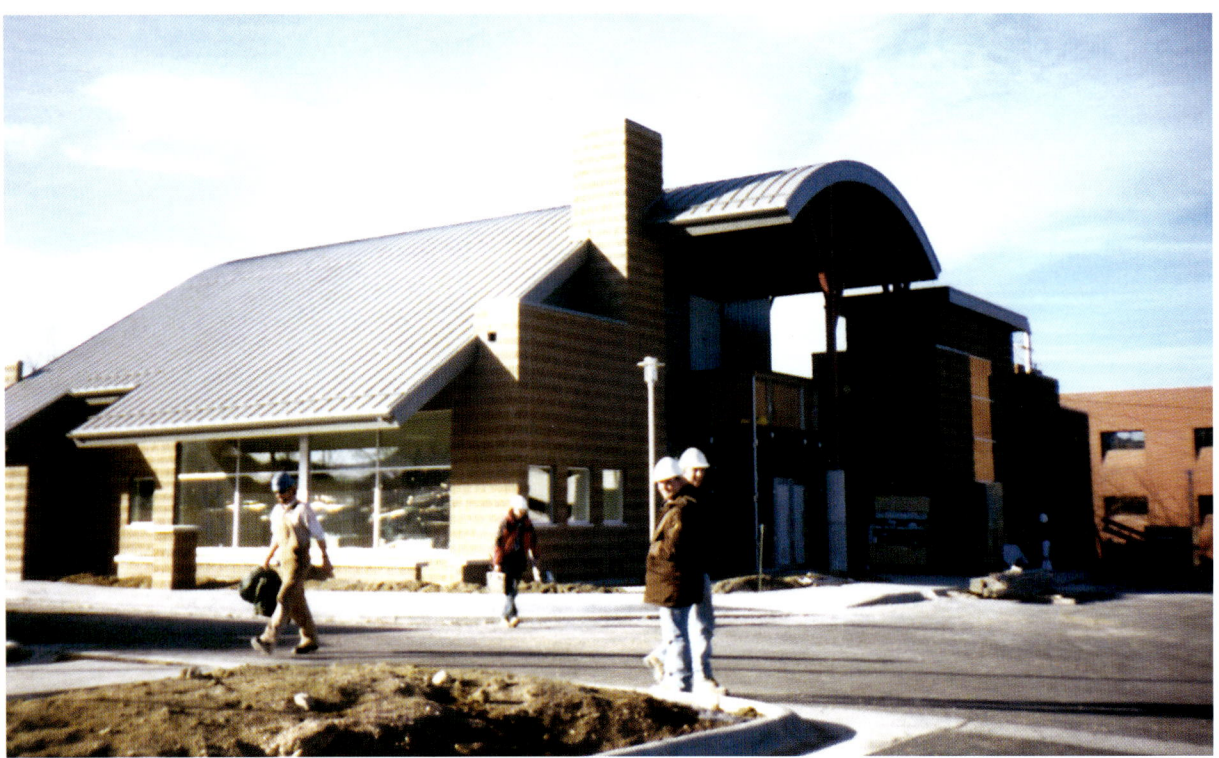

The surgical center was a joint project made possible by Wyoming Medical Center's non-profit structure.

and medical files and allowing visual consultation with patients via camera. The Converse County Memorial Hospital joined the network in 1994.[38]

The hospital created a chaplaincy program in 1994. Dana Schroeder was the head chaplain.[39] He coordinated ministers from the community who visited parishioners in the hospital.

In February 1995, the board announced that they would be shelving the plans for the east building and building an addition to the west of the hospital. The five-story structure would have a new Emergency Department, surgical suites, catheterization laboratories, obstetrics, Intensive Care Unit, and radiology, as well as a second parking structure. Lin Carriger reported that the $45-million cost would be covered by revenue bonds and internal and community fundraising. The board hoped to break ground in the spring of 1996 and have the grand opening in 1998. This new building program bypassed the Nichols Plan, replacing it with ideas that came from community input and the reengineering that had been taking place at the Medical Center.[40]

When Lin Carriger died, senior management created a team that ran the hospital until the board hired Mike Schrader in October 1995. Schrader stepped into a turbulent scene as revenues dropped, Carriger's building plan fell out of favor, and staff malaise grew. One of Schrader's first challenges was an attempt to take over the board by the

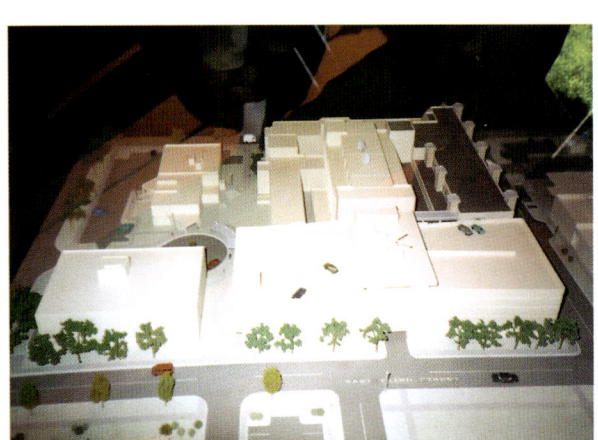

In 1997, architects presented this model of the hospital complex including the new east wing.

112 *Wyoming Medical Center:* A CENTENNIAL HISTORY

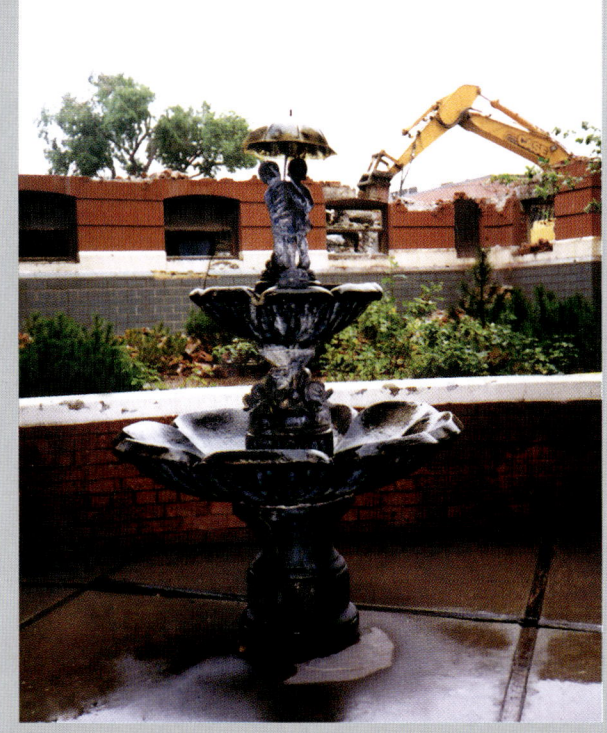
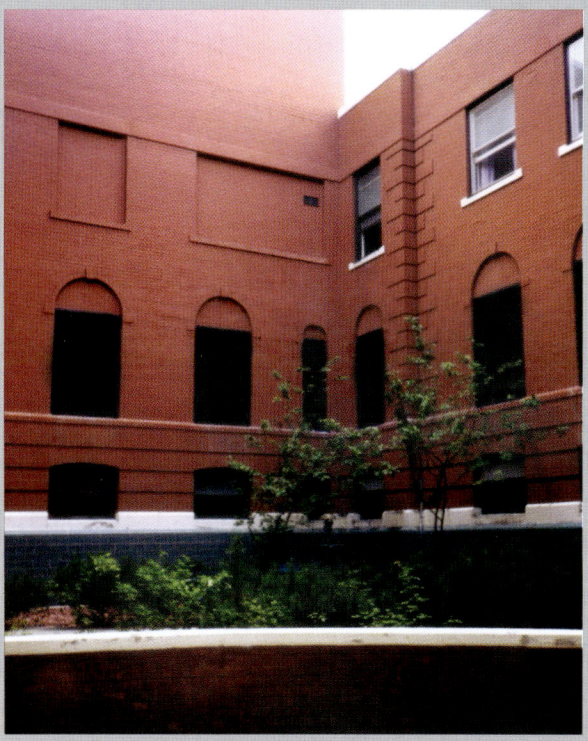
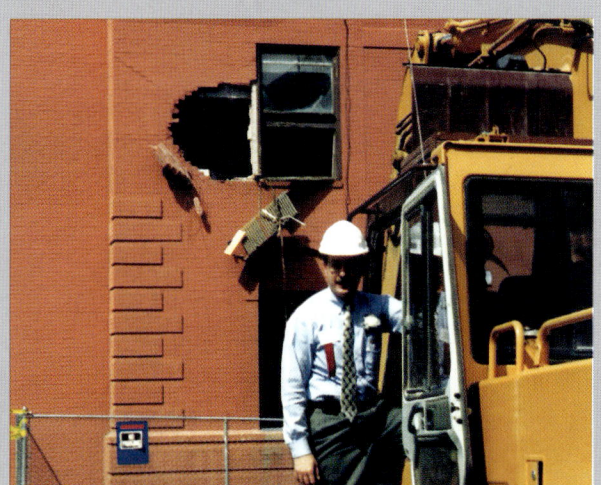
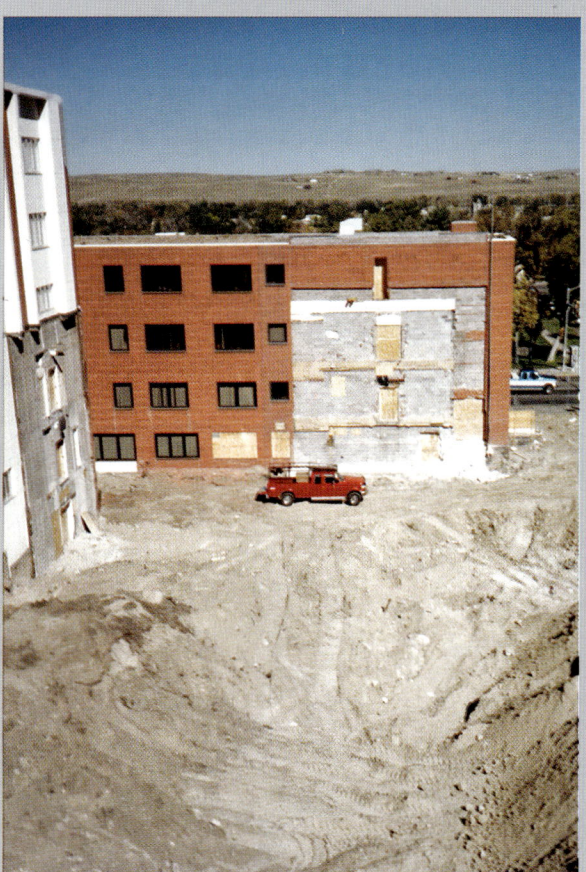
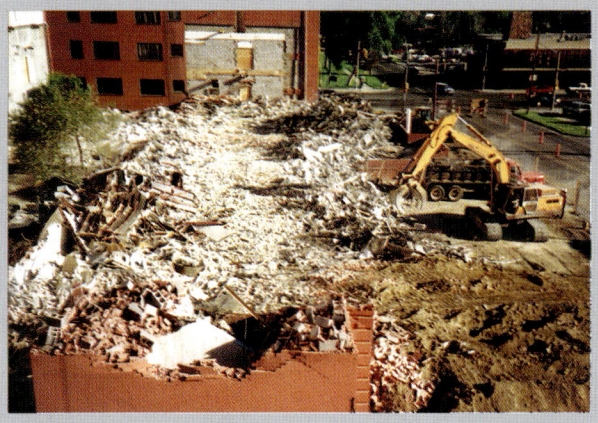

The 1997 demolition of the east wing.

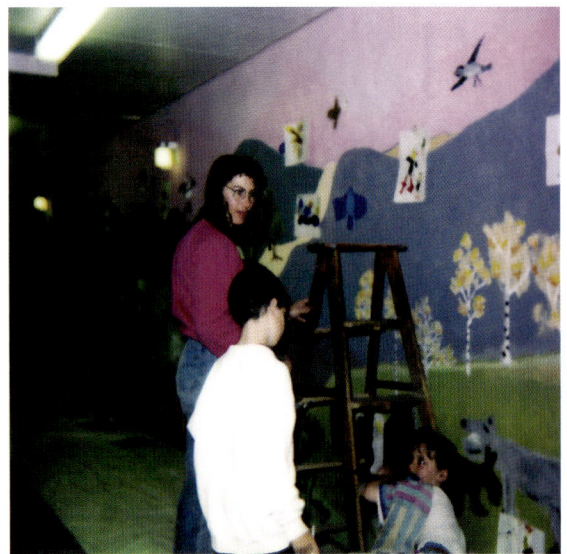

Students from Paradise Valley Elementary School designed and painted the artwork in the hospital's connecting tunnel.

Natrona County Commission. The Commissioners backed down, partly to insure Schrader's arrival. Patient care issues partly caused by employee layoffs earlier in 1995 provided additional problems. Schrader instituted a hiring freeze in 1996 to save existing jobs rather than make more layoffs.

Another issue was where the Medical Center should next expand. Physicians wanted more specialty buildings to the south. The hospital needed a replacement for the 1930s east building while another plan called for building to the west. Carriger had promised Dr. Jerry Youmans and Dr. Louis Roussalis a new office building in exchange for a property swap. When the building project failed because costs ran too high, the deal turned nasty and ended up in a five-year lawsuit.[41] A crisis of confidence followed.

Mike Schrader found that many departments felt that they had been treated badly in the reengineering process. While he looked at the issues he continued to tighten operations because he felt "we cost too much money."[42] This created further unrest. In July, Schrader pledged that he would not raise fees on rooms or services in an effort to rebuild faith with the community.[43]

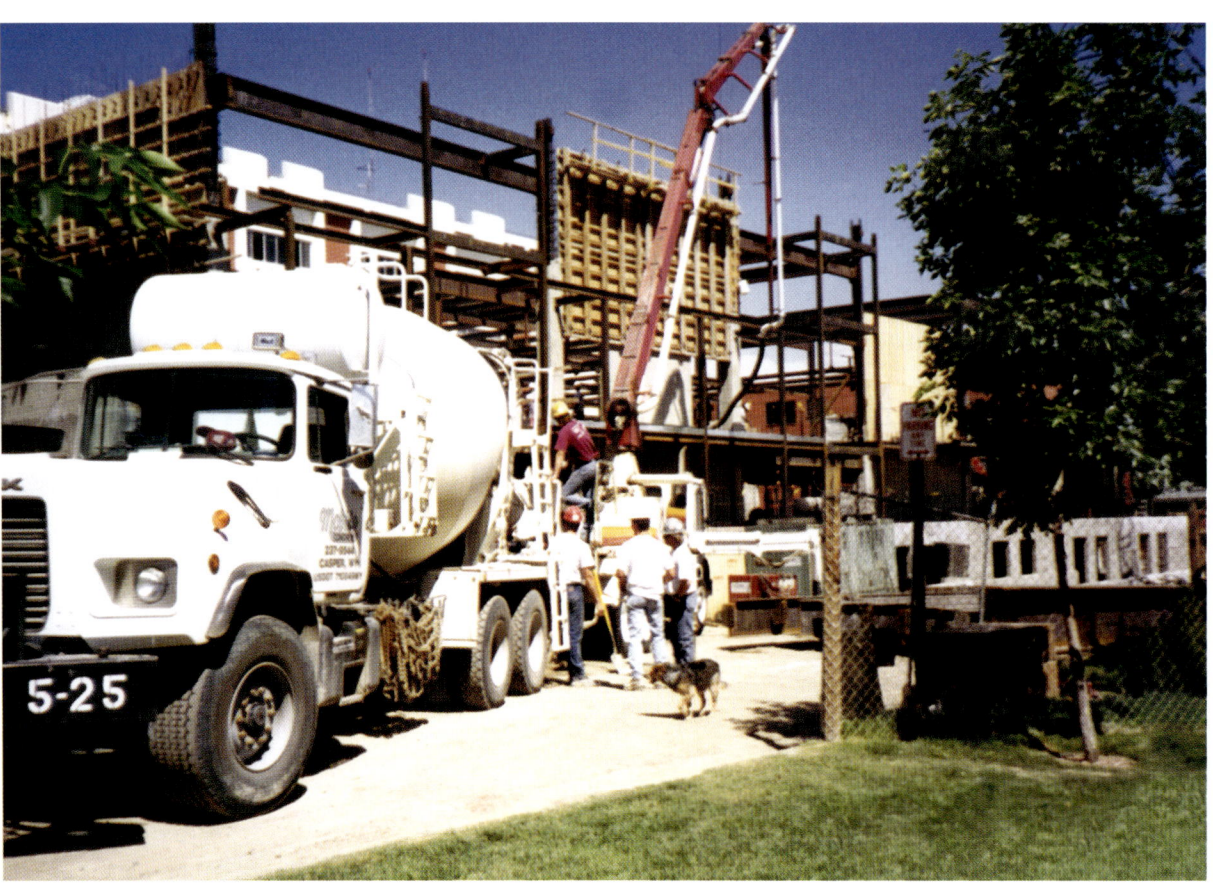

The cement mixers rolled in as the bones of the new wing went up.

114 *Wyoming Medical Center:* A CENTENNIAL HISTORY

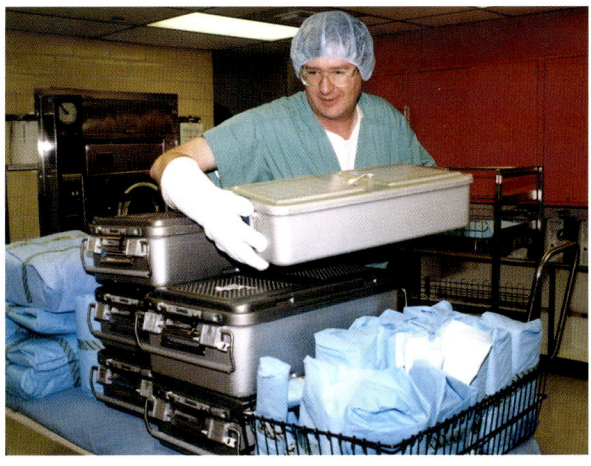
Terry Jensen puts together the supplies going up to the operating room.

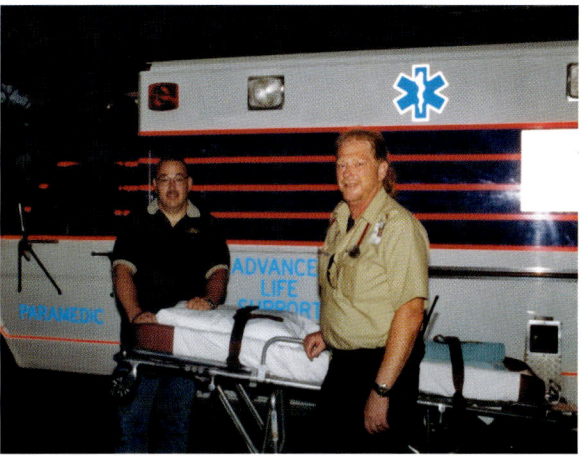
Mike Garwood and Russ Christensen wait for a call next to the ambulance.

In February 1996, frustrated nurses considered unionizing, saying that understaffing was at the core of patient care problems.[44] The tension with the nursing staff reached such a level that the Wyoming State Nurses' Association considered getting involved, but ultimately did not.[45]

Schrader urged a reexamination of the institution's perceived role as the primary regional medical center in Wyoming. In April 1996, he announced that he was not dedicated to the idea of expansion; however, he agreed to revisit the less expensive east wing expansion, although in a much-reduced format. The need for a new Emergency Department and operating rooms had influenced Schrader's decision. Estimates put the cost at $29.1 to $38 million.[46] At the same time, construction continued on the Casper Surgical Center and on office space.[47]

In the midst of all of this, at the end of 1996, Columbia/HCA, a for-profit hospital company based in Nashville, Tennessee, began to look at acquiring Wyoming Medical Center. Schrader declined to negotiate, but Columbia continued to pursue a merger. Nothing came of it.[48]

Some months in 1997 went better than others. On March 7, Dr. Gary Weiss died of a heart attack at age forty-five. Since he was the only cardiac surgeon in Wyoming, this raised the need to recruit another physician. The favorite candidate was Dr. Louis Steplock, who had practiced in Casper but moved to Olympia, Washington. Steplock returned in September.[49] By 1998, he could report that the cardiac team had performed 270 operations with fewer deaths than the national average of 4.5, at a rate of 1.9 percent.[50]

In late March, a water main break contaminated much of Casper's water supply.[51] On May 20, bomb threats led to the total evacuation of the hospital. According to Transport Specialist Rolly Sanftner, the evacuation of more than one hundred patients

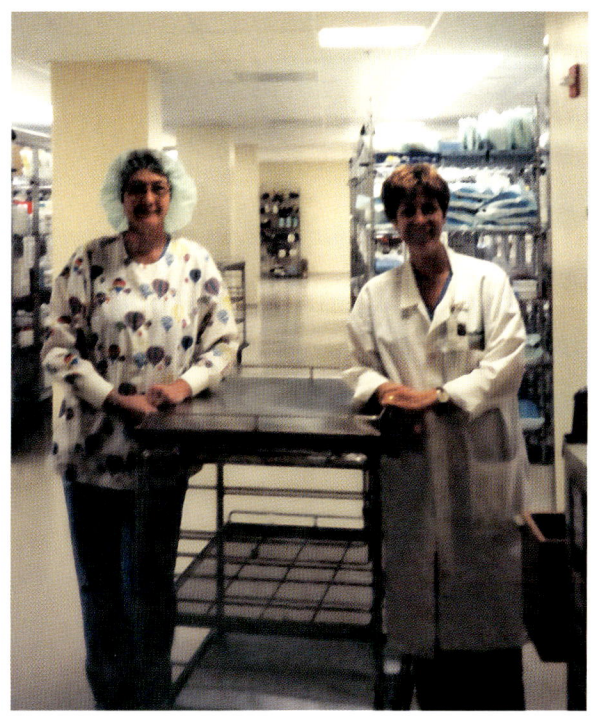
JoAnn Toal and Deb Weaver wait for supplies for the operating room in Central Supply.

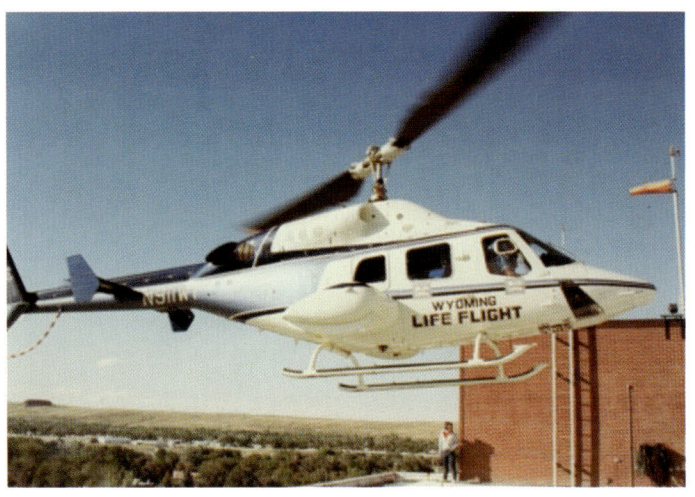

Life Flight begins a run to save yet another life.

took roughly twelve minutes and cleared everyone out except patients and staff in two operating rooms, where surgeons were performing sensitive heart and back surgeries.[52]

On August 26, 1997, the 1930s east wing began to come down. More than a decade of planning was now a reality. In September, the Medical Center announced that they had acquired five houses for the expansion project and were donating them to Habitat for Humanity.[53]

By October, the building plan included a south link lobby from the parking garage to the Medical Center and a tunnel from the buildings south of Third Street to the hospital.[54] In early May 1998, workmen completed the tunnel to the surgical building, which opened in September. Renovation began on the sixth floor of the 1967 building.[55] Project manager Greg Pope reported that remodeling around patient areas required flexibility. He felt that this project was "perhaps the most difficult and complex construction project in Casper's history."[56] The east wing was halfway completed in January 1999, but there was a construction shortfall to consider. In February, the board approved $2 million for an overrun fund.[57]

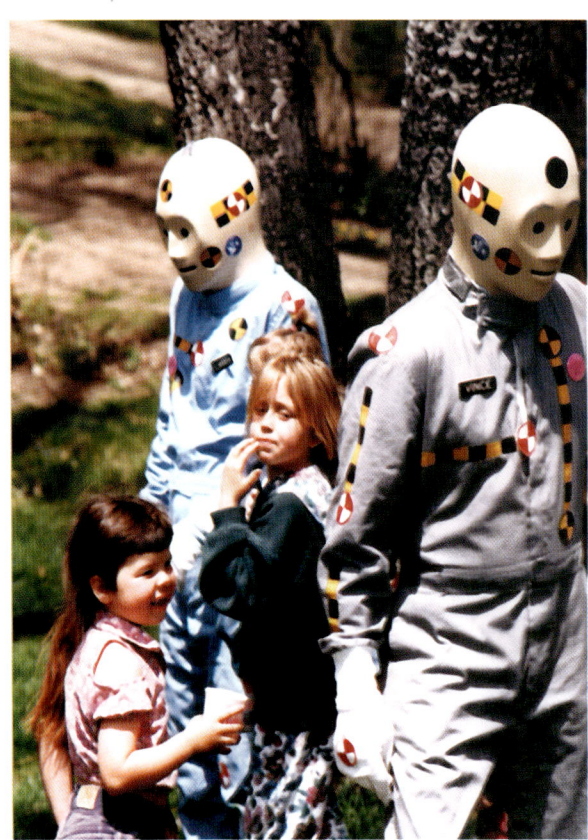 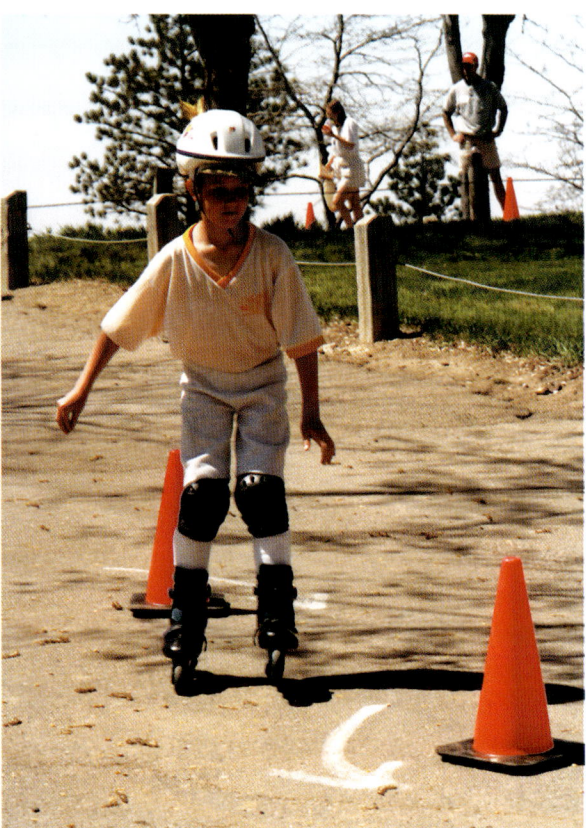

Wyoming Medical Center's Safe Kids Day taught area children about helmets and car safety.

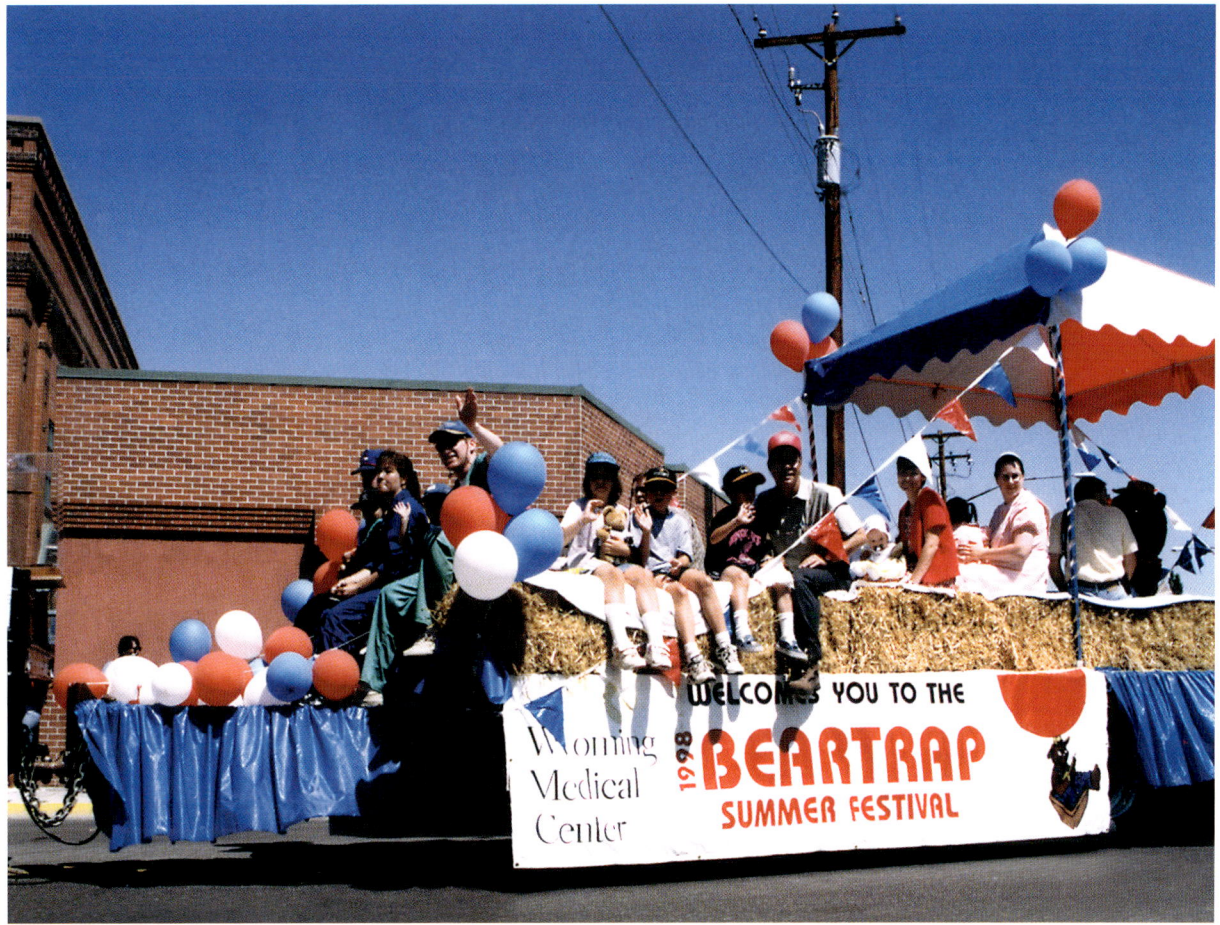

Wyoming Medical Center marketed its sponsorship of the Bear Trap Music Festival.

In January, the Auxiliary gave $5,000 for equipment to test hearing in newborns. They also donated $2,000 to oncology for financial assistance for patients who could not afford to buy post-operative pain medications.[58]

The New Year brought a new logo which was a stylized WMC based on Wyoming's physical features. The logo immediately stirred a controversy for the $8,000 price tag and the fact that it had not been created by a local firm. Schrader indicated that it would stay.[59]

In April, Marriott took over food service at the hospital. Professional dietitians continued to oversee the menu, but this meant a different way of preparing meals and savings of $500,000.[60]

When the City of Casper-Natrona County Health Department moved to a new building, their facility on Third Street became Wyoming Medical Center's Support Services building.[61] In August, when the remodeled sixth floor opened, transfer of patients began from the fourth through sixth floors of the 1967 building. The remodeled space featured improved private and semi-private rooms.[62]

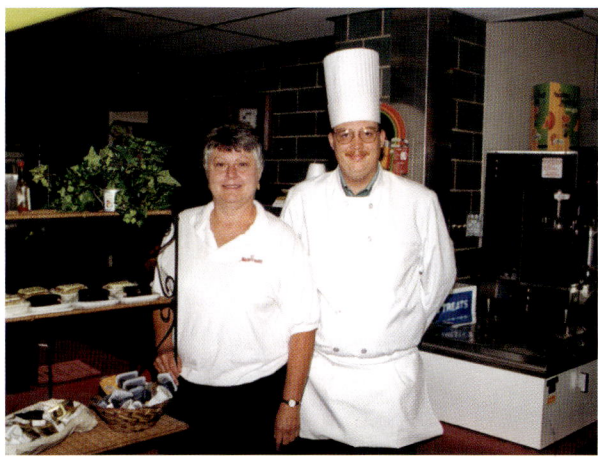

Marriott Food Service took over operation of the hospital cafeteria in 1998.

CHAPTER SIX ❖ *Wyoming Medical Center:* 1986 TO 2010 117

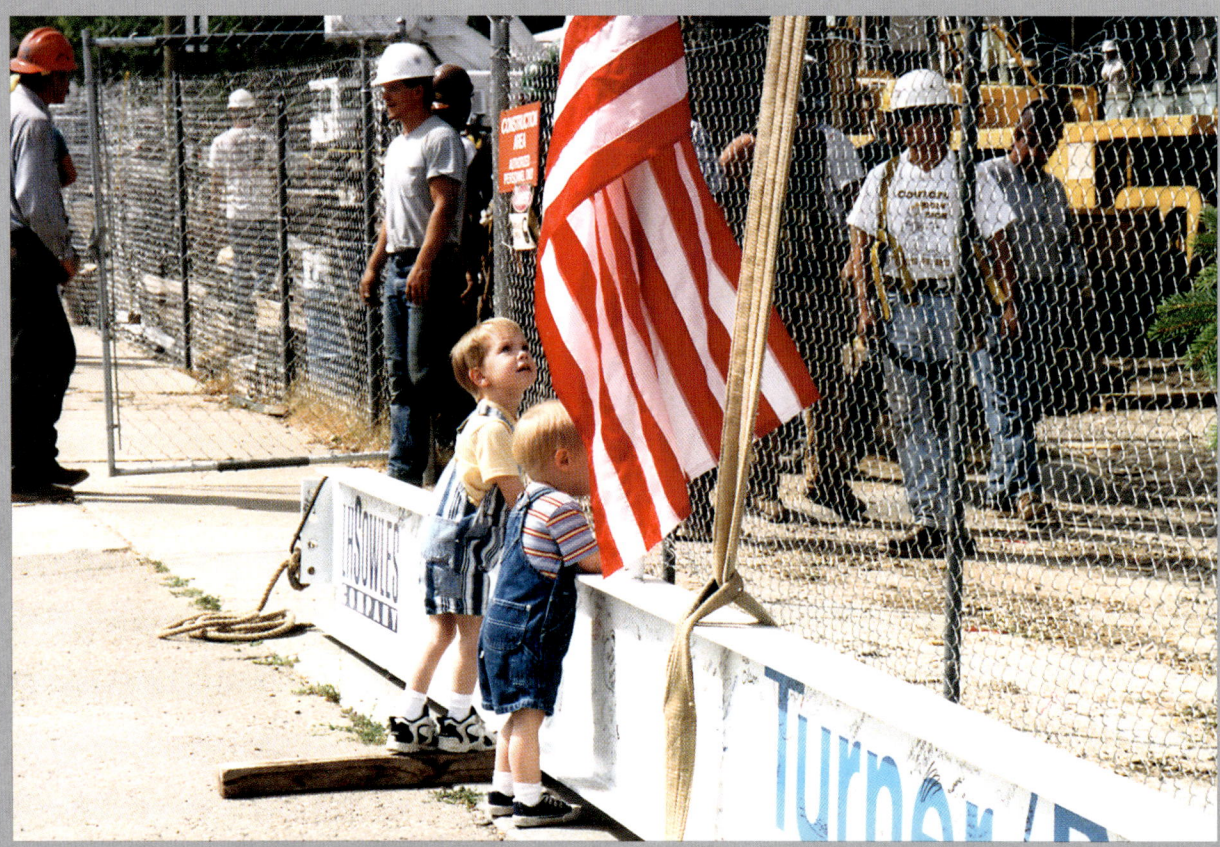

In 1999, two boys watched as the construction continued on the new east wing.

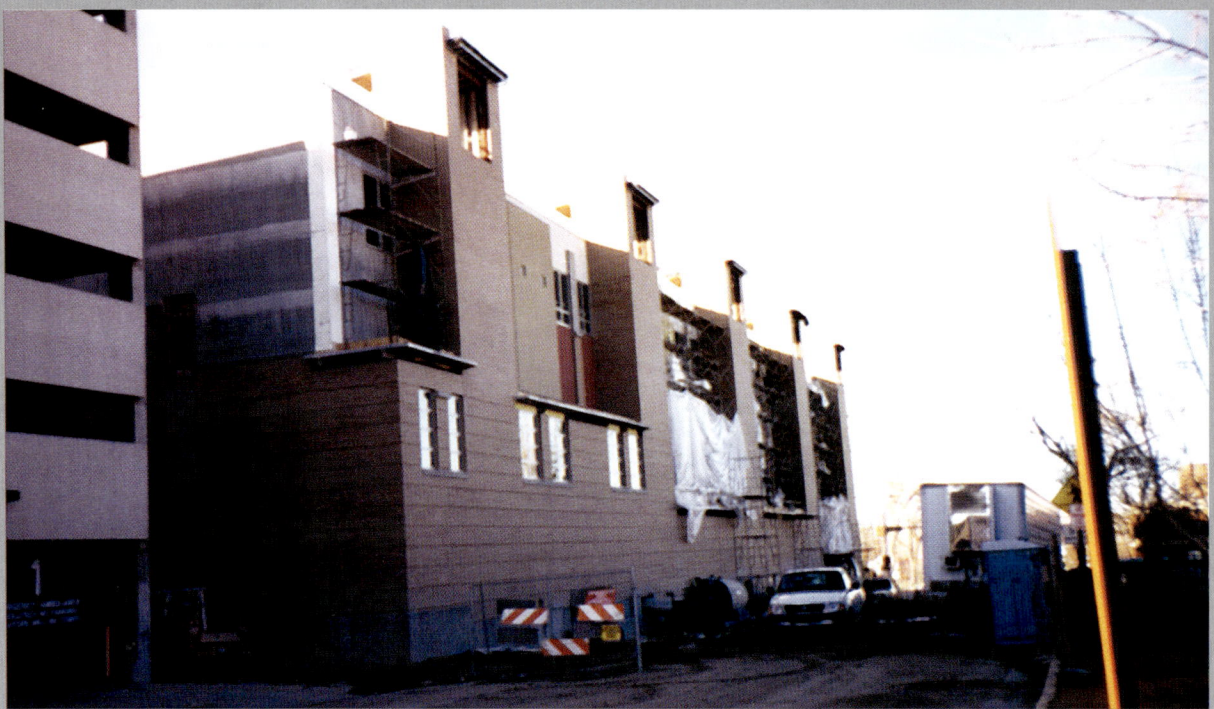

The east wing nears completion in 1999.

118 *Wyoming Medical Center:* A CENTENNIAL HISTORY

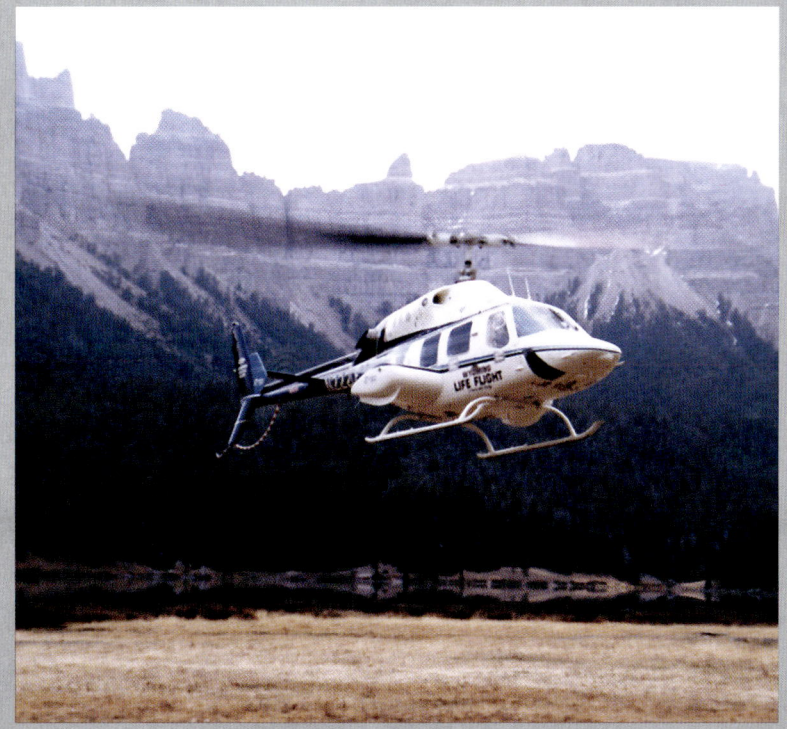

Left: Life Flight takes off from a mountain rescue.

Below: Wyoming Life Flight had become such an institution that the hospital issued Christmas cards with pictures of the flight staff and equipment.

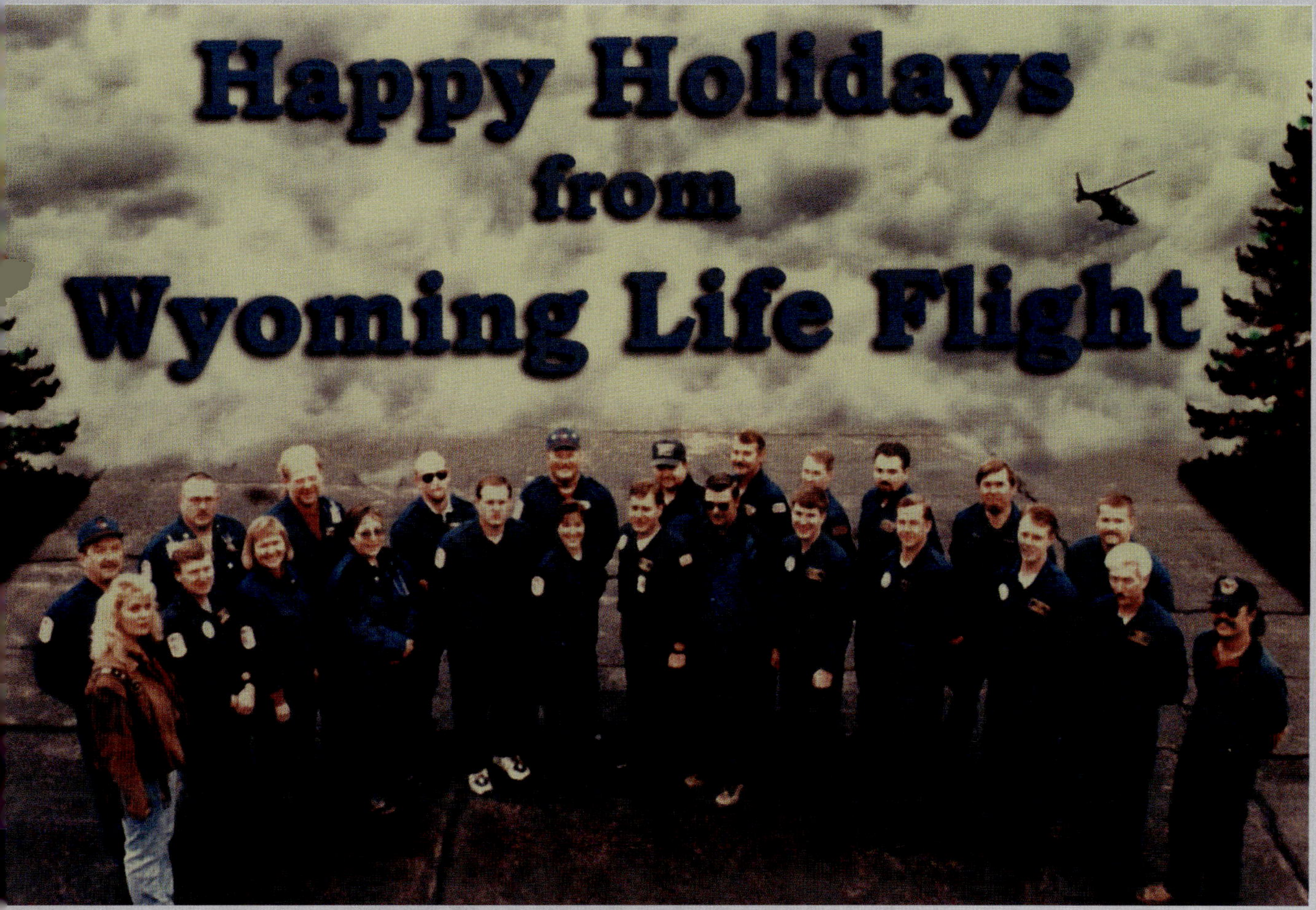

THE FINAL DECADE: PAST MEETS FUTURE

The new decade did not start off with a bang as some had feared. Plans for Y2K problems were thorough, but there was not a single computer-related event at Wyoming Medical Center. The excitement at the hospital instead came from the opening of the new east wing.

A series of articles in the *Casper Star-Tribune* documented the east wing opening. The new operating rooms and recovery rooms were on the third floor of the east wing. Telemetry and ICU were patient- and nurse-friendly as well as state-of-the-art. The ICU had fourteen rooms with a glass wall and closed circuit television for monitoring the patients. Norma Clavier, who had worked in the operating room from 1968 to 1996, noted that the 1960s-era Emergency Department was only four small rooms. More than 2,000 people toured the new ICU and operating rooms. Director of Emergency Services Becky Hanson noted that the new emergency room opened on November 22, 1999, just in time for an influenza epidemic in which 344 cases quickly taxed the resources of the new facility. A total of 2,733 patients visited the Emergency Department in December 1999.[63]

The new Emergency Department opened in 2000.

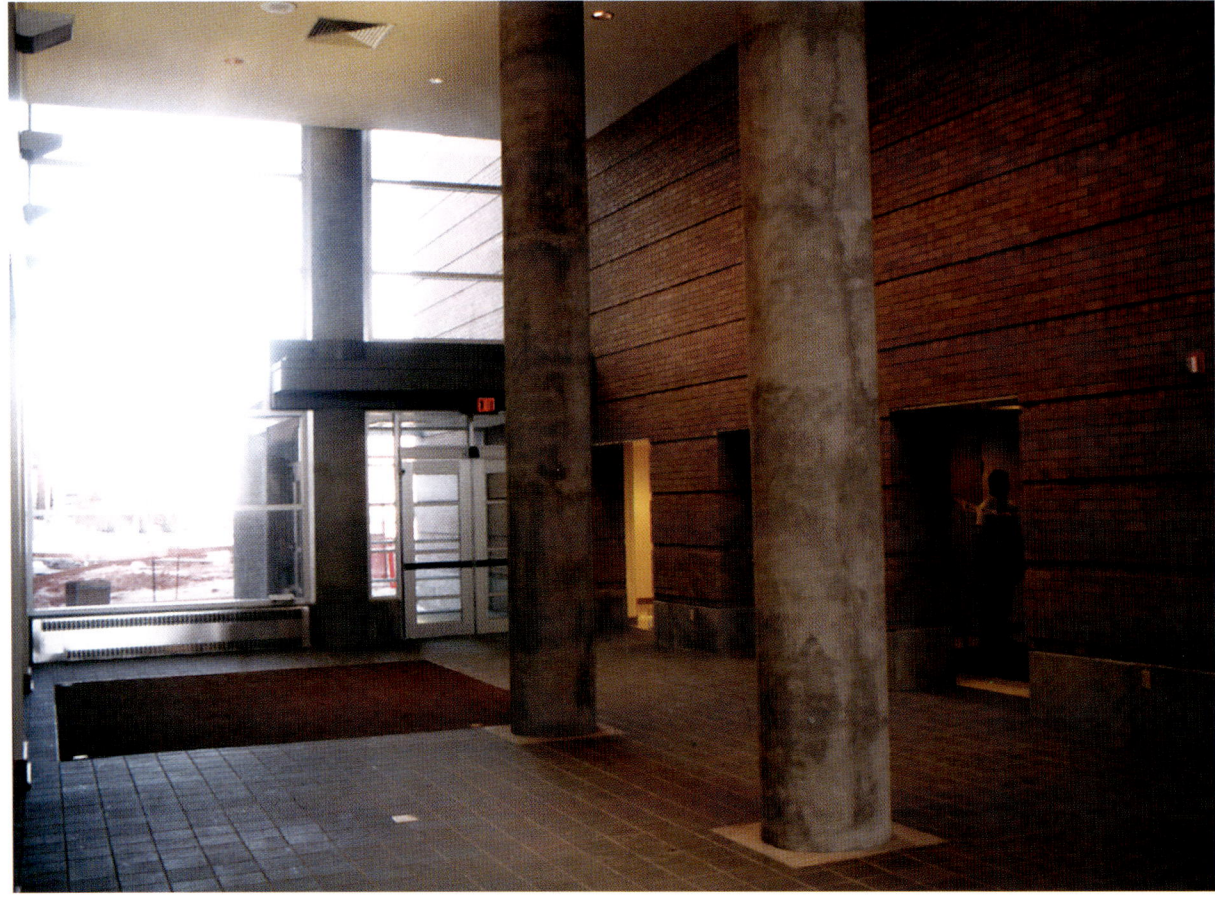

The south link lobby under construction in 2001.

In October 2000, Mike Schrader left Wyoming Medical Center for a job in Colorado Springs. The board appointed Phil Eaton, who had been chief operating officer under Schrader as the interim CEO. Eaton, who had nineteen years' experience in the health care field, served until June 2001, moving on to run the Lander/Riverton hospital.[64] The new CEO was James Gardner, who began work on June 15, 2001.

In October 2000, Wyoming Medical Center applied for regional trauma center designation from the state. The *AMA Journal* ranked the Medical Center sixth in the nation in treatment of heart attack and failure, breast cancer, stroke, pneumonia, and diabetes.[65]

In the new decade, the Medical Center continued to recruit physicians. Longtime ear, nose, and throat physician Dr. Kent Christensen retired and Dr. Eugene Podrasik arrived to replace him. Many areas of general and specialist medicine still needed new practitioners.[66]

Families who wanted to stay close to long-term patients found it difficult to get affordable lodging in Casper. In honor of her husband James, Mary Masterson donated $1 million to Wyoming Medical Center to purchase the Best Western Motel on Yellowstone Highway. Masterson Place would provide low-cost hotel rooms for patients and families. The hospital used the money to renovate the hotel to make it more home-like.[67]

In April, the board and physicians finally agreed on a site plan for a new medical office building and outpatient imaging center. The 50,000-square-foot building was going up at Fifth and Washington streets as a joint venture with Mick McMurry, a local developer.[68] The McMurry Medical Arts Building, opening in the fall of 2005, helped attract more internal medicine physicians to Casper.[69]

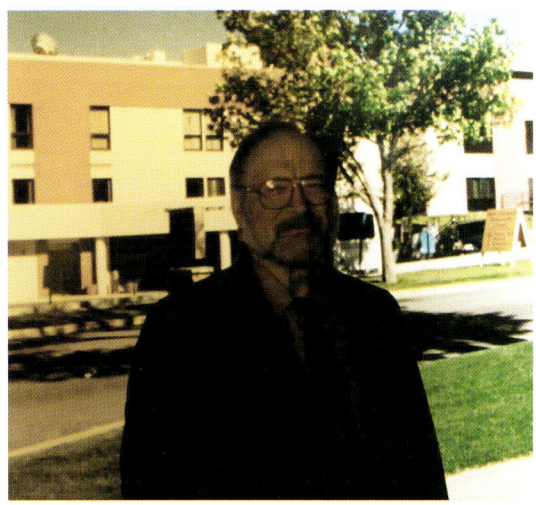

Reverend Ellis Kaster became the head of Chaplaincy Services when Dana Schroeder left.

Finally, it was time for the ribbon-cutting for the new Washington Street entrance to the Medical Center.[70] The $48-million building project included the west addition, the south link lobby, and the new east wing. Officials anticipated that this project would keep the hospital up to date for at least the next decade.

The dedication of the new chapel off the south link lobby marked another milestone for the Medical Center. Dana Schroeder, head of the hospital's pastoral care and Clinical Pastoral Care Education Program, said the chapel was "more evocative than descriptive and doesn't tell you what to believe."[71] The dedication ceremony was also the occasion for installing a new assistant chaplain, Reverend Ellis Kaster.

While Wyoming Medical Center reached out to patients in other parts of Wyoming, it also wanted people to know that its first responsibility was to Casper and Natrona County patients.[72] To keep itself competitive, it froze room rates for 2001–2002. The semi-private rate was $533 per day, ICU was $1,514, and telemetry was $810.[73] Although the Medical Center was in a fairly good financial condition, the high out-of-county

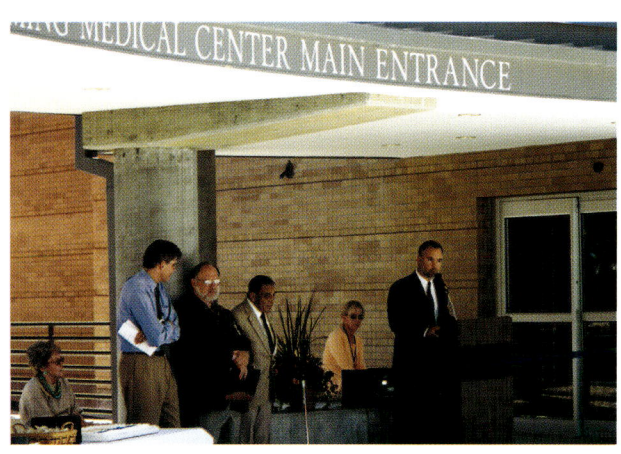

The new west main entrance opened in 2001.

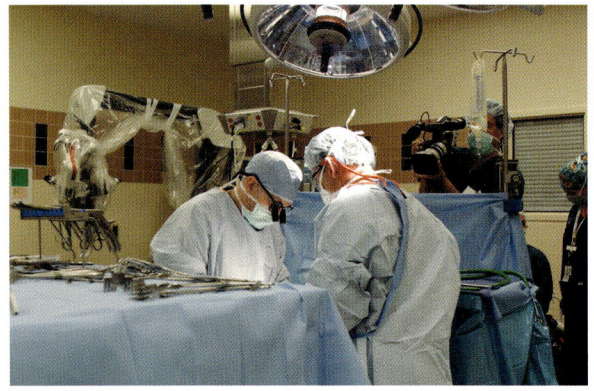
This surgery was performed in one of the new surgical suites.

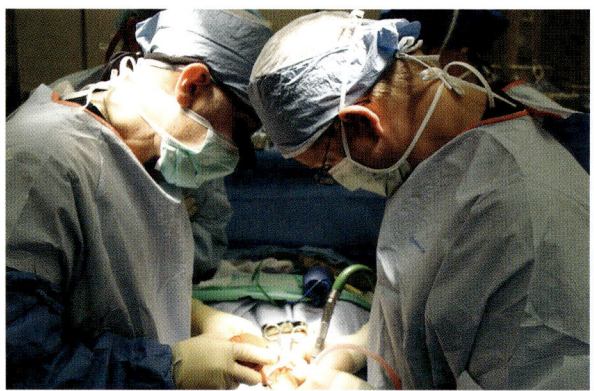
Dr. Brian Wieder and Dr. Joseph Sramek, neurosurgeons, perform a spine surgery.

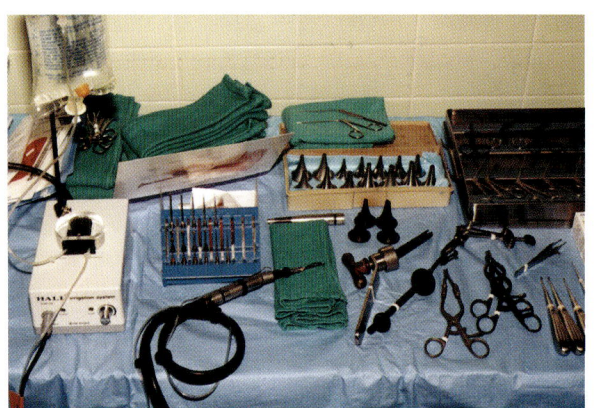
Surgical tools are laid out for an ear, nose, and throat procedure.

charity load became an increasing concern. In early 2002, Wyoming Medical Center announced that it needed other counties to pay for the trauma patients treated in the hospital. Sixty percent of trauma cases were auto accidents that occurred outside of the county. Every time Life Flight responded outside of Natrona County it lost money transporting the patients. The trauma division, including the Emergency Department, had lost $400,000 between June 2000 and June 2001 and the hospital expected that to double in 2002.[74] An additional burden was uncollectible debt, which stood at around $9 million in 1996 but which was expected to be $16 million for 2002.[75]

Wyoming Medical Center had opened their Wyoming Medical Center Community and Family Clinic in 1991, providing free care for poor families. James Gardner convinced the board to close the unprofitable program to help ease the debt load. They sent the patients to the University of Wyoming Family Practice Residency Clinic in Casper.[76]

On November 13, 2002, the Medical Center opened its new Medical and Community Resource Health Library. At the reception, they also celebrated the restoration and rededication of Pershing Geiger's "The Country Doctor" sculpture, now exhibited near the main lobby.[77]

Early in 2003, Wyoming Medical Center Foundation began its newest fundraising event, Connoisseur's Delight. Combining local entertainment and fine dining, it brought out the glitterati of Casper society to support Medical Center programs.[78]

July 26, 2003 was the twentieth anniversary of Life Flight. Brian Cratty, who had flown in the Vietnam War, had been a Life Flight pilot for nineteen years. He figured he had flown around 700 flights a year since he started flying for the hospital.

Jim Gardner experienced management problems in mid-July. Seventeen nurses sent the board a letter of complaint about Gardner's leadership of Wyoming Medical Center. They cited concerns about nurse-to-patient ratios. Gardner noted that the turnover rate for Medical Center nurses was 17 percent, well below the national average.[79] This prompted a no confidence vote on Gardner by physicians on July

27, 2003. Sixty-five of 125 doctors voted against him. In spite of that, the hospital board voted to keep Gardner on.[80] Eventually he left and Pam Fulks replaced him. She served into 2007.

November 11, 2004 marked a milestone when eleven babies were born in eleven hours. That many births required some mothers to recover in the pediatric unit. By the morning of November 12, there were eighteen babies in the nursery. Phyllis Schultz, who helped deliver the babies, commented on the numeric symbolism of the event.[81] In 2005, there were 1,061 babies born at the hospital.

Change and challenge marked 2006. For a second time the hospital applied for magnet status for its nursing program. Director of Critical Care Services Julie Cann-Taylor reported that magnet nursing allowed for more shared governance, more floor autonomy, and more importantly, a greater focus on ethics and positive outcomes in patient care.[82] Although Wyoming Medical Center did not get the coveted status in 2006, it used the process to continue to improve nursing services and patient care.

More patients arriving in the Emergency Department had problems related to methamphetamines, so the Medical Center created a program to educate people about the drug's dangers.[83] At the same time, the Medical Center hired two new, very experienced paramedics when Kim Weikum and Luke Strack transferred in from Katrina-stricken New Orleans.[84]

Later in 2006, the Medical Center upgraded its CT scanner with the acquisition of a Siemens SOMATOM 64-Slice scanner. This allowed for non-invasive detection of heart disease and analysis of other organs.[85]

Wyoming Medical Center provided periodic updates that gave an insight into its operations. In 2007, the online fact sheet gave the following information: There were 5,341 ambulance runs, and Life Flight made 880 emergency and physician runs. A total of 76,075 outpatients visited Wyoming Medical Center, and 35,807 people received care in the Emergency Department. In-patients accounted for another 9,245 people served by the Medical Center. Of those, 1,162 were births and 5,507 were other kinds of surgeries. Wyoming Medical Center also performed 211 open-heart surgeries. There were 1,268 employees, making a total of $73,355,500 that the employees spent in the community. Just 179 Auxiliary members gave 24,404 hours to the Medical Center.[86]

In addition to the services provided in Casper, twelve outreach clinics served Wyoming including the Red Desert Clinic in Rock Springs. Nineteen doctors covering ten specialities provided care in six communities. Wyoming Medical Center provided $7,012,780 in charity care and absorbed $22,084,052 in bad debt and the cost of discounted services.[87]

The Medical Center completed the final piece of the building plan when, in December 2007, the new west end parking structure opened. A small park south

> *In addition to the services provided in Casper, twelve outreach clinics served Wyoming including the Red Desert Clinic in Rock Springs.*

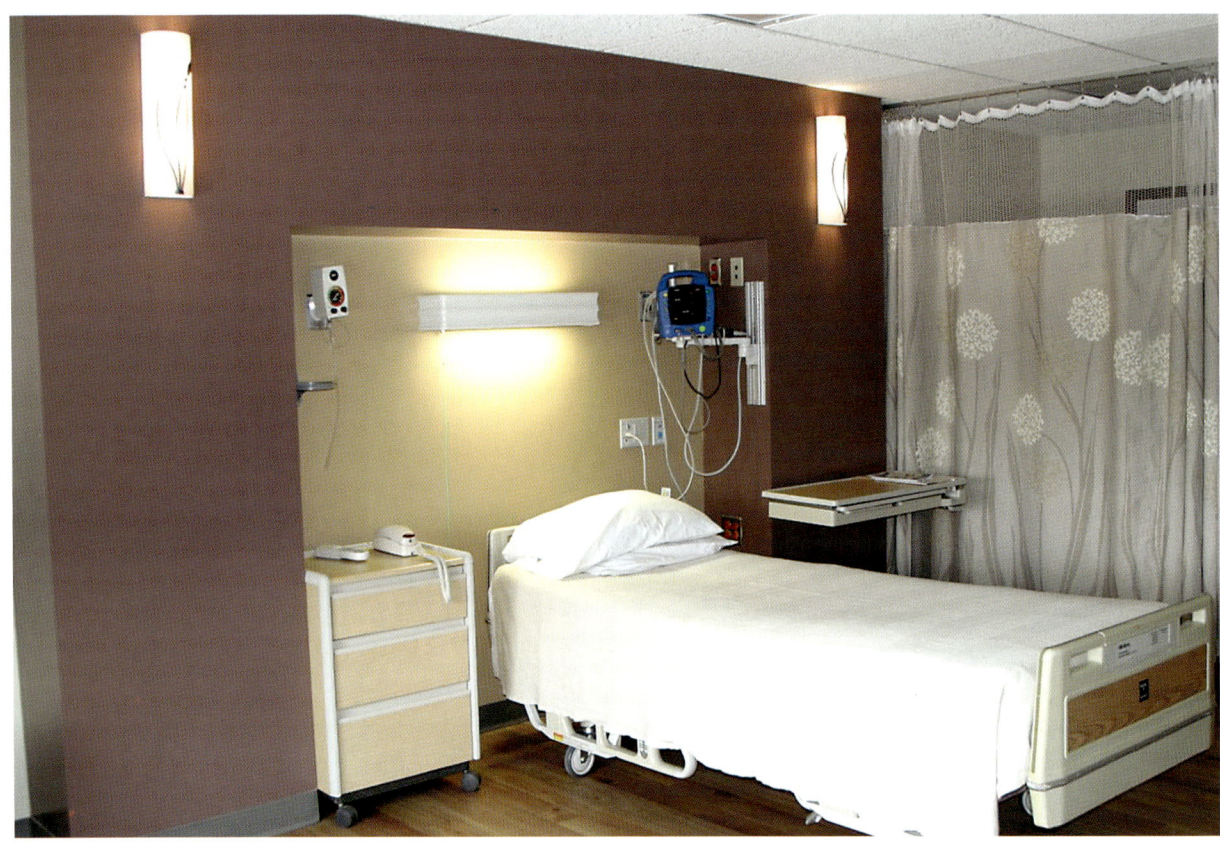

This shows one of the newest private patient suites on the medical unit.

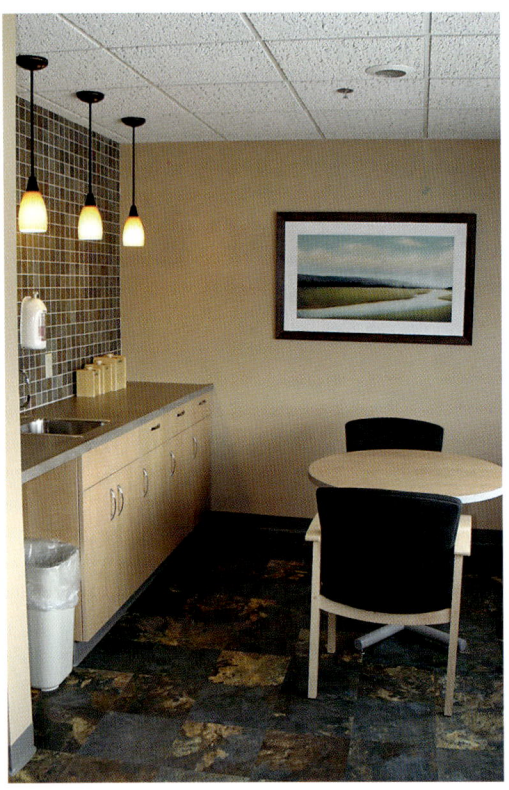

of the structure provided a contemplative space. A temporary covered walkway connected the parking structure to the hospital. The original plan called for tearing down the old parking structure, but that was now on hold.[88]

In March 2007, Pam Fulks, president and CEO of Wyoming Medical Center, wrote her last column in the newsletter. She praised the good work of the institution and shared that her time there had been one of the best experiences of her life. She credited the people of the Medical Center with the continued excellence.[89] Vickie Diamond took over as interim. On September 11, 2007, Bob Turner arrived from Wisconsin to become the next CEO. Turner only stayed a few months and the search was once again on. In April 2008, the board appointed Vickie Diamond the new CEO. Diamond had arrived at Wyoming Medical Center in 2004 and had held a number of positions including senior vice president of patient care services, chief operating officer, and chief nursing officer.

When the Emergency Department had opened in the east wing in 2000, managers figured that it would take almost twenty years to reach capacity in terms of patient load. In 2008, that number reached 39,000. That prompted the Wyoming Medical Center Foundation, in 2009, to begin a capital campaign to raise $6 million

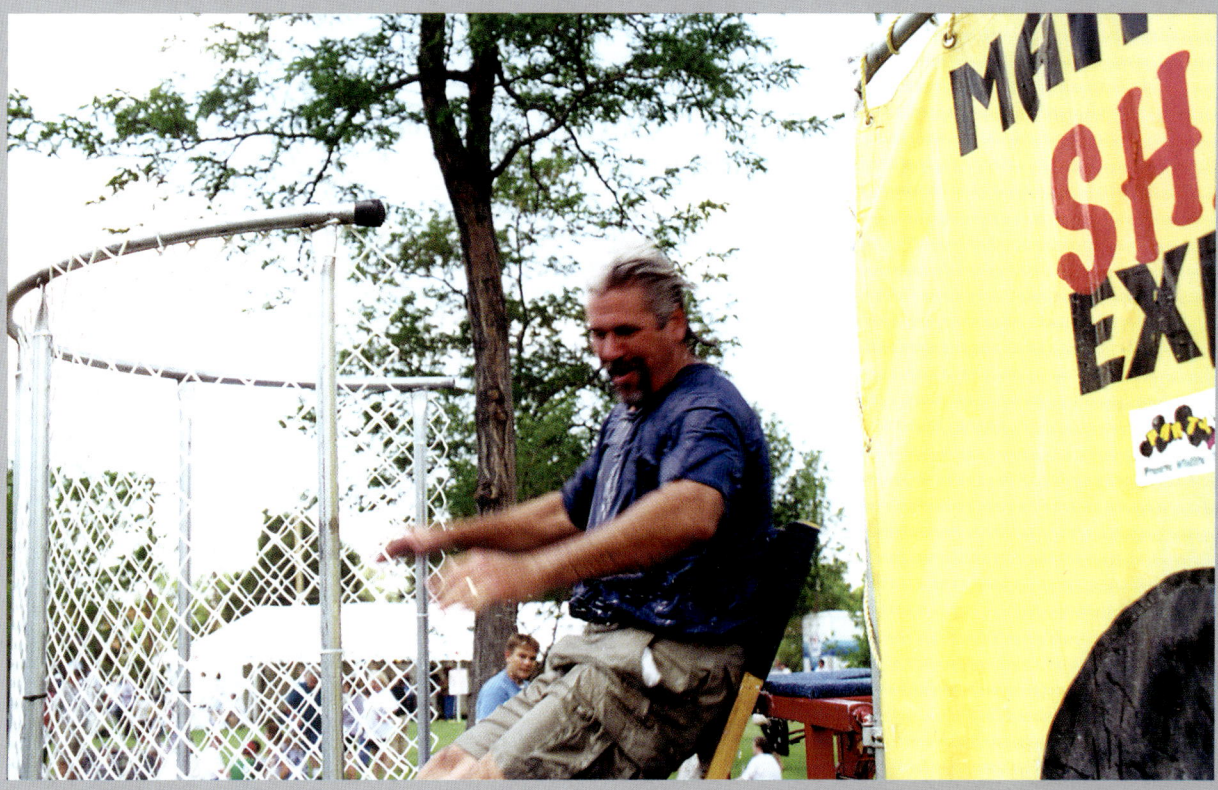

The Wyoming Medical Center summer picnics provided all kinds of fun including dunk tanks.

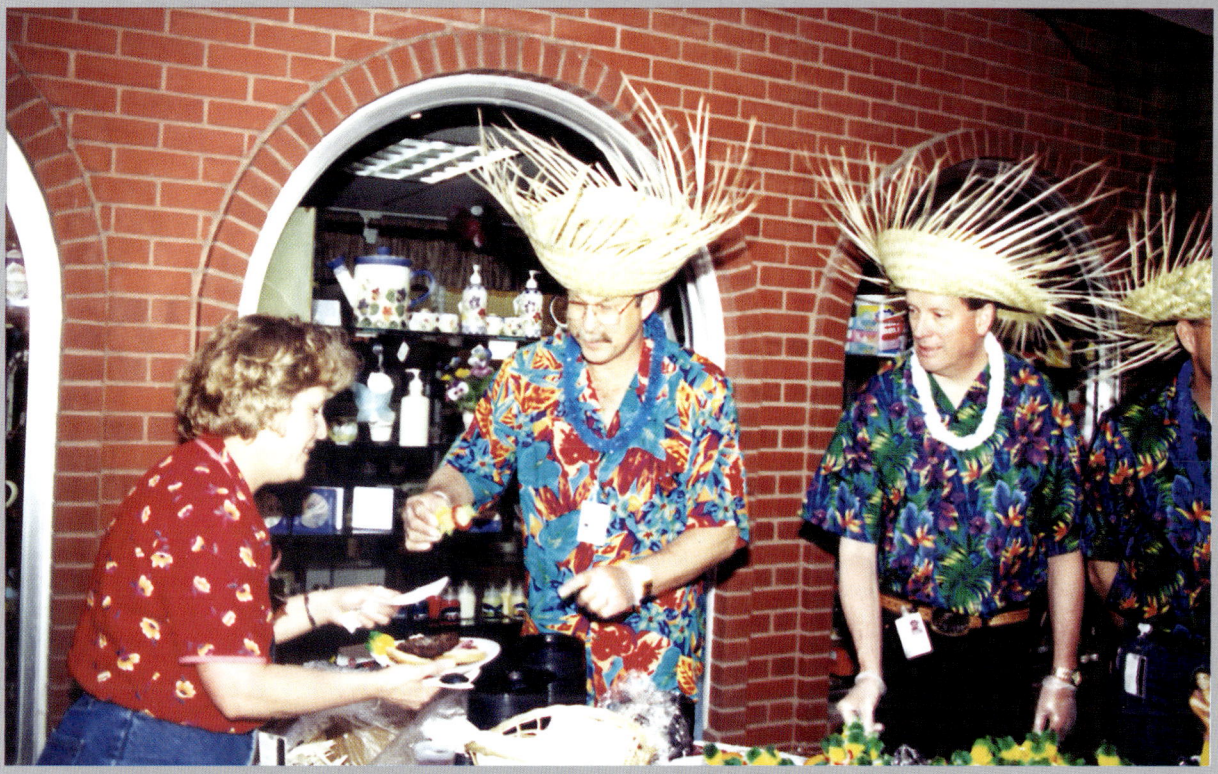

Hospital Week 2005 featured a Hawaiian-themed barbeque for all Medical Center employees.

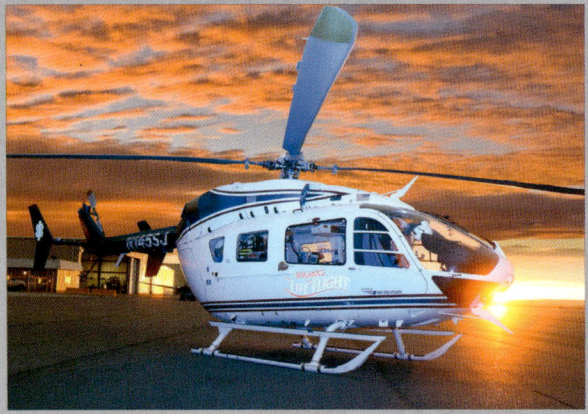
The helicopter glows in a fiery Wyoming sunset.

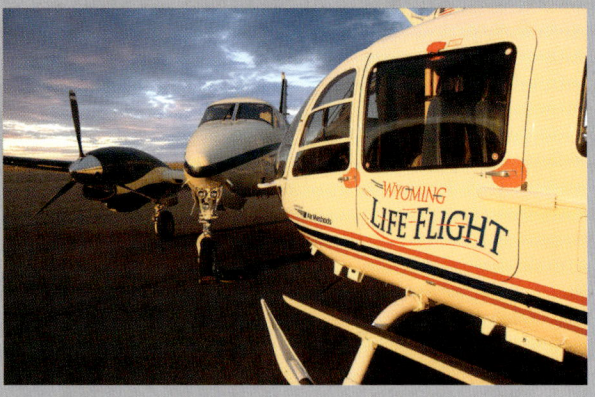
This is Wyoming Medical Center's latest Life Flight helicopter and airplane.

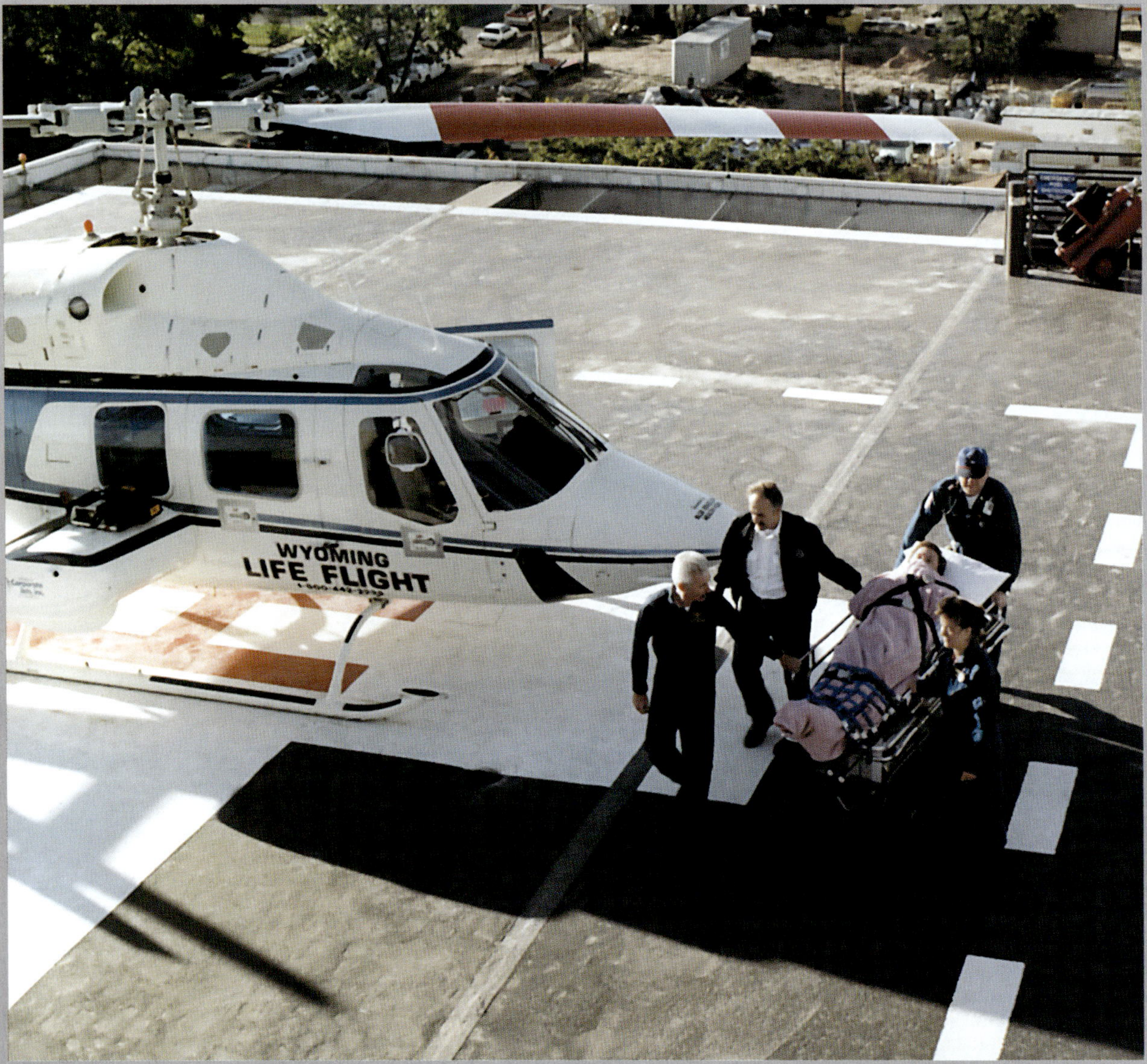

A Life Flight patient arrives at the Medical Center.

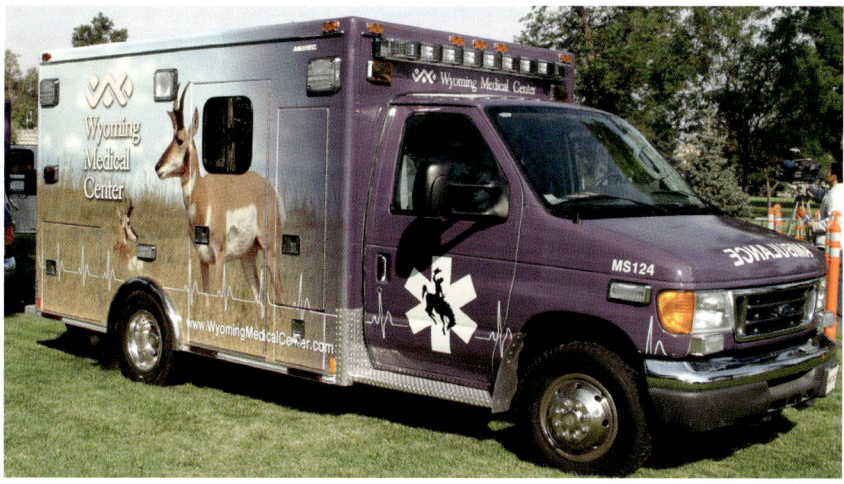
High technology ambulances at Wyoming Medical Center also have new paint jobs reflecting Wyoming's natural wonders.

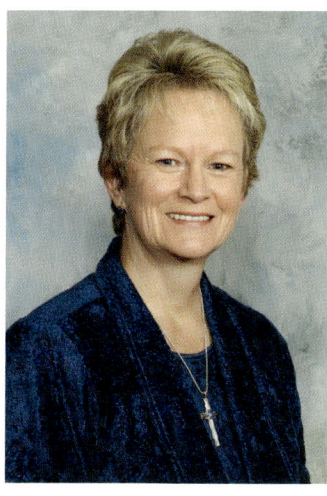
Pam Fulks was CEO during the pivotal mid-2000s, leaving in 2007.

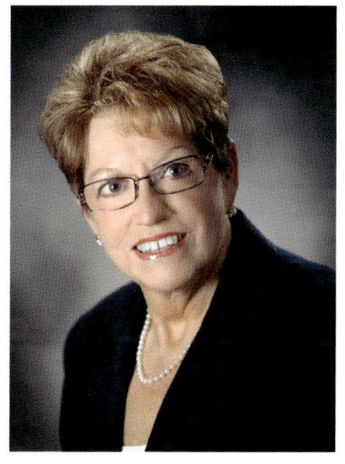
Vickie Diamond, R.N. has been the Wyoming Medical Center president and chief executive officer since 2008.

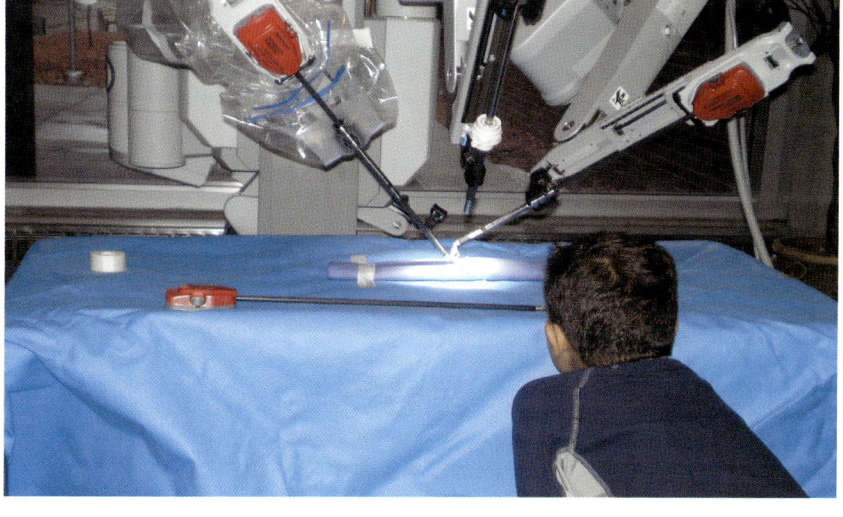
The DaVinci Robotic Surgical System allows a surgeon to perform very precise microsurgery.

to create an expanded and modernized Emergency Department. This was seed money for the $20 million needed for the improvements. The new facility would take up the entire ground floor facing Second Street and contain two parts. One area would deal with severe injuries and the other with less serious illnesses or injuries. This would bring the bed total to thirty-nine.[90]

One ongoing initiative was infection control. For years hospitals had been working closely with employees to reduce instances of staph infections. In 2009, the H1N1 scare brought the public into infection control. Many places installed dispensers of germ-fighting hand cleaner. They urged the public to disinfect their hands before entering and reinforced the idea of cleanliness.[91]

The newest innovation in surgery was the DaVinci Robotic Surgical System. It came to Wyoming Medical Center in 2009 and allowed surgeons to perform minimally invasive microsurgery.

In January 2010, *Highlights* reported that expansion had begun to greatly enlarge the Emergency Department with completion of renovations in 2011.[92] In the summer of 2010, the Auxiliary voted to change their name to Wyoming Medical Center Volunteers. Everything else at Wyoming Medical Center was business as usual in 2010 as the Centennial Committee planned the celebration of the Medical Center's birthday in November.

WHAT HISTORY MEANS

Good history provides both facts and meaning. The facts of Memorial Hospital of Natrona County and Wyoming Medical Center are numerous and show that the community created a hospital in 1911 and that it grew in purpose and meaning over the next century. Meaning is more complicated. Hospitals are important to a community for many reasons. They provide for the health of citizens and of the local economy. They bring prestige and sometimes controversy to a town and a region. When run well, they nurture their employees and keep current with advances in the medical field. Most hospitals also face serious challenges stemming from financial, regulatory, and human sources. It is often a thankless job to be a health care professional or institution, but it also generates great pride and a sense of accomplishment when things go well for patients. This story of Wyoming Medical Center reflects all of that.

In June 2010, Shauna VanderLinden, Marketing and Public Relations representative at Wyoming Medical Center, decided to provide some closure for this book by asking the following question of employees: "What does it mean to you to see our hospital celebrating one hundred years in this community?" The edited and shortened answers below provide a sense of this institution's meaning.

Nora Grierson

"I think it is quite an achievement, and I am proud to work here. I was born at this hospital in May of 1944."

Stuart Ruben, M.D., FACP, CPE
Medical Director, Quality and Regulatory Management
Patient Safety Fellow

"We are effectively and actively participating in the revolutionary changes seen in the last eight years with respect to how medical care is delivered to patients. We have robustly initiated a paradigm shift in the local medical culture to embrace patient safety and measurements of quality. We have survived the trials and tribulations of economic crises while recruiting and retaining new physicians to the community and continuing to improve and expand both services and facility."

Jeanne Wernsmann

"When I was hired by Memorial Hospital of Natrona County in September 1974 my application was handwritten on yellow notepad paper! I was hired via phone without a face-to-face interview. Natrona County was witnessing a major growth with the oil boom. President Nixon had just resigned, the Vietnam War was still fresh in our minds, and we were a liberal bunch of young radicals with heroes such as President Kennedy and Martin Luther King.

"I started my career in the ICU… ABGS were rare, a series of fruit jars connected to a pump created the ability to keep a lung inflated, working nights for the first time in my life, orderlies in the hospital to do 'bed weights,' calling the supervisor for ice to gavage a patient (she would magically bring it in a grocery cart from somewhere), anesthesia managing ventilators, medication cards, kardexes, mercury thermometers, one bank of four heart monitors, nurses in white but mostly yellow dresses and hats, doing an EKG with suction cup attachments and only able to run one lead at a time then to cut and paste it together so the doc could finally read it."

Donna Yount, Aide, OPS

"I was born in this hospital, in the early fifties. Wow! So many years ago. I had my tonsils out here as a youngster, with Dr. Haigler. I remember riding on the cart along with two little boys. One little boy had a hole in his stomach, and was really sick. I worked in the kitchen during my high school years. As an adult I had a few surgeries, knee, and female and of course stitches a time or two. My four children, now adults, were born here. I work as an aide now on an OPS floor, and really like my work. This hospital is like a trusting friend that has always been here in good times and bad. My dad died here, and my mother came here for her chemo while fighting cancer. Yes, a trusted friend, through thick and thin. It is a huge part of my long life."

Mary Jo Daniels, R.N.
Nurse Manager Medical

"This hospital is very special to me, having been born here over fifty years ago and having practiced here as a nurse for over thirty-five years. It is difficult for me to comprehend the changes in health care that have occurred over the last one hundred years. I am proud of the care we have grown to provide our patients, our reputation in the community and the state, and the outstanding staff and physicians that work here. I have the goal of working here until I retire or die, facilitating patient care and making a difference for patients, family, and staff."

Nicole Pouget, MLS, MS
Medical Librarian, Physician and Staff Health Science Library

"As the medical librarian, I am part of a twenty-five-year (at least) tradition at WMC (Wyoming Medical Center). I have been here ten years managing our print and electronic information resources and providing research services to support best clinical care practice. WMC librarians have a history of partnering with clinical and educational facilities throughout the state of Wyoming and beyond to provide our community with the best national and international resources. Traditionally, WMC medical librarians have always insured that rural clinical folks aren't professionally isolated here in Wyoming. In addition to providing research services, the medical librarian also teaches others how and where to perform effective searches for authoritative, quality, and reliable information regarding consumer health needs and evidence-based medicine results for clinical patient needs. As the medical librarian, I have always supported WMC's goal of great patient care and look forward to continuing this tradition during this next century."

Deb Weaver, R.N.

"WOW, what an amazing journey our health care system has made to be now called Wyoming Medical Center… one hundred years. I have been a part of this amazing facility and community for over a quarter of its century! As I retire, my memories are with a smile. I came to the Memorial Hospital of Natrona County in 1982, when the south parking garage was the newest addition to the facility, there wasn't a 'campus,' only the immediate quarter of a block set on Conwell and East Second Street.

"On my day of hire, I was one of three new employees for the 'monthly orientation.' The ICU was an open ward and the ORs a wagon wheel design, with scrub sinks, autoclaves, and sterile supplies all located in the 'hub.' There were NO windows in either department. No one who worked there knew what the weather was, or if it was day or night. That is where I spent the majority of my nursing career.

"It didn't seem as there were many changes until the early 1990s. That was when specialties boomed: cardiac, vascular and neurosurgeries dominated the OR schedule and competed for the nine ICU beds. Space was beginning to be a premium everywhere. Conference rooms were being turned into support spaces and procedure rooms. Staffing shortage wasn't yet in the vocabulary, and morale was friendly. Most all employees knew one another. The ER helped with patient care during night shifts and transported patients to other departments.

"As leadership and administrators evolved, there were many initiatives to improve efficiency, maximize resources, build satisfaction, and assure quality while funding decreased, economics and accessibility became more complicated. We were bound by our dedication to the patient, family, and community.

"Today, I believe Wyoming Medical Center remains a beacon to the state and region. WOW, what a ride! I am proud to have been a part of this magnificent organization, helping make a difference in those we serve. Thank you for inviting me to comment on 'What does one hundred years mean to me?'"

Vanessa Morgan, R.N., CGRN
Manager, OPS/Prehosp/GI Lab

"I was born in this hospital in 1980. My grandmother, uncle, and cousin have all worked here throughout my thirty years, and it still amazes me today how much change I have seen. I am filled with pride to be a born and raised member of the Casper community and a team member at Wyoming Medical Center. I look forward to the changes I will see in the next thirty!"

NOTES

1 Karen Palm. "Easy answers for hard questions," *Hospital Hi-Lites*, Vol. XIII, No. 1, Wyoming Medical Center, July 1988, p. 3.

2 Palm, "Easy answers for hard questions," p. 3.

3 Karen Palm. "Len Gross Appointed New Human Resources Director," *Hospital Hi-Lites*, Vol. XI, No. 7, Wyoming Medical Center, February 1987, p. 3.

4 Karen Palm. "Wanted… R.N.s, Earn $1000 Bounty," *Hospital Hi-Lites*, January 1987, p. 6.

5 Karen Palm. "Maternity Leave Policy Clarified," *Hospital Hi-Lites*, January 1987, p. 2.

6 Karen Palm. "Graduates of residency programs honored at special ceremony," *Hospital Hi-Lites*, Wyoming Medical Center, Vol. XIII, No. 10, April 1989, p. 6.

7 Karen Palm. "Director Elaine Hough: Volunteers are the Hospital's Pipeline to the Community," *Hospital Hi-Lites*, January 1987, p. 5.

8 Karen Palm. "Blue Envelope Donates Funds to WMC Foundation," *Hospital Hi-Lites*, February 1987, p. 1.

9 Karen Palm. "Volunteering has special meaning to Lab staff," *Hospital Hi-Lites*, April 1989, p. 3.

10 Karen Palm. "Raft Teams Celebrate Finish in River Race," and "Paint Your Heart Out," *Hospital Hi-Lites*, Wyoming Medical Center, Vol. XII, No. 2, August 1987, p. 1.

11 Palm, "Blue Envelope Donates Funds to WMC Foundation," p. 1.

12 Karen Palm. "Technological Advances in Radiology Help Diagnose Women's Health Problems," *Hospital Hi-Lites*, Vol. XI, No. 8, Wyoming Medical Center, March 1987, p. 1.

13 Palm, "Easy answers for hard questions," p. 4.

14 Palm, "Easy answers for hard questions," p. 4.

15 Charlene Murdock. "New technology eases nurses' workload," *Hospital Hi-Lites*, Vol. XIII, No. 7, Wyoming Medical Center, January 1989, p. 1.

16 Karen Palm. "Board of Directors elect new members," *Hospital Hi-Lites*, Vol. XIII, No. 2, Wyoming Medical Center, August 1988, p. 1.

17 Ann Burns. "Trash recycling saves dollars; makes sense," *Wyoming Medical Center Hi-Lites*, September 1990, p. 5; Ann Burns. "Wyoming Medical Center incinerates community's medical waste products," *Wyoming Medical Center Hi-Lites*, October 1990, p. 5.

18 Ann Burns. "Marketing and PR Dept. back in full swing," *Wyoming Medical Center Hi-Lites*, August 1990, p. 2.

19 Rebecca Hunt. Interview with Elaine Hough, December 18, 2009.

20 Ann Burns. "The good works of Lin Carriger," *Wyoming Medical Center Hi-Lites*, July 1995, p. 1 and 5.

21 Burns, "The good works of Lin Carriger," p. 1.

22 Rebecca Hunt. Interview with Laurie Sanftner, September 6, 2009.

23 Ann Burns. "WMC welcomes new cardiologist from Canada," *Wyoming Medical Center Hi-Lites*, September 1990, pp. 1–2.

24 Ann Burns. "Casper welcomes new ophthalmologist and general surgeon," *Wyoming Medical Center Hi-Lites*, September 1991, p. 6.

25 Ann Burns. "WMC welcomes Radiation Oncologist, Dr. Robert Tobin," *Wyoming Medical Center Hi-Lites*, August 1991, p. 5.

26 "Women who prefer a woman doctor will get their wish this fall," *Casper Journal*, July 18, 1998.

27 Ann Burns. "Shugart shares firsthand account of Saudi Arabia," *Wyoming Medical Center Hi-Lites*, January 1991, p. 1; Ann Burns. "Scenes from Saudi Arabia," *Wyoming Medical Center Hi-Lites*, February 1991, p. 4.

28 Ann Burns. "1991: a year of progress and growth for WMC," *Wyoming Medical Center Hi-Lites*, January 1992, p. 1.

29 Burns, "1991: a year of progress and growth for WMC," p. 1.

30 Ann Burns. "Guest Relations Program unveiled at WMC," *Wyoming Medical Center Hi-Lites*, May 1991, p. 1.

31 Ann Burns. "Shirley Hunter: A laboratory legend retires," *Wyoming Medical Center Hi-Lites*, February 1992, p. 1.

32 Ann Burns. "Carmel Tice, new pharmacy director, plans for computerization," *Wyoming Medical Center Hi-Lites*, January 1992, p. 5.

33 Ann Burns. "Respiratory Care: On the cutting edge of patient care," *Wyoming Medical Center Hi-Lites*, August 1991, p. 1.

34 Ann Burns. "Preparing for east wing construction," *Wyoming Medical Center Hi-Lites*, November 1992, p. 1.

35 Ann Burns. "Grand openings, name changes and PLT," *Wyoming Medical Center Hi-Lites*, January 1993, p. 7.

36 Ann Burns. "The community responds," *Wyoming Medical Center Hi-Lites*, May 1993, p. 7.

37 Peter Van Houten. "Fixed wing returns to Wyoming Skies," *Wyoming Medical Center Hi-Lites*, October 1995, p. 1 and 10.

38 "Casper and Douglas hospitals link up," *Wyoming Medical Center Hi-Lites*, January 1995, p. 1 and 7.

39 "Medical center dedicates chapel," *Casper Star-Tribune*, July 1, 2001.

40 "Hospital board approves expansion plans," *Wyoming Medical Center Hi-Lites*, February 10, 1995, p. 1.

41 Tom Morton. "Roussalis vs. WMC lawsuit still in play," *Casper Star-Tribune*, April 12, 2000, p. A1 and A14.

42 "N.T.," *Casper Star-Tribune*, January 28, 1996 (from WMC clipping files).

43 "Medical center to keep last year's fees," *Casper Star-Tribune*, July 12, 1996 (from WMC clipping files).

44 "WMC nurses may organize," *Casper Star-Tribune*, February 25, 1996.

45 "Board of Nursing can't settle dispute at WMC," *Casper Star-Tribune*, March 13, 1996.

46 "WMC to review old expansion," *Casper Star-Tribune*, January 11, 1996.

47 "WMC to review old expansion," *Casper Star-Tribune*, January 11, 1996.

48 "HCA is interested in WMC," *Casper Star-Tribune*, December 16, 1996.

49 "WMC board approves heart surgeons' contracts," *Casper Star-Tribune*, July 10, 1997.

50 "WMC sees more heart surgeries," *Casper Star-Tribune*, February 12, 1999.

51 "WMC weathered a rough month," *Casper Star-Tribune*, March 27, 1997.

52 Rebecca Hunt. Interview with Rolly Santfner regarding Wyoming Medical Center, September 6, 2009.

53 "WMC will give five houses to Habitat for Humanity this month," *Casper Star-Tribune*, September 5, 1997.

54 "WMC construction moving ahead," *Casper Star-Tribune*, November 13, 1997.

55 "Renovations at WMC picking up speed," *Casper Star-Tribune*, May 6, 1998.

56 "WMC expansion affects patient care," *Casper Star-Tribune*, July 22, 1998.

57 "WMC revenues up in the first quarter," *Casper Star-Tribune*, January 15, 1999; "WMC board approves $2 million for overruns," *Casper Star-Tribune*, February 12, 1999.

58 "Wyoming Medical Center Auxiliary has given $5,000 to the hospital for special projects," *Casper Star-Tribune*, January 16, 1998.

59 "The medical center will become a sponsor of the Wyoming Health Fair," *Casper Star-Tribune*, February 13, 1998.

60 "Marriott to manage inventory," *Casper Star-Tribune*, April 10, 1998.

61 "WMC takes over health building," *Casper Journal*, April 8, 1999.

62 "WMC opens sixth-floor ward," *Casper Star-Tribune*, August 14, 1999.

63 Laura Azar. "Opening of the new wing at Wyoming Medical Center," *Casper Star-Tribune*, January 11, 2000, pp. B1–2.

64 Hunt, interview with Rolly Santfner, September 6, 2009.

65 "Wyoming patients get good health care," *Casper Star-Tribune*, October 6, 2000; "WMC to apply for trauma designation," *Casper Star-Tribune*, October 12, 2000.

66 "WMC surveys needs for doctors," *Casper Star-Tribune*, January 12, 2001.

67 "Masterson donates $1 million," *Casper Star-Tribune*, January 12, 2001.

68 "WMC site plan approved," *Casper Star-Tribune*, April 25, 2001.

69 Mike Phillips. "Primary care center to open this fall," *Highlights*, Wyoming Medical Center, May 2005, p. 1 and 7.

70 "WMC marks end of $48 million project," *Casper Star-Tribune*, June 30, 2001.

71 "Medical center dedicates chapel," *Casper Star-Tribune*, July 1, 2001.

72 "Wyoming Medical Center sees growth," *Casper Star-Tribune*, August 6, 2001.

73 "Hospital freezes room rates," *Casper Star-Tribune*, June 22, 2001.

74 "WMC wants other counties to share trauma bill," *Casper Star-Tribune*, January 29, 2002.

75 "Rising debt concerns WMC," *Casper Star-Tribune*, February 4, 2002.

76 "WMC-affiliated clinic closure set today," *Casper Star-Tribune*, April 12, 2002.

77 Invitation, Geiger statue rededication, November 11, 2003.

78 Mike Phillips. "Foundation event seeks to prove a simple thesis: Casper's Got Talent," *Highlights*, Wyoming Medical Center, January 2010, p. 1, http://www.wyomingmedicalcenter.com/pdfs/Jan%20Highlights%202010.pdf.

79 "Communication problems at WMC," *Casper Star-Tribune*, July 19, 2003.

80 "Board Keeps Gardner," *Casper Star-Tribune*, July 29, 2003.

81 Mike Phillips. "A whole lot of babies," *Highlights*, Wyoming Medical Center, December 2004, p. 1 and 7.

82 Mike Phillips. "Giddy-up," *Highlights*, February 2006, p. 1 and 7.

83 Mike Phillips. "A focused assault on meth," *Highlights*, February 2006, p. 4.

84 Mike Phillips. "The 25-day shift," *Highlights*, February 2006, p. 5 and 7.

85 Mike Phillips. "A Wealth of Information," *Highlights*, May 2006.

86 Wyoming Medical Center Community Fact Sheet, p. 2, www.wyomingmedicalcenter.com.

87 Wyoming Medical Center Community Fact Sheet, p. 2.

88 Mike Phillips. "Open spaces: Hospital hosts celebration after completion of new parking structure," *Highlights*, December 2007, p. 1.

89 Mike Phillips. "Surrounded by good people," *Highlights*, March 2007, p. 1.

90 Mike Phillips. "Foundation aims at $6 million," *Highlights*, February 2009, p. 2 and 4.

91 Mike Phillips. "Gel in, gel out," *Highlights*, July 2009, p. 1.

92 Mike Phillips. "Expansion begins: New emergency room should be in place in the next 18 months," *Highlights*, January 2010, p. 1.

Selected Bibliography

SECONDARY SOURCES

Alcova Dam, "Reclamation: Managing Water in the West," http://www.usbr.gov/projects/Facility.jsp?fac_Name= Alcova+Dam&groupName=General.

Anderson, Kevin. *Spirit of the Thunderbird: The Growth of Casper College*. Casper: Casper College, 1995.

Beaver, Robin. "He turned lemons into lemonade: Fred Goodstein used his largesse to benefit those who had little," *Made in Wyoming*, http://www.madeinwyoming.net/profiles/goodstein.php.

BP Amoco Timeline, http://trib.com/news/local/article_95dec472-b119-5f7d-8be3-740c6deaf8a1.html.

Casper, Wyoming, Population by Decade, 2010, http://recenter.tamu.edu/data/popmd/pm1350.htm.

Craig, Christopher. Mary Ann Craig, Craig Family genealogy, http://familytreemaker.genealogy.com/users/c/r/a/Christopher-J-Craig/WEBSITE-0001/UHP-0057.html.

Cronin, Vaughn. *Casper*. Casper: Endeavor Books, 2009.

Garbutt, Irving. *History of Casper and Natrona County, Wyoming, 1889–1989*, Vol. 1. Dallas: Irving Media, 1990.

———. *I Was There: Recollections of Ten Decades*. Casper: Casper Journal, 2003.

"General Information and Walking Tour," typescript, 1936.

Hunt, Rebecca and Sandy Durkin. *A Century of Healing: The History of Swedish Medical Center, 1905–2005*. Englewood, CO: Swedish Medical Center, 2005, p. 21.

Johnson, Robert. *A Look Backward, A Step Forward: The Quiet Impact of Fifty Years, City of Casper-Natrona County Health Department, 1954–2004*. Casper: Mountain States Lithography, 2004.

Junge, Mark. *A View from Center Street: Tom Carrigen's Casper*. Casper, WY: McMurray Foundation, 2003.

Larson, T. A. *History of Wyoming*. Lincoln: University of Nebraska Press, 1965.

———. *Wyoming: A History, A Bicentennial History*. New York: W. W. Norton and Co. AASLH, 1977.

"List of Wyoming Airports and Airfields," WPA, Federal Writers' Project, typescript, 1936.

Mokler, Alfred J. *History of Natrona County, Wyoming, 1888–1922*. Chicago: Lakeside Press, 1923 (reprint: Casper, Mountain States Lithography, 1989).

———. "Casper's Post Offices and Postmasters," WPA, Wyoming Writers' Project, typescript, 1936.

Natrona County Tribune, October 29, 1903.

Natrona Tribune, Vol. 3, No. 13, August 31, 1893, p. 4.

Natrona Tribune, Vol. 3, No. 15, August 31, 1893, p. 3.

Orr, Joseph. "Anatomy of a Western Town," WPA, Wyoming Writers' Project, typescript, March 10, 1940.

Phibbs, Brendan, M.D., Donald Becker, M.D., Charles R. Lowe, M.D., Roy Holmes, M.D., Robert Fowler, M.D., Oliver K. Scott, M.D., Kenneth Roberts, M.D., Walter Watson, M.D., and Ralph Malott, M.D. "The Casper Project—An Enforced Mass-Culture Streptococcic Control Program," *Journal of the American Medical Association,* 1958:166 (10):1113–1119.

Rea, Tom. "Mathew Campfield, Barber and Pioneer Survivor," http://www.tomrea.net/Mathew%20Campfield.html.

Roberts, Phil. "Greed, Depression and the End of Wyoming's Cowboy Health Co-operative," *Buffalo Bones,* n.d., http://uwacadweb.uwyo.edu/RobertsHistory/buffalobones.htm.

Sackett, Charline. "Casper, Wyoming," WPA, Wyoming Writers' Project, typescript, 1936.

Schulte, Rhonda. "Centenarian Remembers Childhood Friend, Buffalo Bill Cody," April 6, 2001, http://www.gemstone-memoirs.com/4f274ddf-e8b4-4f6e-8e79-335bad8513e3-9.html.

Sellers, Edson. "Societies and Organizations for Experimental Purposes in Natrona County," WPA, Federal Writers' Project field editor, typescript, 1936.

———. "Fraternal Organizations," WPA, Federal Writers' Project field editor, typescript, 1936.

Smith, Duane and Ronald Brown. *No One Ailing Except a Physician.* Boulder: University Press of Colorado, 2001.

Stebbins, Nancy. "The Casper Chamber of Commerce," WPA, Federal Writers' Project field editor, Platte River Empire District, Casper, typescript, 1936.

———. "Casper's Assets," WPA, Federal Writers' Project field editor, Platte River Empire District, Casper, typescript, 1936.

———. "Casper Mountain: A Year Round Retreat," WPA, Federal Writers' Project field editor, Platte River Empire District, Casper, typescript, 1936.

———. "Casper's Telephone Exchange," WPA, Federal Writers' Project field editor, Platte River Empire District, Casper, typescript, 1936.

———. "KDFN Broadcasting Station," WPA, Federal Writers' Project field editor, Platte River Empire District, Casper, typescript, 1936.

———. "The Natrona County Memorial Hospital," WPA, Federal Writers' Project field editor, Platte River Empire District, Casper, typescript, 1936.

———. "State Home for Dependent Children," WPA, Federal Writers' Project field editor, Platte River Empire District, Casper, typescript, 1936.

———. "Wyoming Air Service," WPA, Federal Writers' Project field editor, Platte River Empire District, Casper, typescript, 1936.

2009 Calendar, Wyoming Heritage Center, Cheyenne: WHC, 2009.

Ward, Henry. *The Story of Casper's Irish.* Plainfield, IL: Bantry Publications, n.d., www.casperirish.com.

"West Across the Skies: Wyoming's Aviation History," online exhibit, http://wyomuseum.state.us/Exhibits/Aviation.asp.

West, Elliott. *Growing Up With the Country: Childhood on the Far Western Frontier.* Albuquerque: University of New Mexico Press, 1989.

Wyoming Medical Center Foundation, 2010, http://www.wyomingmedicalcenterfoundation.org/index.php.

Zamula, Evelyn. "A New Challenge for Former Polio Patients." *FDA Consumer,* 25 (5), 1991, http://www.questia.com/googleScholar.qst?docId=5002167868.

PRIMARY SOURCES

Memorial Hospital of Natrona County Training School for Nurses informational booklet, c. 1930.

MHNC Candy Striper scrapbook, 1968.

National Hospital Day at Memorial Hospital of Natrona County scrapbook, Casper, Wyoming, May 11, 1941.

Natrona County Hospital, School of Nursing ledger books with time sheets and other school records.

Sixth Annual Graduating Exercises, MHNC, May 15, 1937.

WSNA membership book, January 1939–January 1940.

WSNA membership rolls, January 1936–1946.

Wyoming State Nurses' Association (WSNA) memorial program, memorial service at Powell, WY, August 26, 1966.

GOVERNMENT DOCUMENTS

Alcova Dam, "Reclamation: Managing Water in the West," http://www.usbr.gov/projects/Facility.jsp?fac_Name=Alcova+Dam&groupName=General.

Memorial Hospital of Natrona County Board of Trustees Minutes, 1953–1983.

Natrona County Commission Minutes (facsimile copies), December 8, 1921–January 5, 1926.

INTERVIEWS

Hunt, Rebecca. Interview with Elaine Hough regarding Wyoming Medical Center, December 18, 2009.

———. Interview with Laurie Santfner, September 6, 2009.

———. Interview with Rolly Santfner, September 6, 2009.

———. Interview with Tim Weaver, September 7, 2009.

NEWSPAPERS

Bessemer Journal, late 1888–December 12, 1890.

Buffalo News, Buffalo, WY.

Casper Daily Mail, November 1888.

Casper Daily Press, March 3, 1914–.

Casper Daily Tribune.

Casper Derrick, March 1892–March 1906.

Casper Herald.

Casper Record.

Casper Star-Tribune.

Casper Tribune-Herald.

Casper Weekly Mail, 1890–.

Casper Weekly Press.

Denver Medical Times, Vol. 28, No. 1, July 1908.

Hospital Hi-Lites (*Highlights*), Casper: Wyoming Medical Center, 1987–2009.

Laramie Daily Boomerang, Laramie, WY.

Natrona County Tribune, Casper, WY, 1897–1921.

Natrona Tribune, June 1891–1897.

MHNC Outreach, Vol. 1, No. 2, Spring/Summer 1978.

Morton, Tom. "WMC may dodge severe Medicare cuts," *Casper Star-Tribune*, http://trib.com/news/local/article_2c450238-7607-5a17-aad-00dd25f443b4.html.

Rock Springs Rocket, Vol. 9, No. 7, January 7, 1916, p. 1.

Sweetwater Chief, Spring 1890–Fall 1890.

The Wyoming Oil World.

Wind River Mountaineer, Lander, WY.

Wind River Mountaineer, Lander, WY, December 12, 1904, p. 2.

Wyoming State Tribune, Cheyenne, WY.

Wyoming Weekly Review, February 1921.

ARCHIVAL COLLECTIONS

Arrasmith, W. W., M.D. Letter to Miss Leona Mohr, R.N., February 15, 1940.

Blue Envelope Booster, Blue Envelope Health Fund, Vol. 6, Casper, March 1998.

Blue Envelope Cancer Division files.

Blue Envelope notebook of clippings.

Casper City Directories.

The Casper Project: Strep Throat Project, 1958–1959.

Donovan, Agnes K. Biography, manuscript page, Wyoming State Nurses' Association, n.d.

Edness Kimball Wilkins papers, MHNC, Box 8, 1978.

Eschwig, Mary Anne. "Yearly Report of Training School" to the Board of Trustees, MHNC, typescript, 1938.

Fred and J. M. Goodstein linear accelerator donation file, 1978.

Hough, Elaine. "History of the Hospital, 1911–2001," typescript outline.

Hunt, Rebecca. Weaver Family history, typescript, 2005.

Jack Tripeny files: Natrona County Volunteer Health Council, 1960–1963, Natrona County Health Fund.

Larson, T. A. "Highlights of the Wyoming Nurses' Association's First Half Century," typescript, 1959.

"Memorial History of Martha Kimball," WSNA memorial service, typescript, Rawlins, WY, June 19, 1947.

Natrona County Cancer Council Meeting Minutes, October 20, 1965–March 23, 1967.

News release: "25th Annual Health Fair is March 28."

Index

A

Adock, Martha, 68
Allen, Archie, 21
Ambulance service, 53, 75, 89, 91
Ambulance Services, 53, 70
Ambulance. *See* Patient transport.
American Cancer Society, 55
American Red Cross, 22
Anderson, Dr. Harlan, 49
Anesthetics, 51
Arrasmith, Dr. W. W., 41
Athrography, 76
Auxiliary, 48, 55, 59, 70, 72, 73, 77, 83, 95, 102, 104, 117, 123, 128

B

Baker, Dr. James, 46, 71
Balser, Nita, 104
Barber, Dr. Amos, 15
Barton, William, 77
Bawden, Dr. G. S., 25
Beck, Dr. Claude, 69
Becker, Donald, M.D., 53
Becker, Louise, 40
Beechcraft C-90 King Air, MU2, 111
Beller, Dr. Cleve, 82
Benesh, Claretta, 67
Bennett, Dr. W. S., 12, 13
Benson, Joseph, 13
Bird, J. Douglas, 101, 102, 107
Birthing rooms, 39, 94, 95
Blood Assurance Program, 76
Blood bank, 75
Blood services, 84, 102
Blood System of Wyoming, 75

Blue Cross, 53
Blue Envelope Drive Health Fair, 76, 102
Blue Envelope Fund. *See* Blue Envelope Health Fund.
Blue Envelope Health Drive, 58, 75
Blue Envelope Health Fair. *See* Blue Envelope Drive Health Fair.
Blue Envelope Health Fund, 58, 66, 71, 72, 74, 76, 77, 78, 79, 80, 84, 88, 89, 95, 96, 102
Bohler, John, 101
Bohnet, Charlotte, 104
Bostwick, Dick, 78
Bowden, Dr., 56
Bowron, Sara, 46, 48
Boy Scout Council Explorer posts, 88
Boyer, Leona, 68
Brooks ranch, 40
Brooks, Governor B. B., 10, 19
Burns, Ann, 107
Butcher, Casey, R.N., 67
Butler, Alex, 20
Byers, Ned, 94

C

"C" Hill, 20, 65
Cacharelis, O. J., 27
Campfield, Mathew, 10, 14
Cancer care, 72
Cancer center, 74, 79, 84, 102, 109. *See also* Central Wyoming Cancer Center.
Cancer research and treatment, 71, 78
Cancer treatment room, 72

Candy Striper program, 73, 83
Candy Striper, 70, 81
Cann-Taylor, Julie, 123
Cardiac monitors, 71
Carey Cattle Company, 15
Carey, Joseph, 10, 19, 20, 21
Carnahan, Dr. Robert, 49
Carr, James G., Jr., 48, 50, 51, 53, 55, 67, 69, 70, 75, 76, 77
Carrigen, Eleanor, 49
Carriger, Lin, 108, 112
Carter, William, 25
Carubie, Louis, 46
Carubie, Shirley, 49, 61
Casper College, 21, 57, 60, 61, 65, 67, 73, 76, 86, 111
Casper Hospital, 22, 23, 25
Casper Industrial Club, 19
Casper Private Hospital, 25, 26, 28
Casper Project, 53
Casper Red Cross, 27
Casper Surgical Center, 112, 115
Centennial Committee, 128
Central Services, 51, 93, 103
Central Services building, 103, 107
Central Wyoming Cancer Center, 102
Central Wyoming Counseling Center, 72, 84
Central Wyoming Oncology Center, 108, 109, 110
Cesarean-sections, 95
Chapin, Charles, 107
Chaplaincy program, 111, 112
Chaplaincy Services, 121
Chemotherapy, 72, 86
Christensen, Dr. Kent, 74, 121

Christensen, Russ, 115
Cipperly, Dr. Vaughn, 109
City of Casper-Natrona County Health Department, 72, 83, 117
Clavier, Norma, 120
Cleft Palate Clinic, 78
Clinical Pastoral Care Education Program, 121
Cobalt 60 Tele-Therapy unit, 71
Computers, 74
Computerized Tomographic (CT) scanners, 79, 103, 123
Connoisseur's Delight, 122
Converse County Hospital, 15, 27
Converse County Memorial Hospital, 112
Converse, Martha, R.N., 21, 22, 23
Corbett, Dr. John, 69
Cooper, Percy, 71
Cooper, Trula, 78, 106, 107
Cottage Gift Shop, 95
Craig, Mary Ann, 34
Cratty, Brian, 122
CU Hospital. *See* University of Colorado Hospital in Denver.

D

Damon Runyon Foundation, 72
Daniels, Mary Jo, 129
DaVinci Robotic Surgical System, 7, 127
Dean, Dr. T. A., 16, 35
Deane, Jill, R.N., 102
DeClue, Mrs. Katherine, 34
Deming Method, 108
Dennis, Violet, 77
DePaul Hospital, 74
Dialysis center, 73
Dialysis treatment, 73; Dialysis machine, 73
Diamond, Vickie, 124, 127
Dietary Department, 51, 70
Doing, Keith, 71

Donlin, Joe, 71
Dr. Dial, 74, 102
Dryer, Eileen, 75

E

Eaton, Phil, 121
Edelman, Nancy, 75
Edwards, Dix, 76
Electronic Coronary Care unit, 71
Ellbogen, Dr. Martin, 69
Ellison, R. S., 36
Elkin, Dr. Bernice, 74
Emergency Department, 71, 89, 90, 111, 112, 115, 120, 122, 123, 124, 127, 128
Emergency medical technician (EMT), 89, 90, 91
Emergency personnel, 88, 91, 107
Emergency room, 91, 96, 111, 120
Emergency Services, 70, 82, 120
Endoscopic, 74, 109
Eschwig, Mary Anne, R.N., 34, 36, 40, 41

F

Farrell, Dr. Mark, 58, 59
Fellows, Dr. Carol, 79, 86
Fetterman Hospital Association, 15
Fire department, 89, 102
Fisher and Davis Architects, 61
Fisher and Fisher Architects, 50
Fisher, Alan, 69
Fisher, Reece and Johnson, Architects, 86
Fitzgerald, Dr. R. P., 67
Flu; Flu epidemic. *See* Influenza; Influenza epidemic.
Foley, M. J., 36
Fougstadt, Nils, 33
Fowler, Nat, M.D., 96
Fowler, Robert, M.D., 53, 70
Frost, Dr. I. N., 35
Fulks, Pam, 123, 124, 127

G

Gardner, James "Jim", 121, 122
Garner, J. L., M.D., 10, 12
Garwood, Mike, 115
Geis, Dr. N. C., 35
General Rose Memorial Hospital, 74
George, Mrs. Lewis, 68
Gilliam, Dr., 16, 26
Goetz, Barbara, 50, 51, 52
Goodstein family, 73
Goodstein Foundation, 74, 79
Goodstein, Babe, 73, 74
Goodstein, Fred, 73, 74, 79
Goodstein, J. M., 79
Gorder/S Group, 86
Gordy, Dr. Phillip, 74, 76
Greene, Genevieve, 48
Grierson, Nora, 128
Griffin, Alb, 68
Gringauz, Dr. Raisa, 106
Gronning, Debbie, 110
Gross, Len, 101, 102
Guest Relations Program, 110

H

H1N1, 127
Habitat for Humanity, 116
Haigler, Dr. Fred, 53
Hamilton, Wilhelmina, 23
Hanson, Becky, 120
Harmon, Levi, 110
Harold, Jim, 76
Harrison, Grandma, 15
Haselmire, W. B., 48
Hayford, Roy, 111
Heart defibrillator, 68
Heidbrink oxygen tents, 40
Hemry, Kathleen, 48, 78, 84
Hendy, Rob, 89
Henning, William, 21
High Plains Psychiatric Center, 108
Hi-Lites, 79, 107, 110, 111

High Lights, 79
Highlights, 128
Hill-Burton Act, 70, 84
Hill-Burton grant, 70, 84
Hiser, Wesley, 78
Holland, W. M., 36
Holman, Dr., 68
Holmer, Betty, 89
Holmes, Roy, M.D., 53
Home for Dependent Children, 38
Home Health Department, 108
Hospice program, 74, 102
Hough, Elaine, 6, 79, 83, 102
Hubbard, Diane, R.N., 92
Huber, Emrick, 69
Hudgel, Dr., 78
Hunter, Shirley, 111

I

Ideen, Helen, 48, 52
Incubator, 39, 77
Infant resuscitation unit, 68
Influenza, 7, 9, 27, 28, 47; Influenza epidemic, 25, 27, 31, 33, 120
Intensive Care Unit (ICU)/Critical Care Unit (CCU), 83
Intensive Care Unit (ICU), 111, 112, 120, 121, 129, 130
Iron lung, 52
Isolation building, 33

J

Jacobson, Dr. Donald, 71
James, Dr. George, 40
Jensen, Terry, 115
John Tripeny Jr. Streptococcal Control Center, 74
Johnson, Dr. Paul, 107, 109
Johnson, Hillary M., 86
Johnson, Tom, 68
Joint Commission on Accreditation of Hospitals (JCAHO), 69

Jones, Elizabeth, R.N., 102
Jourgensen, Stanley, 53, 70

K

Kahn, Dr. David, 73
Kamp, Dr. Joseph C., 25, 26, 28, 35, 40
Kassis Dry Goods Store, 24
Kassis, Abraham, 23, 24
Kaster, Reverend Ellis, 121
Keith, Dr. Marshall C., 16, 25, 35
Kersting, Juanita, 68
Kidd, William, 107
Kimball, Dr. A. P., 35
Kimball, Justin, 53
Kimball, Martha Converse, 45, 46
Kimball, Wilson S., 10, 14, 16, 22
Knapp, Dr. George, 72
Kolasinski, Joanne, 104
Koontz, Winifred, 40
Kraen, Judith, R.N., 102
Kudolla, Dr. Charles, 53

L

L. D. Liesinger Construction Company, 68
Labor and Delivery unit, 94
Laboratory, 39, 40, 51, 53, 54, 55, 59, 66, 71, 74, 75, 79, 84, 111, 112, 130
Laboratory Department, 59
Larson and Jorgenson, 33
Larson, Lorrie, 110
Lathrop, Homer, M.D., 25, 26, 28, 34, 36, 78
Lathrop, Jean, 45, 46
Lathrop, Virginia, 78
Leeper, Dr. John, 10, 11, 12, 13, 14, 15, 16
Licensed practical nurse (L.P.N.), 50, 57, 60
Licensed practical nurses' training program, 60

Life Flight, 88, 89, 90, 91, 102, 110, 111, 116, 119, 122, 123, 126; Navigation equipment, 91
Lowe, Charles R., M.D., 53, 67
Lowe, Zora, 68
Lund, Dr. Ronald, 71, 76, 79
Lung ventilator, 74
Lyford, Dr. Charles, 86, 107

M

MacGuire, Mary, M.D., 109
Macy, Robert, 86
Magnascanner, 71
Magnetic Resonance Imager (MRI), 103
Mahnke, Dr. Don, 69
Malott, Ralph, M.D., 53
Mammography machine, 103
Manville, Robert, 56, 86
Marketing and Public Relations Department, 79, 107
Marriott, 117
Masterson Place, 121
Masterson, James, 121
Masterson, Mary, 121
Mattson, Dr. Roger, 71, 76
McLellan, Dr. Allen, 35
McMurry Medical Arts Building, 121
McMurry, Mick, 121
Meal-Pac, 50, 54
Medical and Community Resource Health Library, 122
Medical Explorer Post 99. *See* Boy Scout Council Explorer posts.
Medical Staff Research Committee, 69
Mednet, 107
Memorial Hospital Board of Trustees, 36, 45, 50, 51, 52, 55, 56, 57, 59, 66, 69, 73, 74, 75, 77, 78, 86, 91, 96, 101, 106

Memorial Hospital data processing, 84

Memorial Hospital of Natrona County Foundation, 77, 78, 79, 91

Memorial Hospital of Natrona County, 28, 36, 37, 39, 40, 41, 45, 46, 47, 48, 49, 50, 51, 52, 53, 54, 55, 56, 57, 58, 59, 60, 61, 62, 65, 66, 67, 68, 69, 70, 71, 72, 73, 74, 75, 76, 77, 78, 79, 80, 82, 83, 84, 85, 86, 88, 89, 90, 91, 92, 93, 94, 96, 101, 102, 128, 130

Mental health services, 58, 72

Messerschmidt-Boelkow-Blohm Model BO 105CB, 89

Meyers, Tom, 86

Miller, Dana, 92

Miller, Dr. W. W., 10

Mohr, Leona, R.N., 40, 41

Mokler, Alfred J., 10, 11, 12, 13, 37

Moore, Mike, 104

Morad, Dr. N. E., 40

Morgan, Dr. G. T., 16

Morgan, Vanessa, 130

Mothers of Twins, 76

N

Nations, Constance, 67

Natrona County Chapter of the American Cancer Society, 55

Natrona County Commission, 114

Natrona County Health Building, 107

Natrona County Health Fund, 72

Natrona County Heart Association, 57

Natrona County Hospital, 31, 33, 34, 35, 36

Natrona County Medical Society, 35

Natrona County Voluntary Health Council, 58

Nelson, Dr. John, 40

Nelson, Isabella, R.N., 27, 34, 36

Newborn Nursery, 48

Next Generation Child Care Center, 110

Nichols Plan (1986), 107, 112

Nicolaysen, G. G., 71

Nicolaysen, Peter G., 10

Nolan, Dr. M. J., 35

North Casper Junior Orchestra, 46, 50

Northern Wyoming Streptococcal Laboratory, 74

Nursery, 39, 59, 69, 77

Nurses' home. *See* Nurses' residence.

Nurses' quarters. *See* Nurses' residence.

Nurses' residence, 31, 33, 40, 59, 66, 69

Nurses' stations, 71

Nurses' training, 27, 31, 34, 35, 40, 41, 47, 51, 53, 57, 60, 61, 66, 67, 68, 75, 81, 102, 107. *See also* Licensed practical nurses' training program *and* R.N. training.

Nursing program. *See* Nurses' training.

Nursing school. *See* Nurses' training.

Nursing students, 34, 35, 40, 41, 47, 49, 50, 60, 61, 67, 81. *See also* Nurses' training.

O

Obstetrics, 39, 47, 57, 61

O'Connor, P. J., 36

One Cent Sales Tax, 75, 83

Operating room (OR), 39, 54, 56, 59

Ott, Steve, 86

Outreach, 79

P

Paint Your Heart Out, 102, 105

Pair, Nona, R.N., 57, 67

Palato, Jess, 76

Paramedic training, 91

Parking garage, 75, 83, 85, 103

Parking structure. *See* Parking garage.

Parmenter, Patrick, R.N., 102

Partridge, Martha, 45, 46, 48

Pathology, 40, 59

Patient transport: Ambulance, 25, 53, 70, 75, 88, 89, 90, 91, 115, 123, 127; Hearse as ambulance, 53; Pontiac station wagon-style ambulance, 53, 75; Superior Pontiac ambulance, 70; Four-wheel-drive ambulance, 90, 91; Fixed-wing plane, 111; Airplane, 88, 111, 126; Helicopter, 88, 89, 91, 111, 126. *See also* Life Flight.

Patrick, Dennis, 111

Patrick, Dr. Robert, 86

Patton, Hugh, 19

Pediatric ward, 39, 55, 57, 70, 123

Pediatrics, 35, 70

Penley, G. M., 33

Perioperative Nursing Residency Program, 102

Perry, Jack, 40

Pershing Geiger's "The Country Doctor", 122

Personnel Department, 57

Peterson, G. Fred, 86

Phibbs, Brendan, M.D., 53, 57, 75

Philips CT Scanner, 79

Philips Medical Systems, 79

Philips, Mike, 6

Physical therapy training program, 49, 82

Physical therapy, 49, 51, 54, 59, 82

Pink Ladies, 83. *See also* Auxiliary.
Podrasik, Dr. Eugene, 121
Polio. *See* Poliomyelitis.
Poliomyelitis, 49
Poor and Pauper Fund, 31
Pope, Greg, 116
Posker, Jean, 68
Powell, Dr. L. G., 14, 15
Psychiatric program, 59
Psychiatry, 58
Puder, Sandra, R.N., 102
Pursel, Shirley, 46
Pursel, Whitey, 46

Q

Quinlan, Dorothy, 50, 67, 111

R

R.N. training, 61
Radioisotope laboratory, 55
Radioisotopes, 71
Radiology center, 76, 112
Radiology Department, 79
Radiology, 40, 54, 59, 66, 71, 79
Ratcliff, Hardy, 107
Rayner, Dr. Abigail, 92
Reasoner, Dr. Edward, 92
Red Desert Clinic in Rock Springs, 123
Rediesel-Lowe Construction Company, 50
Reeb, James, 73, 83
Reeb, Mae, 73
Reece, John, 86
Reed, Fern, 67
Reengineering, 108, 112
Reichenbach, Dr. H. A., 35
Respiratory therapy technician (RTT) program, 86, 88, 111
Ressler, Jerry, 71
Retzloff, Minnie, R.N., 39, 45
Rheumatic fever program, 57
Rheumatic fever, 53, 71, 95

Riach, Dr. T. A., 35
Rickert, Tom, 111
Right to Life, 84
Ringhouse, Barbara, 108
Roberts, Kenneth, M.D., 53
Rock Springs state facilities, 19, 26
Rohrbaugh, Dr. E. P., 25
Roussalis, Dr. Louis, 69, 114
Ruben, Stuart, M.D., 128
Rucker, Marion, 105
Rucker, Myrtle, 105

S

Salk vaccine, 49
Sanftner, Laurie, 108
Sanftner, Rolly, 115
Satterfield, Darrell, 78
Scherck, Bernadine, 27
Schrader, Mike, 111, 112, 121
Schrann, Lyda, 104
Schroeder, Dana, 111, 112, 121
Schultz, Phyllis, 123
Schuster, Veronica, 72
Schwartz, H. H., 36
Scott, Oliver K., M.D., 53
Sedar, Dick, 78
Sheridan State Hospital, 22
Sheriff's department, 89
Shugart, Bill, 110
Siemens Mevatron XII linear accelerator, 79
Siemens SOMATOM 64-Slice scanner, 123
Simons, Kathy, R.N., 103
Slayler, Dr., 78
Smith, Dr. George, 35
Smoking, 82; Second-hand smoke, 82; Designated smoking zones, 82
South link lobby, 116, 120, 121
Southwest Blood Bank, 75
Spiele, Irene, 68
Spencer, Lewis, 77, 86

St. James, Rosalie, 67
Staph. *See* Staphylococcus.
Staphylococcus, 48, 127
State Board of Charities and Reform, 19, 21
Steen, Ralph, 48
Steplock, Dr. Louis, 115
Strack, Luke, 123
Strep program. *See* Strep Throat Culture Program.
Strep Throat Culture Program, 53, 57, 58, 71, 74, 75, 78, 95, 96
Strep throat laboratory, 84
Strep throat program. *See* Strep Throat Culture Program.
Strep Throat Screening Program. *See* Strep Throat Culture Program.
Strep throat, 53
Stuckenoff, Dr. Harry, 40
Student nurses. *See* Nursing students.
Sullivan, Michael J. "Mike", 77, 101
Sullivan, Murray, 21, 45, 46
Surgical areas, 50, 54
Surgical suites, 59, 112, 122
Swedish Medical Center, 91

T

Talbert, Mrs. Gene, 67
Taylor, JoAnn, R.N., 71
TeKampe, Anne, R.N., 67
Telemedicine, 111
Telemetry, 121
Temporary covered walkway, 124
Thomas, A. J., 33
Thornton, Edna, 68
TI-9100 Loran C Navigator gear, 91
Tice, Carmel, 111
Toal, Joann, 115
Tobin, Mary (Stuckenoff), 40
Tobin, Robert, M.D., 109

About the Author

REBECCA A. HUNT, PH.D.

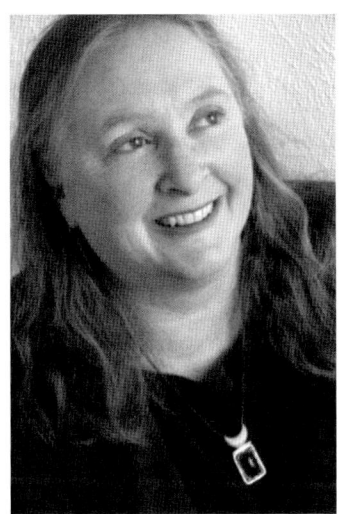

Rebecca Hunt is a historian specializing in the social history of the American West. She is a senior instructor in American and Public History at the University of Colorado, Denver, where she teaches museum studies.

Her Ph.D. is from the University of Colorado in Boulder with a dissertation titled *Urban Pioneers: Continuity and Change in Denver's Ethnic Communities*, focusing on North Denver and Globeville. Rebecca is a part-time archivist/historian for Presbyterian/St. Luke's Medical Center and was the historian for the book *A History of Presbyterian/St. Luke's Medical Center* (2007). Other publications include "Healers on the Hill" and "Swedish Medical Center" in the Summer 2005 *Colorado Heritage* magazine.

Rebecca co-authored *A Century of Healing: The History of Swedish Medical Center* with Sandy Durkin in 2005. This book details the transformation of Swedish National Sanatorium into the Swedish Medical Center.

Rebecca was born at Memorial Hospital of Natrona County in 1952. Although she lives in Denver, she maintains the family home on Casper Mountain. Her next book will be a pictorial history of Natrona County due out in the summer of 2011.

Training program for nurses. *See* Nurses' training.
TriBrook Group Inc., 86
Tripeny, John, Jr., 58, 74
Tuberculosis (TB), 33, 40, 59
Turner, Bob, 124
Turner, Dr. Diane, 109

U

U.S. Public Health Services, 70
Ultra-Sonic unit, 68
United Blood Services of Wyoming, 84
United Fund, 77
United Health Drive, 59
United States Department of Public Health, 71
United Way, 102
University of Colorado Hospital in Denver, 73
University of Wyoming, 61, 67
University of Wyoming Family Practice Residency Clinic, 122

V

Van Rooms, 47
Vance, Michel, R.N., 102
Vanderlinden, Shauna, 6, 128
Volk and Harrison, 69, 70
Volunteer Services, 102
Volunteers, 48, 58, 71, 81, 84, 88, 94, 95, 96, 102, 104, 128

W

W. R. Coe Memorial Hospital, 67
Walott, Dr., 35
Walters, Eleanor, 50
Washington Street entrance, 121
Watson, Walter, M.D., 53, 70
Weaver, Alyce, 25
Weaver, Debora, R.N., 115, 130
Weaver, Sam, 24, 25
Weaver, Sara (Bowron), 48, 53
Weaver, Tim, 90, 91
Weaver, Warren, 46, 48
Weaver, Wayne, 46
Webb, Frances Seely, 27
Weikum, Kim, 123
Weiss, Dr. Gary, 115
Wernsmann, Jeanne, 128
Western Wyoming Community College, 86
Wetherbee, Jerry, 86
Wheeler, Lois, R.N., 57
Whiston, Dr. Gordon, 49
Wiley, G. O., 36
Wiley, Mary Anne Eschwig, 77
William Barton Memorial Computerized Tomographic Center, 79
Williams, Dr. L. J., 74
Williamson, Hank, 111
Willis, Dr. A. L., 35
Winship, Mrs., 68
Wisk, Hans, 76
Wolfe, Tom, 111
Women's Army Medical Corps, 47
Women's Auxiliary, 48, 55, 59, 70, 73. *See also* Auxiliary.
Wood, Dr. Charles, 86
Wymedco, 103
Wynn, Dr., 35
Wyoming Blue Cross, 53
Wyoming Farm Bureau, 53
Wyoming Highway Patrol, 89
Wyoming Hospital Association, 86
Wyoming Hospital Service, 53
Wyoming Imaging Center, 103
Wyoming Medical Center, 67, 53, 96, 101, 102, 103
Wyoming Medical Center Community and Family Clinic, 122
Wyoming Medical Center Foundation, 102, 103, 122, 124
Wyoming Medical Center Volunteers, 128. *See also* Auxiliary *and* Volunteers.
Wyoming Medical Center's Support Services building, 117
Wyoming National Guard, 110
Wyoming State Health Department, 70
Wyoming State Hospital, Casper Branch, 16, 19, 21, 26, 31
Wyoming State Hospital, Rock Springs, 21, 26
Wyoming State Hospital, Sheridan, 26
Wyoming State Nurses' Association (WSNA), 22, 23, 31, 34, 115
Wyoming Tuberculosis Association, 55

X

X-ray Department, 35, 59
X-ray films, 40
X-ray machines: Victor X-ray machine, 36, 40; Portable X-ray machine, 40, 68; X-ray therapy unit, 74
X-ray technology, 76, 81
X-rays, 13, 55, 76, 111

Y

Y2K, 120
Youmans, Dr. Jerry, 114
Yount, Donna, 53, 129
Ysebaert, John, 110

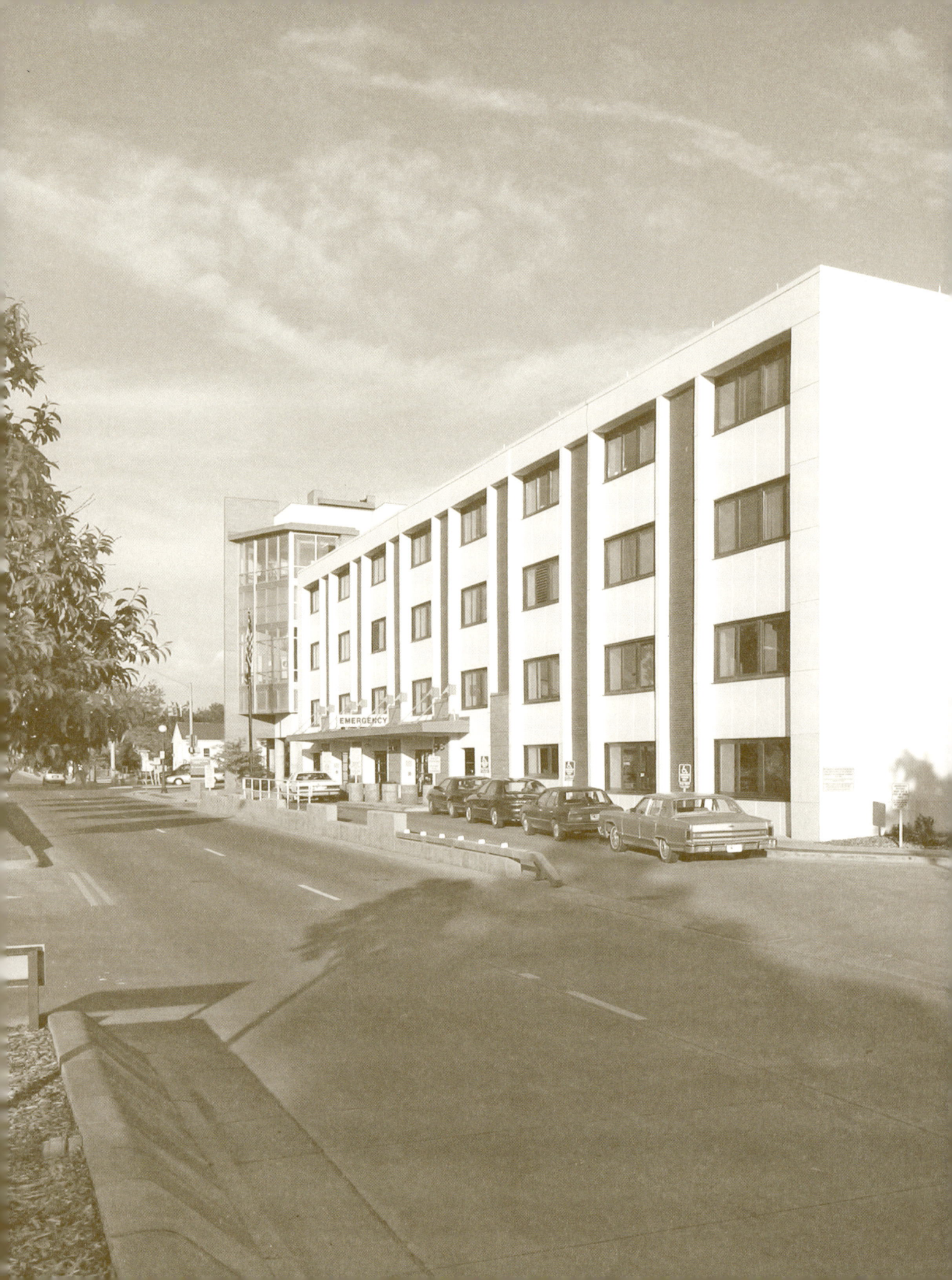